Teratogen Update
Environmentally Induced Birth Defect Risks

Teratogen Update
Environmentally Induced Birth Defect Risks

Editors

John L. Sever

Infectious Diseases Branch
National Institute of Neurological and Communicative
Diseases and Stroke
Bethesda, Maryland

Robert L. Brent

Stein Research Center
Jefferson Medical College
Thomas Jefferson University
Philadelphia, Pennsylvania

Alan R. Liss, Inc., New York

Address all Inquiries to the Publisher
Alan R. Liss, Inc., 41 East 11th Street, New York, NY 10003

Printed in the United States of America

Library of Congress Cataloging-in-Publication Data

Teratogen update.

Includes Index.

1. Fetus—Abnormalities—Etiology. 2. Fetus—Diseases—Etiology. 3. Environmentally induced diseases. I. Sever, John L. II. Brent, Robert L.
RG627.5.T47 1986 618.92′0043 86-7219
ISBN 0-8451-4208-9

Contents

Publisher's Note

The chapters in this volume were rewritten or reproduced from articles which appeared in several publications over the past ten years. A list of the chapters and the publications in which they originally appeared is given below.

Chapter Name	Original Source
DRUGS	
Clinical Aspects of Thalidomide Embryopathy—A Continuing Preoccupation	Teratology 32:133–144(1985)
Fetal Alcohol Syndrome	Teratology 13:345–348(1976)
DES—Transplacental Teratogen—And Possible Carcinogen	Teratology 13:101–104(1976)
Warfarin Embryopathy	Teratology 14:205–210(1976)
Fetal Hydantoin Effects	Teratology 33:349–353(1986)
Fetal Trimethadione Syndrome	Teratology 17:103–106(1978)
Aminopterin and Methotrexate: Folic Acid Deficiency	Teratology 17:353–358(1978)
Antituberculous Drugs	Teratology 20:133–138(1979)
Tetracycline Staining of Teeth	Teratology 15:127–130(1977)
Bendectin	Teratology 27:277–281(1983)
Vitamin A Congeners	Teratology 33:355–364(1986)
Penicillamine	Teratology 33:127–131(1986)
INFECTIONS	
Congenital Rubella—An Encapsulated Review	Teratology 14:111–114(1976)
The Congenital Rubella Syndrome	Teratology 31:297–307(1985)
Congenital Cytomegalovirus Infection	Teratology 17:179–182(1978)
Congenital Toxoplasmosis	Teratology 15:213–218(1977)
Congenital Varicella	Teratology 15:329–330(1977)
Venezuelan Equine Encephalitis: Its Relation to Severe Cerebral Malformations	Teratology 16:359–362(1977)
Congenital Syphilis	Teratology 16:217–224(1977)
CHEMICALS	
Methylmercury Poisoning	Teratology 12:311–314(1975)
Congenital Minimata Disease: Intrauterine Methylmercury Poisoning	Teratology 18:285–288(1978)
PCBs and Cola Colored Babies: Japan, 1968, and Taiwan, 1979	Teratology 26:259–261(1982)
PHYSICAL, NUTRITIONAL AND OTHER FACTORS	
Smoking and Pregnancy	Teratology 32:473–481(1985)
Small Head Size After Atomic Irradiation	Teratology 14:355–358(1976)
Radiation Teratogenesis	Teratology 21:281–298(1980)
Malformations in Infants of Diabetic Mothers	Teratology 25:385–394(1982)
Iodine Deficiency	Teratology 31:309–311(1985)
Hyperthermia	Teratology 33:365–371(1986)
TERATOLOGY	
The Complexities of Solving the Problem of Human Malformations	Prevention of Physical and Mental Congenital Defects, Part A: The Scope of the Problem. Maurice Marois (ed). Alan R. Liss, Inc., pp. 55–68(1985)
Methods of Evaluating the Alleged Teratogenicity of Environmental Agents	Prevention of Physical and Mental Congenital Defects, Part C: Basic and Medical Science, Education, and Future Strategies. Maurice Marois (ed). Alan R. Liss, Inc., pp. 191–195(1985)
Medicolegal Aspects of Teratology	Mead-Johnson Symposium #7:65–76(1975)
Litigation-Produced Pain, Disease and Suffering: An Experience With Congenital Malformation Lawsuits	Teratology 16:1–14(1977)
The Irresponsible Expert Witness: A Failure of Biomedical Graduate Education and Professional Accountability	Pediatrics 70:754–762(1982)*

*Reprinted with permission of the publisher.

Contributors

Charles A. Alford
Department of Pediatrics
The University of Alabama at Birmingham
Birmingham, AL 35294 **[93]**

Robert L. Brent
Stein Research Center
Thomas Jefferson University
920 Chancellor Street
Philadelphia PA 19107 **[xiii, 145, 189, 199, 203, 215, 229]**

Sidney Q. Cohlan
Department of Pediatrics
New York University School of Medicine
530 First Avenue
New York, NY 10016 **[51]**

Richard A. Doherty
Department of Pediatrics
University of Rochester School of Medicine and Dentistry
Rochester, NY 14642 **[119]**

David A. Fuccillo
Department of Virology
Microbiological Associates
5221 River Road
Bethesda, MD 20816 **[101]**

Allen S. Goldman
Center for Craniofacial Anomalies
University of Illinois College of Medicine at Chicago
800 S. Wood Street
Chicago, IL 60680 **[35]**

John H. Grossman III
Department of Obstetrics and Gynecology
George Washington University School of Medicine and Health Sciences
Washington, DC 20037 **[113]**

James W. Hanson
Department of Pediatrics
University of Iowa
College of Medicine
Iowa City, IA 52242 **[29]**

Masazumi Harada
Department of Epidemiology
Institute for Medical Genetics
Kumamoto University Medical School
Kumamoto 862 JAPAN **[123]**

Lewis B. Holmes
Embryology-Teratology Unit
Children's Service
Massachusetts General Hospital, and
Department of Pediatrics
Harvard Medical School
Boston, MA 02114 **[53, 131]**

Frances O. Kelsey
Center for Drugs and Biologics
Food and Drug Administration
Rockville, MD 20857 **[61]**

Sheldon B. Korones
Department of Pediatrics
Section on the Newborn
University of Tennessee
Center for Health Sciences
Memphis, TN 38163 **[77]**

The number in brackets is the opening page number of the contributor's article.

John W. Larsen, Jr.
Department of Obstetrics and Gynecology
George Washington University School of Medicine and Health Sciences
2150 Pennsylvania Avenue N.W.
Washington, DC 20037 **[97]**

Robert W. Miller
Clinical Epidemiology Branch
National Cancer Institute
The National Institutes of Health
Bethesda, MD 20892 **[141]**

James L. Mills
Epidemiology Branch
National Institute of Child Health and Human Development
The National Institutes of Health
Bethesda, MD 20205 **[165]**

John J. Mulvihill
Clinical Epidemiology Branch
National Cancer Institute
The National Institutes of Health
Bethesda, MD 20892 **[13, 141]**

Claus G.H. Newman
Leon Gillis Unit
Queen Mary's Hospital
Roehampton
London SW 15, ENGLAND **[1]**

Barbara R. Pober
Embryology-Teratology Unit
Children's Service
Massachusetts General Hospital, and
Department of Pediatrics
Harvard Medical School
Boston, MA 02114 **[131]**

David W. Reynolds
Suite 414 Women's Medical Plaza
2006 Brookwood Medical Center Drive
Birmingham, AL 35209 **[93]**

Walter J. Rogan
Epidemiology Branch
National Institute of Environmental Health Sciences
Post Office Box 12233
Research Triangle Park, NC 27709 **[127]**

Franz W. Rosa
HFN 730, Food and Drug Administration
Rockville, MD 20851 **[61, 71]**

John L. Sever
Infectious Diseases Branch, IRP
National Institute of Neurological and Communicative Disorders and Stroke
The National Institutes of Health
Bethesda, MD 20205 **[xiii, 81]**

Mary Ann South
Infectious Diseases Branch, IRP
National Institute of Neurological and Communicative Disorders and Stroke
The National Institutes of Health
Bethesda, MD 20205 **[81]**

Sergio Stagno
Department of Pediatrics
The University of Alabama at Birmingham
Birmingham, AL 35294 **[93]**

Howard Ulfelder
Vincent Memorial Hospital
(Gynecological Service of the
Massachusetts General Hospital)
Boston, MA 02114 **[19]**

Josef Warkany
Children's Hospital Research Foundation
Elland Avenue and Bethesda
Cincinnati, OH 45229 **[23, 39, 45, 177, 181]**

Bernard Weiss
Environmental Health Sciences Center
University of Rochester School of Medicine and Dentistry
Rochester, NY 14642 **[119]**

Franz Wenger
Edificio El Saman - 8°
Calle 73A, No. 2B-45
Maracaibo, VENEZUELA **[107]**

Martha M. Werler
Embryology-Teratology Unit
Children's Service
Massachusetts General Hospital
Boston, MA 02114 **[131]**

Ann L. Wilk
Center for Drugs and Biologics
Food and Drug Administration
Rockville, MD 20857 **[61]**

Sumner J. Yaffee
Center for Research for Mothers and Children
National Institute of Child Health and Human
Development
The National Institutes of Health
Bethesda, MD 20205 **[35]**

Elaine H. Zackai
Clinical Genetics Center
The Children's Hospital of Philadelphia
University of Pennsylvania
School of Medicine
Philadelphia, PA 19104 **[35]**

Introduction

The "Teratogen Update" reports on human teratogens were started in the journal *Teratology* in 1975. The articles were intended to "summarize the clinical manifestation, etiology, pathogenesis, treatment, and prevention of the phenomena." In the last ten years over twenty-five Teratogen Updates have been submitted to *Teratology*.

Because of the widespread interest in the articles it was decided to ask the authors to bring the papers up to date and republish the articles together as a book. The authors have complied with the request and several new Teratogen Updates have been added. A Summary Table of Human Teratogens has been prepared. The chapters have been grouped into four sections: Drugs; Infections; Chemicals; and Physical, Nutritional and Other Factors. Agents which are considered to be teratogenic for humans have been included. Three of these agents are each covered in two papers—rubella, methylmercury and radiation. Several agents are not covered because the papers on these topics have not yet been completed for the journal—valproic acid, lithium, progestagens, androgens, and maternal phenylketonuria. A review paper on the status of anesthetic agents is also in preparation. These papers will appear in future issues of the Journal. Bendectin, although not a human teratogen, was included because of the special interest associated with this medication, and an article on the association of non-genital malformations with progestagens will be included in a future issue for the same reason.

For the reader interested in teratology—the complexities of solving the problem, methods of evaluating teratogenicity and medicolegal problems in teratology, we have included five related articles.

This compilation of articles should be useful not only to the investigators and clinicians who spend most of their time investigating or dealing with teratological problems, but also to the many health professionals who are only occasionally confronted with questions relating to teratology. The neonatologist and maternal fetal medicine physician may be the first contact that patients have when asking about teratogenic risks or when confronted with a malformed child. Information is provided to these families at this time, not necessarily by the physician but by other health professionals or trainees staffing the maternal-fetal medicine division. The physician or health professional who has the first contact with the family of a malformed child has the burdensome responsibility of providing accurate information concerning the causes of congenital malformations and to make sure that the family is properly informed. Misinformation can have serious consequences both emotionally and medicolegally.

Royalties paid on the sales of this book will be donated to the Teratology Society.

John L. Sever
Robert L. Brent

Summary Table of Human Teratogens

Agent	Most common major defects
I. DRUGS	
1. Thalidomide	• Limb reduction deformities Girdle hypoplasia Ear anomalies
2. Alcohol	• Growth retardation Reduced palpebral fissures Microcephaly, mental retardation
3. Diethystilbesterol	• Vaginal adenosis Cervical erosion and ridges Adenocarcinoma of the vagina (rare)
4. Warfarin	• Hypoplasia of nasal cartilage Various CNS defects Stippled epiphyses
5. Hydantoin (Dilantin)	• Growth retardation Dysmorphic craniofacial features Microcephaly, mental retardation
6. Trimethadione	• Developmental delay V-shaped eyebrows, low ears Cleft lip or palate
7. Aminopterin and methotrexate (Folic acid deficiency)	• Abortion Hydrocephalus Growth retardation, mental retardation
8. Antituberculos drugs (Streptomycin)	• Hearing loss
9. Tetracycline	• Stained teeth Hypoplasia of enamel
10. Valproic Acid	• Neural tube defects
11. Retinoic Acid (Vitamin A)	• Abortion Craniofacial dysmorphism Neural tube defects
12. Lithium	• Ebstein's heart defects Other cardiac defects
13. Antithyroid	• Hypothyroidism Goiter
14. Androgens and high dosages of masculinizing progestigens	• Masculinization
15. Penicillamine	• Skin hyperelastosis
II. INFECTIONS	
1. Rubella	• Deafness Cataracts Heart defects
2. Cytomegalovirus	• Growth retardation Mental retardation Hearing loss
3. Toxoplasmosis	• Hydrocephalus Blindness Mental retardation
4. Varicella	• Skin scarring Muscle atrophy Mental retardation

(continued)

Summary Table of Human Teratogens *(continued)*

Agent	Most common major defects
5. Venezuelan equine encephalitis	• Brain destruction Cataracts Death
6. Syphilis	• Abnormal teeth and bones Mental retardation
III. CHEMICALS	
1. Methylmercury	• Cerebral atrophy Spasticity, seizures Mental retardation
2. PCB	• Growth retardation Skin discoloration
IV. PHYSICAL, NUTRITIONAL AND OTHER FACTORS	
1. Smoking	• Abortion Intrauterine growth retardation
2. Ionizing radiation (Exposures above the diagnostic range)	• (Dependent on stage of pregnancy) Abortion Major organ malformations (18–36 days) Microencephaly and mental retardation (8–15 weeks)
3. Diabetes	• Congenital heart disease Caudal hypoplasia syndrome
4. Iodine deficiency	• Goiter Mental retardation Growth retardation
5. Maternal phenylketonuria	• Abortion Microcephaly Mental Retardation

Clinical Aspects of Thalidomide Embryopathy—A Continuing Preoccupation

C.G.H. NEWMAN
Leon Gillis Unit, Queen Mary's Hospital, Roehampton, London SW15, England

ABSTRACT There is much misinformation in the medical community regarding the thalidomide syndrome. Some physicians and scientists are unaware of the fact that organs other than the limbs were frequently affected. Some believe that thalidomide could produce any type of limb reduction defect. Most were aware of the very narrow period of early organogenesis during which the thalidomide-type malformations could be produced. Important features include the fact that limb reduction defects were primarily preaxial, included concomitant girdle hypoplasia when limb reductions were severe, were almost universally bilateral and did not include distal transverse-type defects often called "hemimelia". While it can be said that some spontaneous (non-thalidomide) malformations can mimic the thalidomide syndrome, it can also be said that many limb reduction defects can be determined not to have been produced by thalidomide. The risks of the various defects can be estimated following exposure, with most certainty for limb defects, with less certainty for other defects. Many defects were not associated with exposure to thalidomide such as cleft lip and severe mental retardation.

The thalidomide epidemic started in 1959 and the drug was withdrawn in 1961. Despite the passage of nearly 23 years, the most recent medico-legal proceedings concerning compensation of possible thalidomide victims in the United States of America were completed only in 1984. These proceedings emphasised the difficulties involved in assigning a specific cause to patterns of human malformation and clearly demonstrated the need for the definition of a recognisable syndrome. Thalidomide embryopathy, therefore, still retains a medico-legal and historical relevance but potentially a much greater interest in that the syndrome as defined produced a variety of malformation patterns all of which have occurred naturally, though some with extreme rarity.

Dr. William McBride ('77) briefly covered the history, some of the clinical manifestations, and some experimental data. The present paper will focus more closely on the clinical aspects.

The author's opinions are based on his personal examination of over 100 thalidomide victims, on his participation in the United Kingdom medical assessment panel concerning thalidomide-affected children, and on the analysis of the records of a further 180 United Kingdom thalidomide victims examined according to a standard protocol; also on his examination of something like 300 children with different types of congenital limb reduction defects, with a distinction between thalidomide and non-thalidomide types very much in mind.

TERMINOLOGY

Before describing the clinical effects, some comment on terminology is necessary. While Greek terms are time-honoured in medicine and there is no ambiguity about "amelia," the term "phocomelia" (seal-limb), "hemimelia" (partial absence—either transverse distal loss or longitudinal defects with loss of preaxial or postaxial ray), "peromelia" (maimed-limb), "dysmelia" (limb abnormality), or "ectromelia" (total or partial limb deficiency) are sometimes used without definition and can be most misleading. The most recent suggestion regarding terminology

(Working Group of the International Society for Prosthetics and Orthotics, '75) is effective though somewhat cumbersome at times. The author prefers to use the shortest unambiguous terms that can be readily defined. However, when describing an individual patient in detail, the ISPO terminology should be used.

EPIDEMIOLOGY

Unfortunately our knowledge concerning many aspects of the epidemic remains incomplete. There were no properly controlled or prospective series, and much of the information concerning exposure was based on postal enquiry, with, subsequently, considerable evidence concerning the unreliability of patients' recollections of whether they had or had not taken thalidomide or any other drug. The dramatic limb reduction defects naturally attracted the greatest attention, and the possibility of an undetected increase in minor isolated defects (for example, squint, minor degrees of deafness, hernia) remains. Only estimates are available regarding how many women actually took the drug during the sensitive period in pregnancy.

RISK OF EXPOSURE

Evidence based on retrospective analysis allowed the construction of a timetable of clinical effects associated with exposure at definitive times during embryogenesis (Lenz and Knapp, '62; Kreipe, '67). There is no evidence why one or another defect appears when one or either or both may be observed in different patients exposed at similar periods, and animal experiments do not appear to have shed much light on this. Individual coincidence of blood level and embryonic timing could explain this. There is also no clinical or experimental evidence that thalidomide was capable of damaging the foetus when administered after the sensitive period of 38–50 days after the first day of the last menstrual period.

There is only indirect evidence concerning how many mothers took the drug yet had babies that showed no evidence of thalidomide defect. Relatively few definite cases of exposure at the critical period with no detectable effect on the foetus have been described (Pembrey et al., '70; Kajii et al., '73), probably as a result of the absence of any large-scale prospective investigation. An overall risk factor for sensitive-period exposure leading to malformation of approximately one in two to one in ten is probably correct. Weicker et al. ('62), investigating this aspect close to the epidemic, considered that the risk factor was of the order of 20%. Thalidomide is one of the most potent teratogens known, yet probably a majority of mothers and foetuses resisted the effects of the drug. Digestive status and the pH sensitivity of thalidomide (Williams, '68) and uteroplacental or genetic factors in mother and foetus may all have played a part.

SYNDROME DEFINITION

On the basis of descriptions (variably detailed) based on well over 2,500 cases in Europe, Japan and Taiwan, and Canada, a definitive pattern was evidenced, fitting in well with animal experimentation, particularly on primates. In the author's personal experience, cases with a positive history of thalidomide have all fitted in with the described pattern. Nevertheless, children with atypical features have been found in the literature, though largely without any definitive evidence of exposure. When a drug is very widely used and fails to prevent other types of defect, sporadic defects will at times coincide, and infants who might have been affected but escaped the effects of the drug can continue to be affected by whatever other factors operate. These exceptions, therefore, do not upset the overall definition of a well-defined syndrome. Professor Poswillo (personal communication, '83) has confirmed that such atypical defects occurred but with a frequency no greater than in control groups during thalidomide studies on animals.

THALIDOMIDE SYNDROME

For convenience, abnormalities affecting the limbs and limb girdles, spine, special senses and the central nervous system, the heart and circulation, internal organs, and the genito-urinary system will be considered separately, though they often coincide. Thalidomide patterns will be contrasted with phenomena occurring sporadically or as part of known syndromes.

Limbs and limb girdles

Relative to differing exposure times—but not, apparently, to dose and only to some extent to unknown factors—there is a pattern of increasingly severe reduction deformity as described by Henkel and Willert ('69). The effects are grossly symmetrical, though opposite limbs are often unequally affected to some degree (Siguira et al., '79; Lenz, '71). Upper limb defects in thalidomide embryopathy are mostly associated with lower limb defects and rarely occur alone; in only very few cases was a single arm affected, primarily if the defect was not severe.

The thumbs are affected by hypoplasia (in the least degree sometimes only of the thenar muscles). As a variety of hypoplasia the thumb may be converted into a triphalangeal finger in line with the others. Rarely it is duplicated. The big, toe, however, is commonly duplicated, and it may also be converted into a triphalangeal digit. The same process may affect the index finger or second toe with hypoplasia to disappearance. Disappearance is more frequent in the upper, duplication more frequent in the lower, limb digits. Affected feet have five to eight digits, hands often only four or fewer. The forelimb long bones and part of the carpus/tarsus supporting the preaxial first and second digits are next variably reduced to the point of absence with the companion long bone less affected and sometimes fused to its more reduced partner in the forearm and more rarely in the leg. The hand (or foot) will deviate to the unsupported side as well as showing further deformity as a result of stiffening of joints and contractures, least marked on the ulnar or fibular side. Skin and nails remain unaffected, although some soft tissue syndactyly may occur. By way of contrast in non-thalidomide radial aplasia with thrombocytopenia, the thumb remains even when there is total absence of the radius. In Holt Oram syndrome, however, the upper limb reduction pattern is very similar to that of thalidomide, although the legs are unaffected (Figs. 1–8).

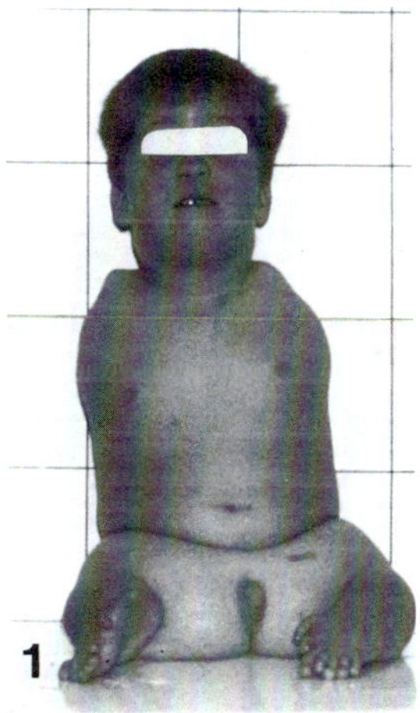

Fig. 1. Thalidomide amelia: projecting acromioclavicular joints. Polydactylic lower phocomelia.

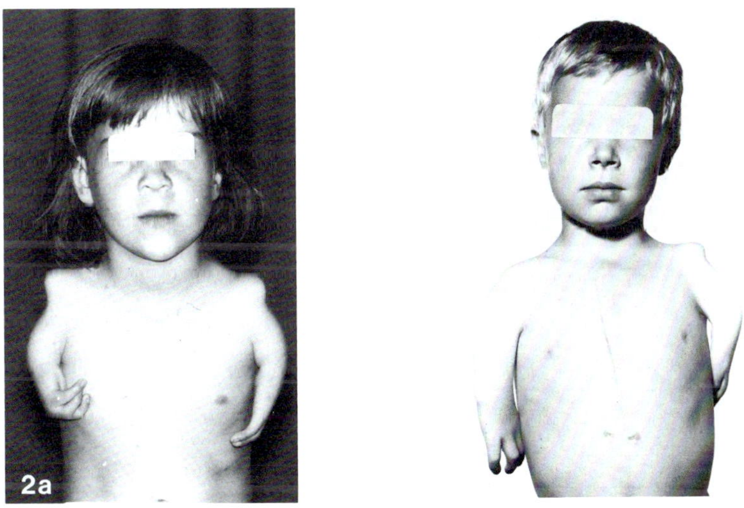

Fig. 2. A. Thalidomide upper phocomelia. Projecting acromioclavicular joints. Preaxial digits lost. B. Non-thalidomide, but phenotype very similar. Holt Oram syndrome, after repair of atrial septal defect. Note prominent acromioclavicular joint.

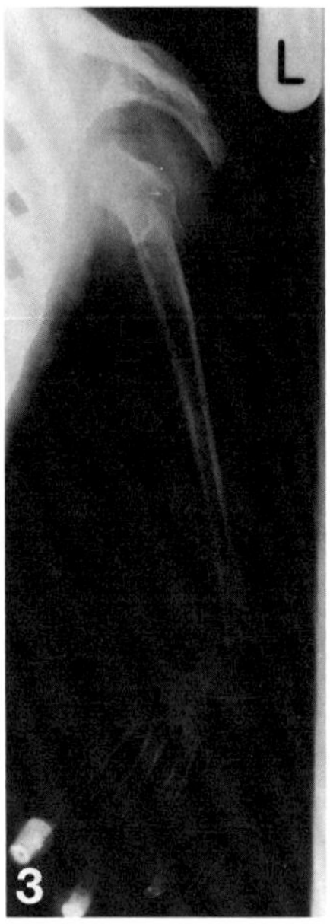

Fig. 3. Prominent acromioclavicular joint, deficient glenoid process, severe reduction of humerus, radial aplasia, loss of first and second ray. Ulna and three postaxial fingers remain.

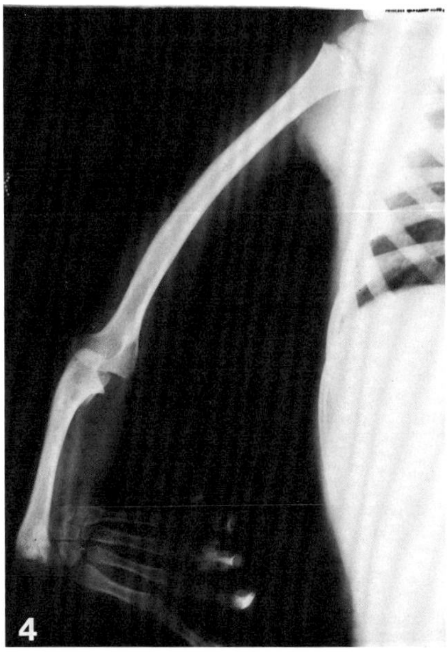

Fig. 4. Thalidomide preaxial defect with virtual radial aplasia and loss of thumb.

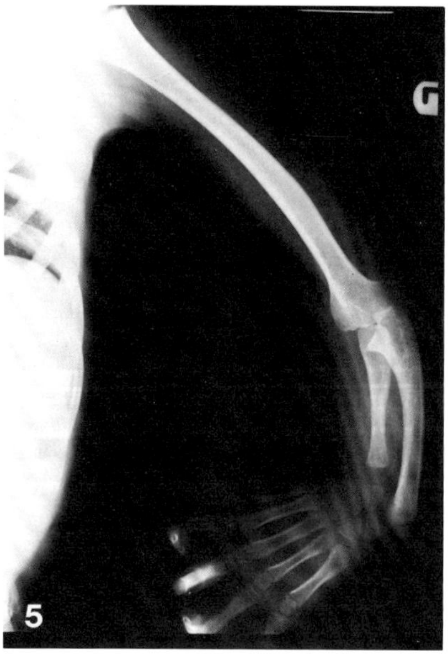

Fig. 5. Thalidomide preaxial defect with radius more affected than ulna and hypoplastic thumb.

With increasingly severe malformation of the preaxial side of the forelimb, changes are also observed at the shoulder and hip. In the shoulder there may be simple capsular defects leading to shoulder subluxation; in more severe examples, hypoplasia of the upper humerus and glenoid process, leading to a flail shoulder generally when the deformity has progressed to a flipperlike limb; and with very great severity resulting eventually in only one or two fingers attached to a pendulous and very short limb with only a few long bone remnants, the best preserved sometimes still retaining a resemblance to an ulna. With extreme severity, amelia results with perhaps one or two virtually functionless digits attached to the trunk. The shoulder contour in thalidomide amelia or severe reduction defect becomes sharpened owing to prominence of the acromioclavicular joint with deficiency of the glenoid process and of the upper end of the humerus. In non-thalidomide reduction defects short of amelia, the shoulder contour mostly remains normal and a digit may resemble a thumb in the postaxial-type defects. If amelia occurs in

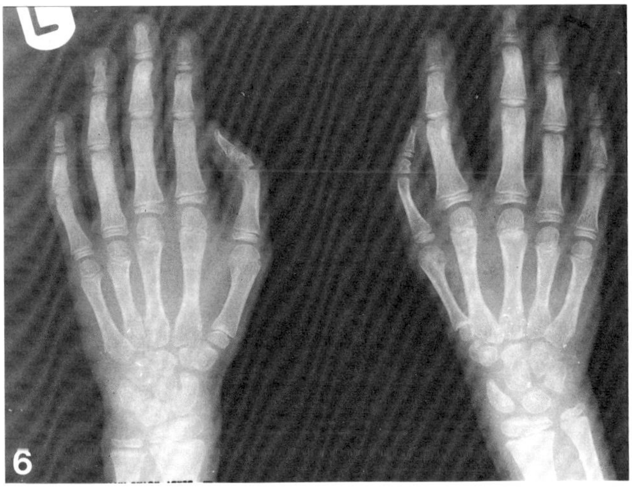

Fig. 6. Triphalangism of thumbs with some hypoplasia (thalidomide).

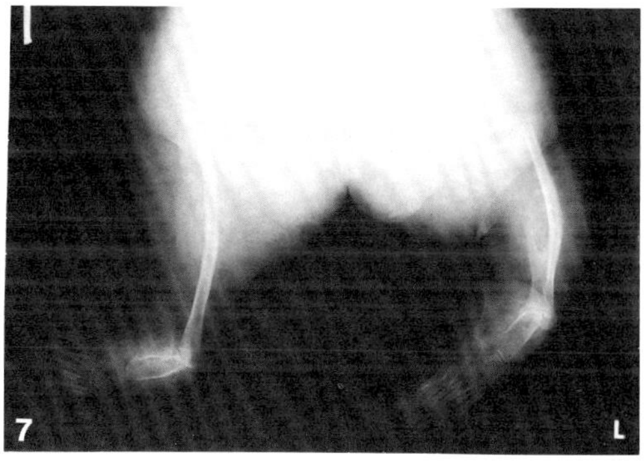

Fig. 7. Thalidomide. Only the fibula remains (R), fused to a tibial remnant (L). Six-digit (L) foot.

non-thalidomide cases, it is usually one-sided with at least a portion of limb on the other side. Also, the glenoid process may or may not be deficient. In examples of amelia, therefore, where there is a clear glenoid process, one can be sure that this is not an example of thalidomide syndrome (Figs. 9,10).

Transverse fusion of the forearm bones in non-thalidomide-affected limbs may occur distally in the relatively common transverse below elbow distal deficiencies, but not with postaxial defects affecting the fifth, or fourth and fifth digits on at least one limb. In this type of upper limb defect, elbow fusion with bizarre radial extension of the humerus and one or two digits often attached laterally and short of the distal end of the limb may occur. Femoro-tibial remnant fusion also occasionally occurs in postaxial deficiency, evidenced by loss at least of the fifth toe and part of the foot or a similar postaxial defect in the upper limb on at least one side. In thalidomide de-

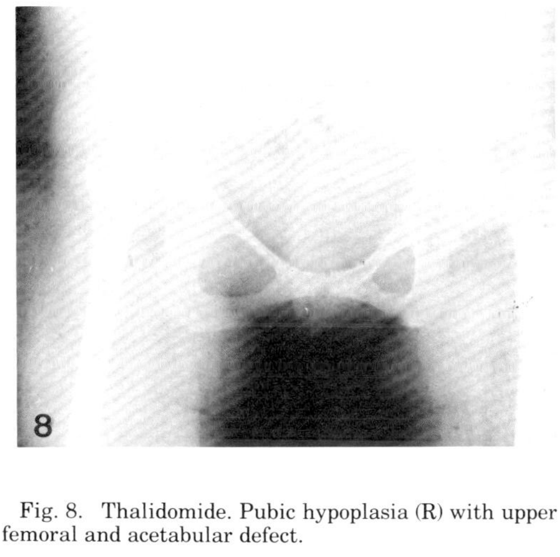

Fig. 8. Thalidomide. Pubic hypoplasia (R) with upper femoral and acetabular defect.

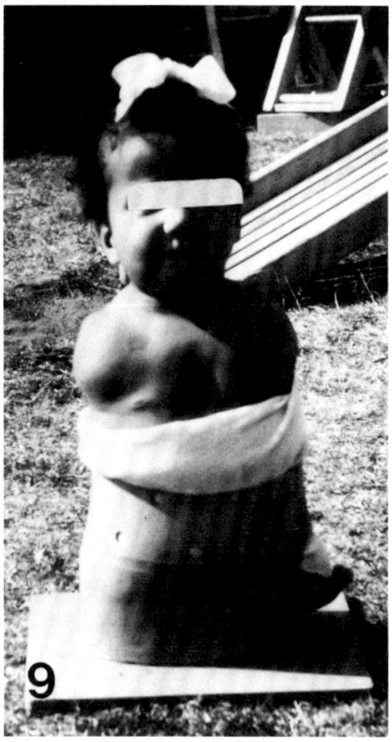

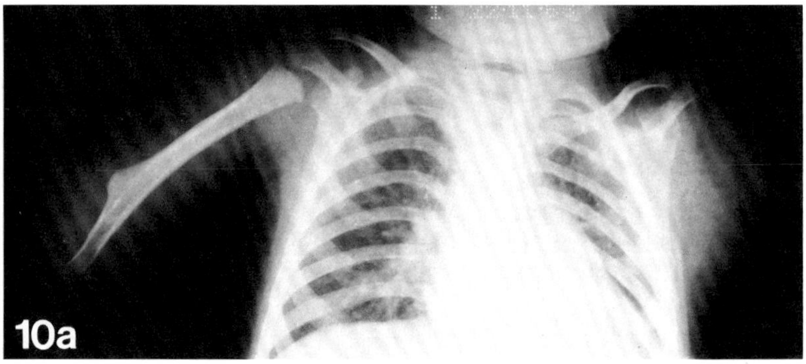

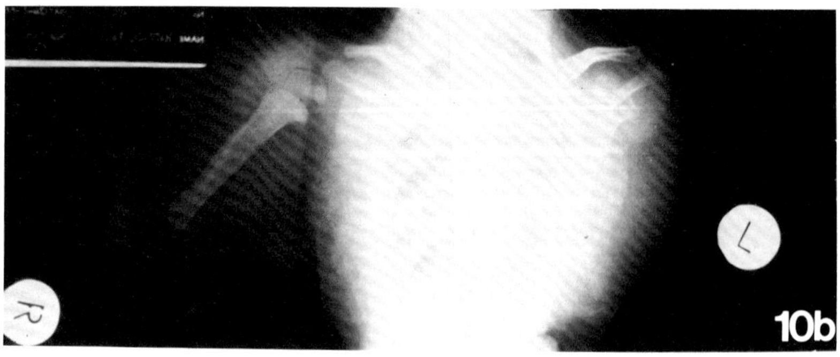

Fig. 9. Non-thalidomide amelia. Normal glenoid process and shoulder contour retained.

Fig. 10. A. Non-thalidomide. Distal transverse deficiency and amelia (FFU). Genoid process persists. B. Non-thalidomide. Further example, similar to A. Glenoid process persists on the left.

fects, the emphasis on preaxial forelimb defects with the occurence of proximal defects with persistence of distal postaxial structures occurs regularly and more or less symmetrically, and longitudinal elbow or knee fusion is not found.

In the leg quite minor defects, for example, slight shortening of the femur and laxity of the knee joint, may escape attention unless carefully looked for. Typically, thalidomide induces tibial hypoplasia and foot deformity with abnormality of the big and second toe, often associated with proximal femoral defects which may occur alone without defects below the knee. This type of femoral hypoplasia may also occur as part of the postaxial femur-fibula-ulna (FFU) syndrome (Lenz and Feldman, '77) and is therefore in itself not diagnostic. There may be prolonged ossification delay of the upper end of the femur, sometimes with fracture or modelling defect of the femoral head or neck, often with coxa vara. In severe cases a very late ossifying mass corresponded to the more proximal femoral elements, with femoral condyles and a dislocated fibula close to the pelvic girdle supporting a malformed and polydactylic foot. Lower amelia also occurred but was rare. The *pelvic girdle* showed acetabular hypoplasia ranging to complete absence of the acetabulum, also hypoplasia of the pubic bone. The symphysis pubis, however, remains normal (Fig. 8).

In non-thalidomide instances of amelia (upper or lower) there is generally asymmetry at least of the upper or lower limbs, and when at least one limb remains this will frequently show a pattern quite distinct from that found in thalidomide, for example, a distal transverse loss above the knee or elbow, or postaxial emphasis with the postaxial structures absent or more reduced than the preaxial ones (Fig. 11).

In the FFU syndrome there may be severely shortened limbs with few remaining digits, or complete amelia, or a much less severely affected limb. There is, therefore, a superficial resemblance to some types of thalidomide embryopathy, but the fundamental differences described above remain. The FFU syndrome is well described by Kuhne et al. ('67) and by Lenz ('69), also again by Lenz and Feldmann ('77) (Figs. 11–15).

In the thalidomide literature there are a very small number of puzzling and atypical case reports. Interpretation is made more difficult in some instances by confusion in labelling abnormal forelimb bones, for example, fibula for tibia in the chapter by Klaus Knapp in the book edited by Chester A. Swinyard ('69) (legends to Figures 153 and 155, pp. 334 and 335, respectively), where the fibula is said to be aplastic, yet where, especially in Figure 153, it is clearly the tibia that is missing. It is correctly described by the same author in the similar illustration especially of the left leg in the paper by Knapp and Lenz ('62, their Fig. 9). However, an error in the legend to a figure cannot be the explanation in a case reported by E. Odette Hagan ('65) where there was a "very likely" exposure to thalidomide and the baby suffered from severe preaxial upper limb reduction deformity fully compatible with the syndrome but with a fibular aplasia in the lower limb proved anatomically. Other defects were compatible with a thalidomide effect. Equally atypical is the Japanese report of two fraternal twins [cases 41, male, and 41, female, of Tabuchi et al. ('63)], both of whom had, among other malformations, aplasia of the appendix, cleft palate, very hypoplastic upper limbs with some residual digits, and predominantly fibular deficiency

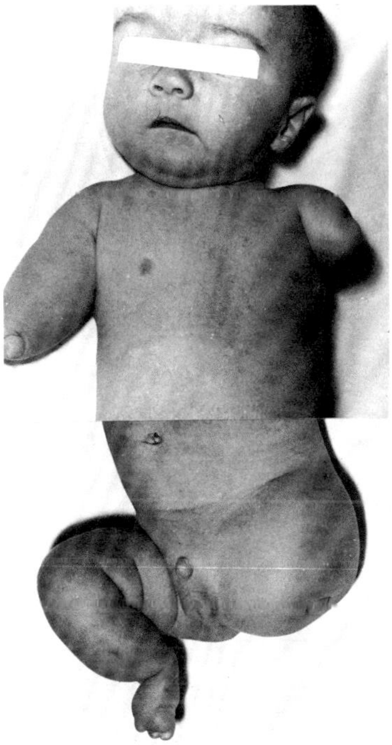

Fig. 11. Non-thalidomide. The foot shows a postaxial ray defect. FFU complex.

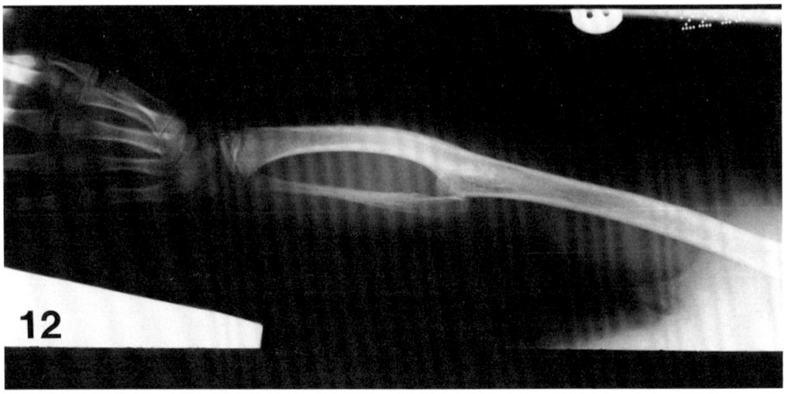

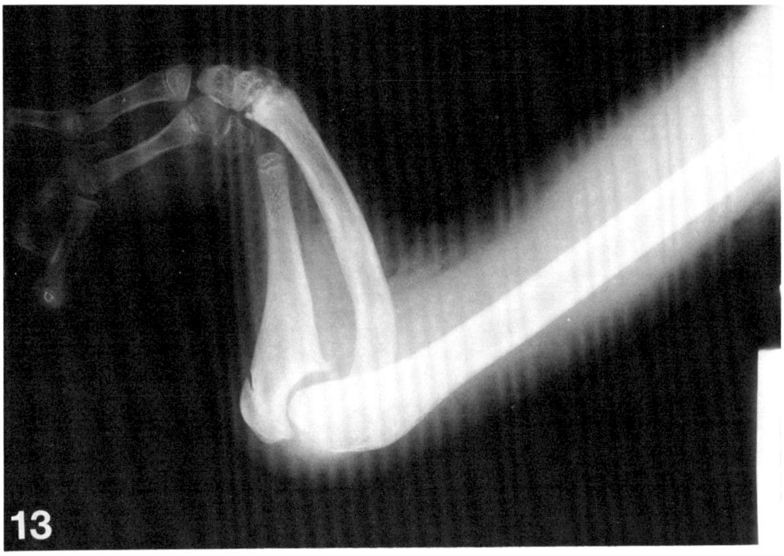

Fig. 12. Non-thalidomide postaxial defect. Ulnar hypoplasia with humeroradial fusion (FFU).

Fig. 13. Non-thalidomide postaxial ray deficiency (FFU).

in the boy's left leg. Admittedly, the upper limb defects are not typical and their malformations could have been a coincidental postaxial defect syndrome. An environmental cause is, however, likely when fraternal twins are both affected, and thalidomide exposure had occurred but at an undetermined time. Nevertheless, in the very extensive thalidomide literature, there are very few such cases. These are the only ones I have been able to find where the likelihood of exposure during the sensitive period was strong, yet some of the defects were predominantly postaxial.

There are few described conditions combining preaxial with postaxial defects. Robert's syndrome, pseudo-thalidomide, radio-fibular phocomelia, or SC syndrome—which are all synonymous—is one, and an autosomal recessive condition. There is also bilateral fibular defect associated with hypoplasia of metacarpals and phalanges, in which the thumb is more affected than the postaxial rays (Lenz, '79). Such mixed types are, nevertheless, very

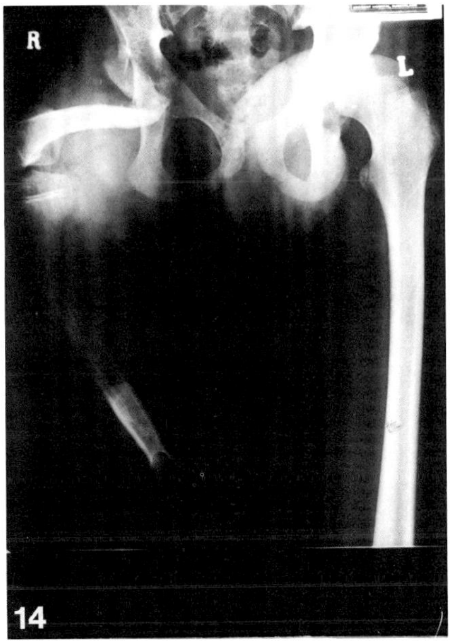

Fig. 14. Non-thalidomide postaxial and upper femoral deficiency. (Right foot has been amputated; FFU.)

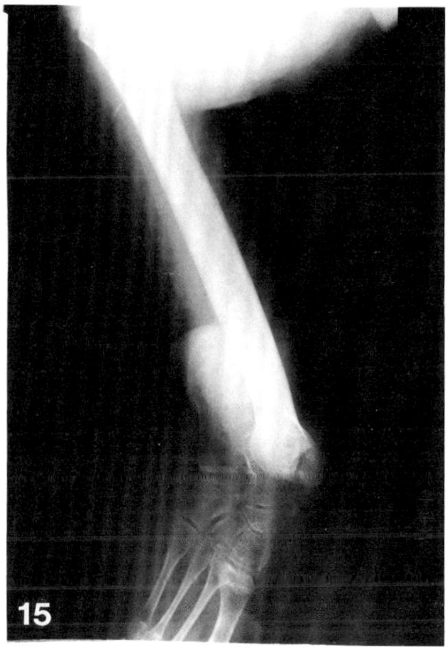

Fig. 15. Non-thalidomide postaxial defect. Fibular aplasia and loss of fifth ray (FFU).

much rarer than the purely preaxial varieties of malformation, as in thalidomide, and the postaxial types, as in the FFU pattern.

Spine

There is an increased incidence of defects that otherwise occur without thalidomide exposure, for example, spina bifida occulta, meningomyelocele, and changes such as those caused by Sheuermann's disease. In addition, in individuals with severe lower limb reduction defects, there may be progressive ossification of the anterior spinal ligaments (Edwards and Nichols, '77), converting the sacral and lumbar vertebral bodies into a solid mass of bone. There may be spondylolisthesis and also sacral defects with loss of a number of distal segments. *Rib* defects have not been observed, but no careful analysis has, as far as the author is aware, been undertaken. Their incidence is described in many other syndromes, for example, those listed in Smith ('82).

Growth

An analysis of over 200 children demonstrated truncal shortness but a normal growth rate. This shortness was independent of any apparent vertebral defects (Brook et al., '77).

Skull and teeth

Minor changes are described, such as deficiency in number or hypoplasia of teeth (Axrup et al., 1966; Stahl, '68; Hammarström et al., '70). Facial asymmetry and some changes of the basisphenoid are also described, but these changes, while they occur more commonly than would be expected by chance in thalidomide victims, are not sufficiently distinctive to be useful for diagnosis. There is no evidence of any foraminal stenosis or other changes that might affect the issuing cranial nerves. The cranial nerve lesions are, in fact, more central. There are changes, however, in the petrous temporal bone that are associated with the semicircular canal and cochlear hypoplasia in association with deafness and disturbances of balance.

Special senses and cranial nerves

No abnormalities have been described affecting the sense of smell. The *nose* may have a hypoplastic bridge and expanded tip. Choanal atresia also occurred, affecting one or both nostrils, constituting a neonatal emergency.

The *eyes* may show refractive errors, abnormalities of the pupil and of extrinsic muscle function, and colobomas, and they may be severely affected with microphthalmos and cataracts, resulting in blindness (Cullen '64; Rafuse et al., '67; Zetterström, 1966). All three oculomotor nerves may be affected. There is frequently associated *facial nerve* paralysis and *deafness* (Smithells, 1965). The latter is conductive or neural or both, with defects of the *external ear* (hypoplasia, atresia) with partial or complete anotia, *middle ear* (fusion and defects of ossicle chain), or of the *cochlea* and *semi-circular canals*. Thalidomide ear defects are commonly symmetrical, whereas in non-thalidomide patients they are more commonly unilateral (Livingstone, '65; Takemori et al., '76; Mündnich et al., '74). Quite minor ear defects such as long narrow auditory canals can cause a good deal of trouble from blockage from wax. They can also suggest a thalidomide causation when, for example, this defect coincides with radial aplasia or hypoplasia in a potentially affected individual. It is interesting that radial defects can also be associated with deafness and external ear malformation, for example, in the lacrimo-auriculo-dentodigital (LADD) syndrome, in which there may also be dental, congenital heart, and eye abnormalities. This syndrome, however, is inherited as an autosomal dominant. Similarly, deafness may be a feature of the Fanconi anaemia syndrome associated with preaxial defects (recessive inheritance) and narrow ear canals may coexist with the radial aplasia—thrombocytopenia syndrome, also recessively inherited. It is clear, therefore, that thalidomide can mimic some hereditary syndromes in some detail.

Cranial nerve abnormality may be associated with the Marcus Gunn or "jaw-winking" phenomenon, or the crocodile tear syndrome, possibly due to malconnections centrally in the nucleus ambiguus. Paralysis may also occur affecting the *palate*. *Tongue* abnormalities are most commonly due to a marked tongue-tie with a V-shaped anterior notch, and not to neural defects. The skeletal defects in the ankyloglossia syndrome are not thalidomidelike, nor are those occasionally found in association with congenital cranial nerve defects (Moebius syndrome).

Epilepsy probably occurs with some increase in incidence (Stephenson, '76), and this was already predicted in the study by Horstmann ('66) on the basis of EEG findings. The increase, however, is small.

The 4% incidence of *mental retardation* in the UK series is most likely not a direct thalidomide effect but secondary to sensory deprivation and additional handicap.

Additional and internal abnormalities

The incidence of these abnormalities is well described in the literature, for example, Kreipe ('67), Ruffing ('77), and Quibell ('81). There were *laryngeal* and *tracheal* abnormalities and abnormal lobulations of the *lungs* (Bilateral trilobed lungs). The laryngeal abnormalities on occasion gave rise to problems with intubation during anaesthesia.

Heart and circulation and blood vessels

A midline capillary naevus extending along the dorsum of the nose and present on the philtrum was prominent in infancy in many patients but faded as the child grew older. No other haemangiomata occurred related to embryopathy. *Congenital heart disease* occurred with considerable frequency and was a major cause of death [30% incidence at birth, 6% incidence in survivors (Ruffing, '77)]. The commonest defects were of the conotruncal region. Patients with the Holt Oram syndrome cannot be distinguished from thalidomide victims in the absence of a family history, although points of difference arise. For example, lower limb defects are not found in Holt Oram syndrome, and atrial septal defects are far more common than in the thalidomide syndrome. By contrast, isolated upper limb defects are relatively rare in thalidomide embryopathy. It could yet be that some individuals considered to be thalidomide victims will prove to have the Holt Oram syndrome if some of their own children are affected. Up to the present the author is aware of more than 60 thalidomide-affected parents who have had a child, and none has had a congenital limb reduction handicap.

Abdomen

Upper *intestinal atresias* required early surgery. Congenital absence of the gall bladder and of the appendix, the latter reviewed by Shand and Bremner ('77), may occur in thalidomide embryopathy, and with great rarity independently. *Inguinal hernias* and *delayed testicular descent* were also common, the latter particularly so in children with severe lower limb defects (Newman, '77). The author has come across only one patient with subsequent and probably related sterility, but unfortunately considerations of confidentiality and reluctance to reopen a potentially distressing situation has resulted in a continued lack of more than anecdotal data.

Kidney defects occurred such as abnormal rotation, pelvic position, horseshoe kidney, hydronephrosis, and double ureter. *Double vagina* and *anal atresia*, *rectal-vaginal fistula*, and *anal stenosis* also occurred with significantly increased frequency.

It can be seen that the vertebral-anal-cardiac-tracheal-esophogeal-renal-limb (VACTERL) association of defects can copy many of the defects characteristic of thalidomide embryopathy, although the detail is often different. For example, the limb defects may not be preaxial, tracheo-oesophageal fistula was very rare in thalidomide embryopathy and the vertebral defects can include hemivertebrae, not seen with increased frequency in thalidomide.

Late defects

No late defects have occurred, or at any rate none have been described, other than progression of previously established lesions as in the spine or kidney. Difficulties in balancing were described late by some young people, as was crocodile tear syndrome, probably because of increasing awareness on the part of the professionals. Excessive sweating, noticeable when the children were very young, appears to be less of a problem now, but this may merely be because of greater acceptance or because the surface area increases with growth.

Is there a definitive thalidomide syndrome that is sufficiently exclusive to indicate thalidomide ingestion in a patient without known access? The answer is probably no, since thalidomide phenocopies continue to occur, though very rarely, and probably have always occurred, the uncertainty being due to variable detail in the descriptions found in the literature. The implication that the drug must have been responsible can be given something of a mathematical probability by calculating the likelihood and timing of access and of affecting the foetus on the one hand, against the usually rare sporadic incidence of the observed abnormalities on the other. In assessing a cause-and-effect relationship retrospectively, inevitably there were some individuals exposed to the drug who demonstrated defects of different types, for example, Poland syndrome, transverse terminal defects or postaxial defects as in the FFU syndrome. None of these defect patterns increased in incidence during the years of thalidomide availability nor were produced by thalidomide in experimental animals, yet inevitably difficult decisions had to be made where litigation for compensation was undertaken. It is, therefore, necessary to distinguish clearly between correlations based on scientific evidence and those based on the skill of an advocate or on popular sympathy. While it is impossible to prove a negative, there is no evidence that thalidomide-caused defects outside the described pattern, and the success of the construction of a sensitive period with retrospective data indicates a rather clear cause-and effect relationship. This, of course, was supported by the animal experimentation particularly in primates.

Hopefully there will never be a similar man-made epidemic in the future. The possibility nevertheless exists, and one can only hope that recognition and response can be accelerated and made more effective. Nationwide notification of congenital malformations with sufficient detail is a prerequisite but is not yet established in many countries whose services are otherwise advanced; and more effective training in epidemiological methods to establish study and control populations for prospective analysis at the earliest possible opportunity would also be a high priority. Hopefully some lesson has been learned from the tragedy, and the experience may yet provide future insights as the study of naturally occurring defects advances.

LITERATURE CITED

Axrup, K., M. d'Avignon, K. Helgren, C.-O. Henrikson, I.-O. Juhlin, K.S. Larsson, G.E. Persson, and E. Welander (1966) Children with thalidomide embryopathy: Odontological observations and aspects. Dental Digest *72*(9):403–405, 423–425.

Brook, C.G.D., S.N. Jarvis, and C.G.H. Newman (1977) Linear growth of children with limb deformities following exposure to thalidomide in utero. Acta Paediatr. Scand., *66:*673–675.

Cullen, J.F. (1964) Ocular defects in thalidomide babies. Br. J. Ophthalmol., *48:*151.

Edwards, D.H., and P.J.R. Nichols (1977) The spinal abnormalities in thalidomide embryopathy. Acta Orthop. Scand. *48:*273–276.

Hagan, E. Odette (1965) Congenital malformations in a thalidomide baby: A post mortem anatomical study. Can. Med. Assoc. J., *92:*283–286.

Hammerström, L., C.-O Henrikson, and K.S. Larsson (1970) Anomalies of the teeth in a child with upper phocomelias. Oral Surg. *29*(2):191–196.

Henkel, L., and H.E. Willert (1969) Dysmelia. A classification & pattern of malformation in a group of congenital defects of the limbs. J. Bone Joint Surg., *51*(B):399–414.

Horstmann, W. (1966) Heinweise auf zentralnervöse Schäden im Rahmen der Thalidomid-Embryopathie. Z. Kinderheilkunde, *96:*291–307.

Kajii, T., M. Kida, and K Takahashi (1973) The effect of thalidomide intake during 113 human pregnancies. Teratology, *8*(2):163–166.

Knapp, K., and W. Lenz (1962) Die Formen der Thalidomid-Embryopathie. Roentgen. Eur., *5:*105–127.

Kreipe, U. (1967) Miszbildungen innerer Organe bei Thalidomidembryonpathie. Arch. Kinderheilkunde, *176:*33–61.

Kuhne, D., W. Lenz, D. Petersen, and H. Schonenberg (1967) Defekt von Femur und Fibula mit Amelie, Peromelie oder ulnaren Strahldefekten der Arme. Ein Syndrom. Humangenetik *3:*244–263.

Lenz, W.D. (1969) Bone defects of the limbs—An overview. Birth Defects: Original Article Series, *V*(3):1–6. (National Foundation.)

Lenz, W.D. (1971) How can teratogen action be established? S. Med. J. Suppl., *1:*41.

Lenz, W., and U. Feldmann (1977) Unilateral and assymmetrical limb defects in man: Deliniation of the femur-fibula-ulna complex in birth defects. Birth Defects: Original Article Series, *XIII*(1):269–285. (National Foundation.)

Lenz, W., and K. Knapp (1962) Die Thalidomid-Embryopathie.Dtsch. Med. Wochenschr., *87:*1232–1242.

Livingstone, G. (1965) Congenital ear abnormalities due to thalidomide. Proc. R. Soc. Med., *58:*493–497.

McBride, W.G. (1977) Thalidomide embryopathy. Teratology, *16:*79–82.

Mündnich, K., J.H.F. Batstone, D.O. Maisels, B.H. Colman, and W. Edwards (1974) Congenital abnormalities of the ear. Proc. R. Soc. Med., *67:*1197–1206.

Newman, C.G.H. (1977) Clinical observations on the thalidomide syndrome. Proc. R. Soc. Med., *70:*225–227.

Pembrey, M.E., C.A. Clarke, and M.M. Frais (1970) Normal child after maternal thalidomide ingestion in critical period of pregnancy. Lancet, *1:*275–277.

Quibell, E.P. (1981) The thalidomide embryopathy. An analysis from the UK. Practitioner, *225:*721–726.

Rafuse, E.V., M. Arstikaitis, and H.P. Brent (1967) Ocular findings in thalidomide children. Can. J. Ophthalmol., *2:*222–225.

Ruffing, L. (1977) Evaluation of thalidomide children. Birth Defects: Original Article Series, *XIII*(1):287–300. (National Foundation.)

Shand, J.E.G., and D.N. Bremmer (1977) Agenesis of the vermiform appendix in a thalidomide child. Br. J. Surg., *64:*203–204.

Siguira Y., K. Tsuchiya, M. Kida, and M. Arima (1979) Thalidomide dysmelia in Japan. Cong. Anom., *19:*1–19.

Smith, D.W. (1982) Recognizable patterns of human malformation. In: Major Problems in Clinical Pediatrics, Vol. VII, 3rd. edition. W.B. Saunders Company, Philadelphia.

Smithells, R.W. (1965) The thalidomide legacy. Proc. R. Soc. Med., *58:*491–492.

Stahl, A. (1968) Clinical, orthodontic and radiological findings in the jaws and face of children with dysmelia associated with thalidomide embryopathy. Dent. J., *18:*631–638.

Stephensen, J.B.P. (1976) Epilepsy. A neurological complication of thalidomide embryopathy. Dev. Med. Child Neurol., *18:*189–197.

Swinyard, C.A., ed. (1969) Limb Development and Deformity: Problems of Evaluation and Rehabilitation. Charles C. Thomas, Springfield, Illinois.

Tabuchi, A., A. Yamada, H. Umisa, T. Shintani, M. Horikawa, K. Shirasuna, and M. Sawasaki (1963) Phocomelia-like deformity and thalidomide preparations. Hiroshima J. Med. Sci., *12:*(1):11–35.

Takemori, S., T. Yoshisato, and J.-I. Suzuki (1976) Thalidomide anomalies of the ear. Arch. Otolaryngol., *102:*425–427.

Weicker, H., K.D. Bachmann, R.A. Pfeiffer, and J. Gleiss (1962) Thalidomid-embryopathie. Dtsch. Med. Wochenschr., *33:*1597–1607.

Williams, R.T. (1968) Thalidomide—A study of biochemical teratology. Arch. Environ Health, *16:*493–502.

Working Group of the International Society for Prosthetics and Orthotics (1975) The proposed international terminology for the classification of congenital limb defects. Dev. Med. Child Neurol. (Suppl. 34), 17(3).

Zetterström, B. (1966) Ocular malformations caused by thalidomide. Acta Ophtalmol., *44:*391–395.

TERATOGEN UPDATE: ENVIRONMENTALLY INDUCED BIRTH DEFECT RISKS, PAGES 13–18 (1986)

Fetal Alcohol Syndrome

JOHN J. MULVIHILL
Clinical Epidemiology Branch, National Cancer Institute, Bethesda, Maryland 20892

MANIFESTATIONS

Major features (Figs. 1–4) are prenatal and postnatal growth retardation, mental deficiency, small head size relative to height, and minor anomalies of the face, eye, heart, joints, and external genitalia. Mental retardation is the most serious defect and probably the most sensitive manifestation of maternal alcohol abuse. Ocular anomalies include epicanthal folds, convergence defects, ptosis, microphthalmia, and palpebral fissures that are below average in length. Skeletal and cardiac defects, usually mild, include campodactyly, clinodactyly, decreased range of motion, and spontaneously closing ventricular septal defect.

Minimal diagnostic criteria are physical and mental retardation with associated minor birth defects and a characteristic history of chronic maternal alcoholism. Mothers are often multiparous with severe alcoholism of several years' duration, involving any type of beverage—wine, beer, or spirits. The patient may be seen first by obstetricians recognizing alcoholism in their patients, by neonatologists evaluating "intrauterine growth retardation," by pediatricians confronted with a patient with growth failure or learning disability, or by social workers involved because of familial negligence. The syndrome can be readily distinguished from others with similar features, such as the Cornelia de Lange, Smith-Lemli-Opitz, trisomy 18, familial blepharophimosis, and fetal hydantoin syndromes.

Over time, the frequency of features (Fig. 4) has not changed, but additional characteristics found in over 50% of patients are:

Growth and development.. Poor coordination, hypotonia, neonatal irritability, and hyperactivity are seen in early life (Landesman-Dwyer et al., '78). Newborns have been called "short for weight rather than light for length" (Anon., '76). Average I.Q. of 20 children was 65 (Streissguth et al., '78a).

Ocular. Ptosis and strabismus are common. Standards for palpebral fissure length in white newborns (Jones et al., '78) should facilitate the objective search for short fissure length, a very specific feature.

Facial. The most common diagnostic characteristics of the syndrome, besides short palpebral fissure, are midfacial hypoplasia, long flat philtrum, and long convex upper lip with thin vermilion border.

Other. As specialists examine affected children, additional defects are recognized. Possibly life-threatening anomalies may be commoner than thought at first; renal hypoplasia (DeBeukelaer et al., '77; Qazi et al., '79) and atrial and ventricular septal defects (Dupuis et al, '78) seem the commonest visceral malformations. Malignancy, mostly embryonal neoplasms, has ocurred in ten patients, including two who also had fetal hydantoin syndrome (Bostrom and Nesbit, '83; Cohen, '81; Zaunschirm and Muntean, '84).

EPIDEMIOLOGY AND ETIOLOGY

Since the firm delineation of the fetal alcohol syndrome (FAS) by Jones et al. ('73), reports of many cases affecting several races with an equal sex ratio have appeared in English (Mulvihill et al., '76). Of 23 children of clearly alcoholic women in the Perinatal Collaborative Project, six with the FAS (26%) were found. The risk of a fetus' being affected may be directly related to the amount of alcohol it is exposed to, but the actual dose and duration of exposure required are unknown. The susceptible period probably spans the major part of gestation. It is speculative whether polymorphic and developmental isozymes of alcohol dehydrogenase alter fetal susceptibility or whether ethanol is, indeed, the sole agent. Other substances in alcohol, such as aldehydes and heavy metals, may cross the placenta. The social and medical complications of alcoholism, like inadequate nutrition, altered metabolism, and irregular medical care, may potentiate the prime teratogen. Most mothers in the Johns Hopkins series were underweight and had a history of poor diet. Folic acid deficiency may be a mechanism for teratogenesis, since alcohol

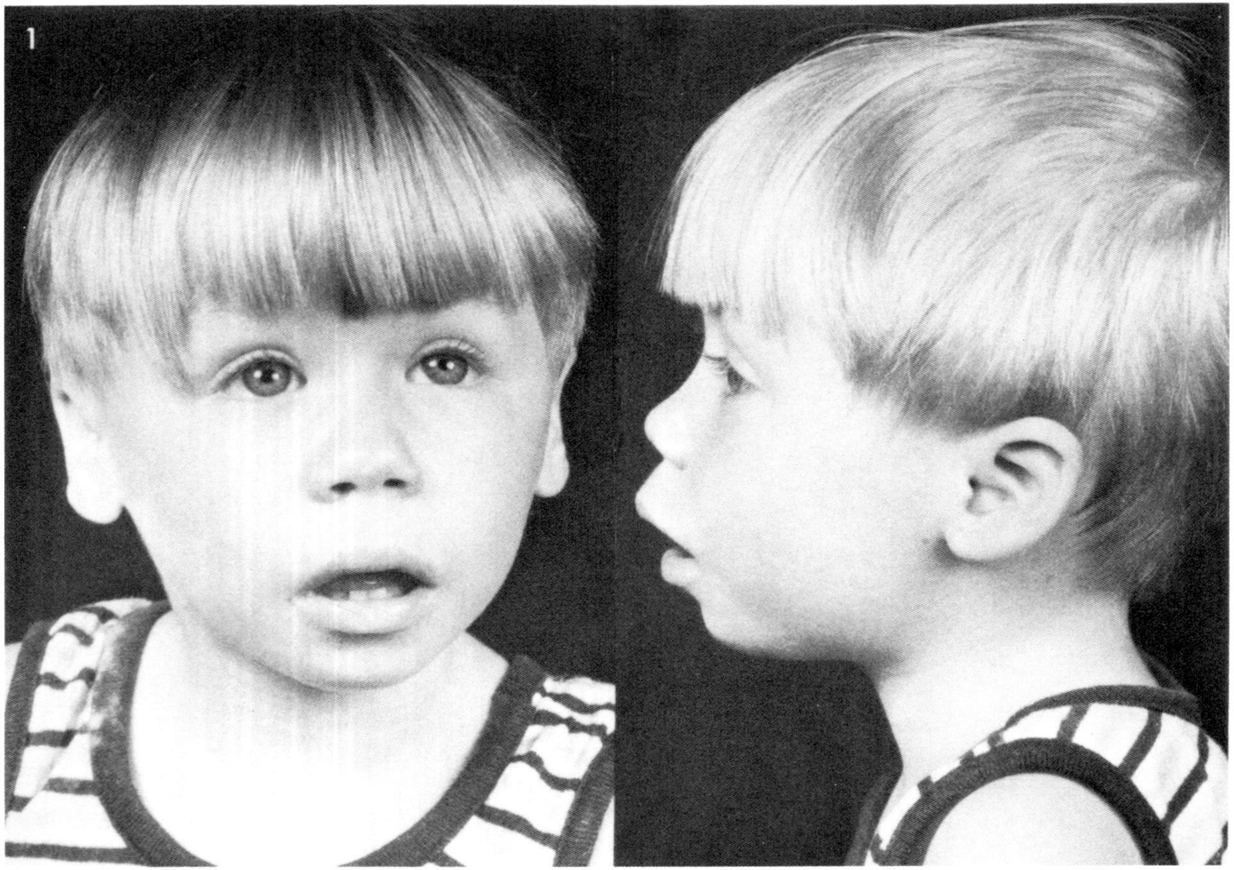

1

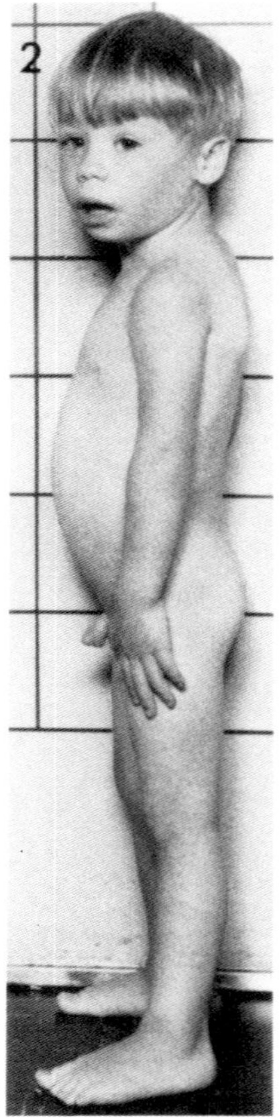

2

Figs. 1–2. A 3½-year-old-boy with growth retardation, small head circumference for height, mild ptosis, micrognathia, and hypoplastic midfacial structures (epicanthal folds, broad nasal bridge, upturned nares, and long philtrum). Each palpebral fissure is 20 mm long, about 2 SD below the mean for age; pinnae have prominent anthelices and long helical roots with pits; penis bows upward. The palate, bones, joints, and palmar creases are normal, as is the heart, despite a history of murmur in infancy.

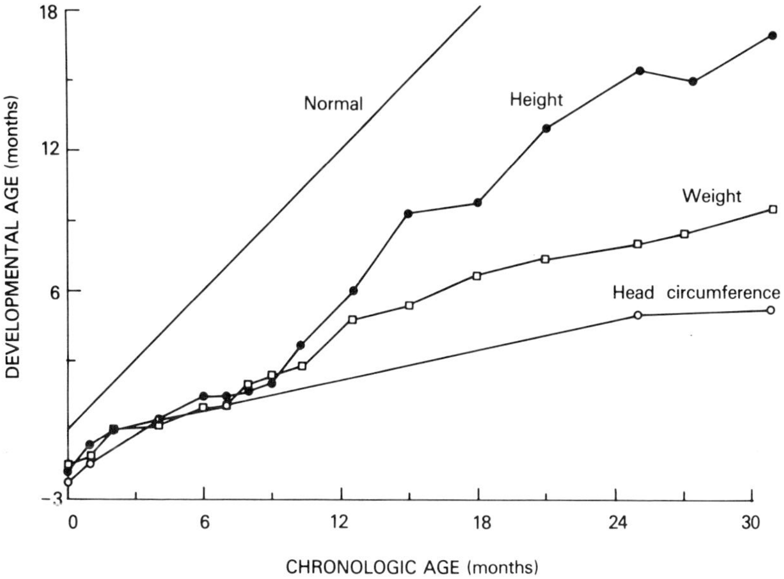

Fig. 3. Patient's growth was typical of FAS. At birth he was small for gestational age, with length more severely retarded than weight; in infancy growth remained below the 3rd percentile but weight was more impaired than height.

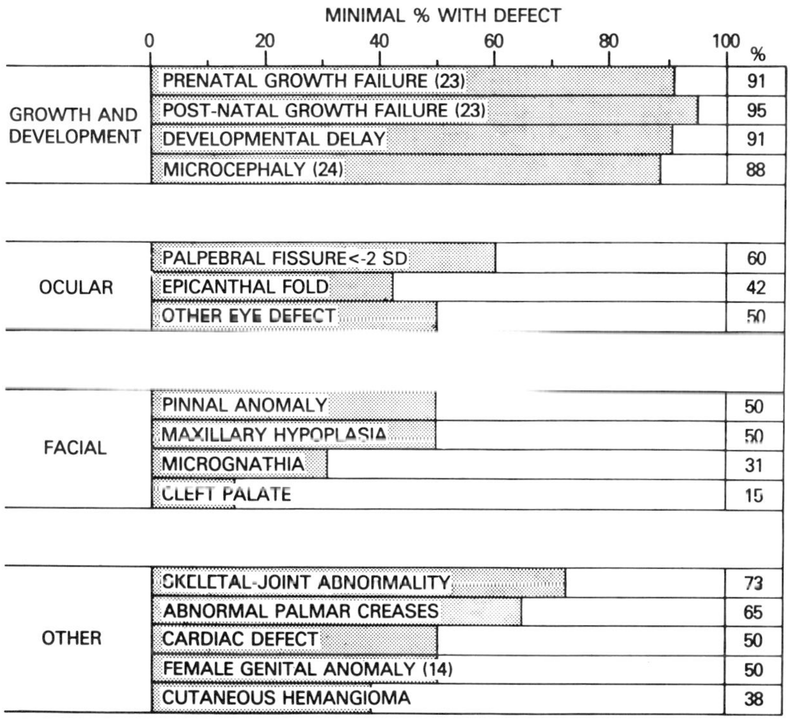

Fig. 4. Minimal frequency of defects, based on 26 published cases (or fewer, as given in parentheses).

and diphenylhydantoin interfere with folate metabolism and the malformation syndromes ascribed to each agent share many features.

Six of ten prospective surveys reported lower birth weights in offspring of drinkers compared to controls (Rosett and Weiner, '85). One showed the rate of malformations in children of heavy drinkers to be greater than the controls (Ouellette et al., '77). No cases of fetal alcohol syndrome were initially recognized (perhaps because specific characteristics were not sought), but one was found on reexamination (Streissguth, '78). Other investigators prospectively identified heavy drinkers by the fifth month of pregnancy; their 163 newborns were paired with nursery controls and examined by a pediatrician unaware of the drinking history but skilled in recognizing the syndrome. Fetal alcohol syndrome was recognized in two offspring of heavy drinkers and suggestive features were seen in seven others; two control babies had suggestive signs (Hanson et al., '78).

Majewski ('78) defined three grades of alcohol embryopathy and Shaywitz et al. ('80) suggested an "expanded fetal alcohol syndrome," comprising hyperactivity and defects of attention span and learning, with normal intelligence and minimal other birth defects. Very unusual brain pathology, consisting of neuroglial heterotopia in the leptomeninges and interruption of neuronal migration, was found in babies born to alcoholic women even when external signs of the full syndrome were lacking (Clarren et al., '78). With minimal expression of the syndrome ill-defined, its frequency must await prospective studies, but it has been called the third most frequent cause of mental retardation. Similarly, the most susceptible period of gestation and minimal toxic dose are undetermined. Dermatoglyphics (Fig. 5) suggest the twelfth week as the most susceptible. Several animal models have been proposed (Chernoff, '77; Weathersbee and Lodge, '78), and one teratologic study in rats incriminated acetaldehyde (O'Shea and Kaufman, '79).

Over 400 cases of FAS were reported by 1978 (Clarren and Smith, '78; Majewski '78). The syndrome is now a subject of a three volume text (Abel, '81–'82), a periodically updated Literature Search from the National Library of Medicine (Kenton, '83), and various symposia (Ashley, '81; Messiha and Tyner, '83). Clinicians have come to rely on the thin vermilion border and hypoplastic philtrum as the most specific diagnostic signs. The diagnosis can be difficult in the absence of a history of maternal alcoholism, all the more so since the features resemble those seen in offspring of mothers with untreated phenylketonuria (Lipson et al., '81). Zinc deficiency (Flynn et al., '81) and acetaldehyde (Véghelyi, '83) have been suggested as the prime teratogen, rather than ethanol, on the basis of human and/or experimental models (Porter et al., '85)

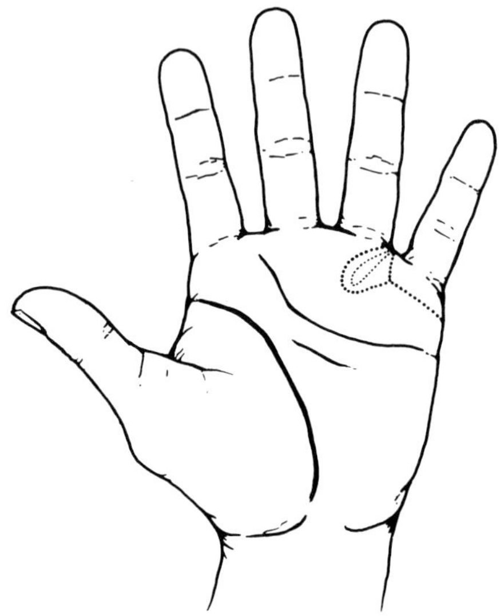

Fig. 5. Characteristic palmar crease abnormalities consist of prominent thenar crease, nearly absent proximal transverse crease, and abrupt turning of distal transverse crease into second interdigital space. Fourth interdigital loop with termination of dermal ridge line D in that space is the most consistent but nonspecific dermatoglyphic anomaly (redrawn form Tillner and Majewski, '78).

TREATMENT AND PREVENTION

Prognosis awaits full documentation. Growth and mental deficiency seem to persist into adult life (Streissguth et al., '78a, '85). In childhood, I.Q. may vary widely as individuals are followed (Streissguth et al., '78b). The public has been informed in a thorough nonalarming fashion that could serve as a model for other newly discovered health hazards. The U.S. National Institute of Alcohol Abuse and Alcoholism has recommended that pregnant women drink no more than one ounce of absolute alcohol (two cocktails) a day. The National Clearinghouse for Alcohol Information (c/o NIAAA, Rockville, MD 20852) is a source of current medical and public information on the syndrome (Chafetz, '75).

CLINICAL ADVICE

Women at risk of pregnancy must be warned of the hazards to the fetus of alcohol abuse. Fetal harm can occur throughout pregnancy. Further, women should be told of the uncertainty of the scientific evidence concerning whether or not there is a threshold level of minimal or moderate alcohol use below which no embryotoxicity occurs. The safest advice is total abstinence, but most commentators allow the equivalent of a glass of wine per day (Neugut, '81; Fabro and Brown, '82; AMA Council on Scientific Affairs, '83; Edwards, '83).

HISTORICAL FOOTNOTE

Although recent priority of recognition has been widely assigned to Lemoine in 1968 (Clarren and Smith, '78), his compatriot Alexandre Lamache ('67) deserves credit. He recognized children of alcoholics to have "low weight, growth retardation, often anorexia, and, of course, these physical troubles occur together with more or less marked problems of either character, behavior, or academic failure. . . ." The term "Jones-Smith syndrome" would recognize the rediscoverers of the disorder and emphasize its common occurrence. Despite Majewski's logical suggestion of "alcohol embryopathy," "fetal alcohol syndrome" has become an index term at the National Library of Medicine.

LITERATURE CITED

Abel, E.L. (1981–1982) Fetal Alcohol Syndrome. 3 Volumes. CRC Press, Inc., Boca Raton, Florida.

AMA Council on Scientific Affairs (1983) Fetal effects of maternal alcohol use. JAMA, *249:*2517–2521.

Anon. (1976) Fetal alcohol syndrome. Lancet, *1:*1335.

Ashley, M.J. (1981) Symposium: Alcohol and the fetus. Can. Med. Ass. J., *125:*141–166.

Bostrom, B., and M.E. Nesbit, Jr. (1983) Hodgkin disease in a child with fetal alcohol-hydantoin syndrome. J. Pediatr., *103:*760–762.

Chafetz, M.E. (1975) A biomedical information source: The National Clearinghouse for Alcohol Information. Fed. Proc., *34:*2001–2004.

Chernoff, G.F. (1977) The fetal alcohol syndrome in mice. Teratology, *15:*223–230.

Clarren, S.K., E.C. Alvord, Jr., S.M. Sumi, A.P. Streissguth, and D.W. Smith (1978) Brain malformations related to prenatal exposure to ethanol. J. Pediatr., *92:*64–67.

Clarren, S.K. and D.W. Smith (1978) The fetal alcohol syndrome. N. Engl. J. Med., *298:*1063–1067.

Cohen, M.M., Jr. (1981) Neoplasia and the fetal alcohol and hydantoin syndromes. Neurobehav. Toxicol. Teratol., *3:*161–162.

DeBeukelaer, M.M., C.L. Randall, and D.R. Stroud (1977) Renal anomalies in the fetal alcohol syndrome. J. Pediatr., *91:*759–760.

Dupuis, C., P. Dehaene, P. Deroubaix-Tella, A.P. Blanc-Garin, C. Rey, and C. Carpentier-Courault (1978) Les cardiopathies des enfants nés de mère alcoolique. Arch. Mal. Coeur, *71:*565–572.

Edwards, G. (1983) Alcohol and advice to the pregnant woman. Br. Med. J., *286:*247–248.

Fabro S. and N.A. Brown (1982) In utero alcohol exposure: Threshold for effects? Reprod. Toxicol.: A Medical Newsletter, *1(3):*11–14.

Flynn A., S.I. Miller, S.S. Martier, N.L. Golden, R.J. Sokol, and B.C. Del Villano (1981) Zinc status of pregnant alcoholic women: A determinant of fetal outcome. Lancet, *1:*572–574.

Hanson, J.W., A.P. Streissguth, and D.W. Smith (1978) The effects of moderate alcohol consumption during pregnancy on fetal growth and morphogenesis. J. Pediatr., *92:*457–460.

Jones, K.L., J.W. Hanson, and D.W. Smith (1978) Palpebral fissure size in newborn infants. J. Pediatr., *92:*787.

Jones, K.L., and D.W. Smith (1973) Recognition of the fetal alcohol syndrome in early infancy. Lancet, *2:*999–1001.

Jones, K.L., D.W. Smith, C.N. Ulleland, and A.P. Streissguth (1973) Pattern of malformation in offspring of chronic alcoholic mothers. Lancet, *1:*1267–1271.

Kenton, C. (1983) Maternal alcohol consumption and fetal and newborn effects, including the fetal alcohol syndrome (FAS). National Library of Medicine Literature Search No. 83-22, 304 ref. National Institutes of Health, Bethesda, Maryland, 21 p.

Lamache, A. (1967) Réflexions sur la descendance des alcooliques. Bull. Acad. Nat. Med., *151:*25–26.

Landesman-Dwyer, S., L.S. Keller, and A.P. Streissguth (1978) Naturalistic observations of newborns: Effects of maternal alcohol intake. Alcoholism, *2:*171–177.

Lipson, A.H., J.S. Yu, M.T. O'Halloran, and R. Williams (1981) Alcohol and phenylketonuria. Lancet, *1:*717–718.

Majewski, F. (1978) Über schädigende Einflüsse des Alkohols auf die Nachkommen. Nervenarzt, *49:*410–416.

Messiha F.S. and G.S. Tyner (1983) Fetal alcohol syndrome. Neurobehav. Toxicol. Teratol., *5:*169, 259–272.

Mulvihill, J.J., J.T. Klimas, D.C. Stockes, and H.M. Risemberg (1976) Fetal alcohol syndrome: Seven new cases. Am. J. Obst. Gynecol., *125:*937–941.

Neugut R.H. (1981) Epidemiological appraisal of the literature of the fetal alcohol syndrome in humans. Early Hum. Dev., *5:*411–429.

O'Shea, K.S. and M.H. Kaufman (1979) The teratogenic effects of acetaldehyde: Implications for the study of the fetal alcohol syndrome. J. Anat., *128:*65–76.

Ouellette, E.M., H.L. Rosett, N.P. Rosman, and L. Weiner (1977) Adverse effects on offspring of maternal alcohol abuse during pregnancy. N. Engl. J. Med., *297:*528–530.

Porter, R., M. O'Connor, and J. Whelan, eds. (1984) Mechanisms of Alcohol Damage *In Utero.* Pitman, London.

Qazi, Q.H., A. Masakawa, D.H. Milman, B. McGann, A. Chua, and J. Haller (1979) Renal anomalies in fetal alcohol syndrome. Pediatrics, *63:*886–889.

Rosett, H.L., and L. Weiner (1985) Alcohol and pregnancy: A clinical perspective. Ann. Rev. Med., *36:*73–80.

Shaywitz, S.E., D.J. Cohen, and B.A. Shaywitz (1980) Behavioral and learning difficulties in children of nor-

mal intelligence born to alcoholic mothers. J. Pediatr., *96:*978–982.
Streissguth, A.P. (1978) Fetal alcohol syndrome: An epidemiologic perspective. Am. J. Epidemiol., *107:*467–478.
Streissguth, A.P., S.K. Clarren, and K.L. Jones (1985) Natural history of the fetal alcohol syndrome: A 10-year follow-up of eleven patients. Lancet, *2:*85–91.
Streissguth, A.P., C.S. Herman, and D.W. Smith (1978a) Intelligence, behavior, and dysmorphogenesis in the fetal alcohol syndrome: A report on 20 patients. J. Pediatr., *92:*363–367.
Streissguth, A.P., C.S. Herman, and D.W. Smith (1978b) Stability of intelligence in the fetal alcohol syndrome: A preliminary report. Alcoholism, *2:*165–170.
Tillner, I. and F. Majewski (1978) Furrows and dermal ridges of the hand in patients with alcohol embryopathy. Hum. Genet., *42:*307–314.
Véghelyi, P.V. (1983) Fetal abnormality and maternal ethanol metabolism. Lancet, *2:*53–54.
Weathersbee, P.S. and J.R. Lodge (1978) A review of ethanol's effects on the reproductive process. J. Reprod. Med., *21:*63–78.
Zaunschirm, A., and W. Muntean (1984) Fetal alcohol syndrome and malignant disease. Eur. J. Pediatr., *141:*256.

DES—Transplacental Teratogen—And Possible Carcinogen

HOWARD ULFELDER
Vincent Memorial Hospital (Gynecological Service of the Massachusetts General Hospital), Boston, Massachusetts 02114

MANIFESTATIONS

Both gross and microscopic anomalies of development of the uterus and vagina have been detected in women exposed during the first 18 weeks of fetal life to stilbestrol or one of its chemical congeners. Moreover, the likelihood of teratogenic effects was inversely proportional to the fetal age at first exposure.

Abnormalities of three types have been described—vaginal adenosis, cervical erosions, and ridges. Adenosis is the generic term for histologically demonstrable glandular epithelium or its mucinous products in the vaginal wall. It usually consists of a single layer of columnar cells, but occasionally epithelial cells are also present; they are sometimes ciliated and resemble the lining cells of the endometrial cavity or tubal canal. Cervical erosions are visible areas of red tissue extending for variable distances from the canal out over the exocervix. In a pure sense the term erosion is a misnomer, since the epithelium is intact. Histologically, it is not squamous but columnar and indistinguishable from that which lines the canal, with which it is continuous. Ridges (also called hoods, coxcomb cervices, cervical pseudopolyps, etc.) are genuine morphological aberrations of the upper vagina and cervix that may partially constrict the canal, or deform the cervix, or partition it into central and peripheral circumforontial segments. Association between all or several of these abnormal findings is the rule. In young women not exposed to stilbestrol in fetal life only smaller cervical erosions occur normally and this in less than 50% of individuals.

EPIDEMIOLOGY

Historically the teratological stilbestrol disorders were first noted in 1971 in association with an almost unique tumor clear cell adenocarcinoma of the vagina in adolescent girls. Much of our original information was acquired through careful study of several hundred of these cancer cases collected and documented in a registry.

A meticulous current study of diethylstilbestrol adenosis—known as the (DESAD) project—of over 3,000 young women exposed in fetal life provides us with dependable statistical information that can be extrapolated to the population at large, somewhat in contrast to the reports of selected material from individual doctors or clinics, which is heavily weighted with symptomatic or referred patients. The risk of this cancer is now estimated to be less than one in a thousand; DESAD reports that none of 1,275 asymptomatic women identified through review of their mothers' obstetrical records had cancer on physical examination.

Congenital morphological changes, on the other hand, were detectable in 34%. These vaginal epithelial changes (VEC), by which are meant all mucosal abnormalities including adenosis, are noted with a frequency that correlates with the week of pregnancy during which medication was first administered; there is a marked decrease in anomalies if DES was first given after the 20th week. VEC also correlates with increasing total dose and length of time administered, but these, of course, also of necessity reflect time of onset of medication.

The prevalence of vaginal epithelial changes falls off significantly after the age of 26 years, which suggests that many of these anomalous lesions heal spontaneously with normal-appearing stratified squamous epithelium. This assumption is fortified by another observation on the DESAD cohort of girls examined solely because their mothers took DES in pregnancy. In these "record review" women epithelial dysplasia has been found with great rarity (0.4%) and when present it has been mild or moderate at the worst. No instance of severe dysplasia or carcinoma-in-situ has been found in this population.

DIAGNOSIS

Because the abnormal epithelium is poor in glycogen the cervical erosions and patches

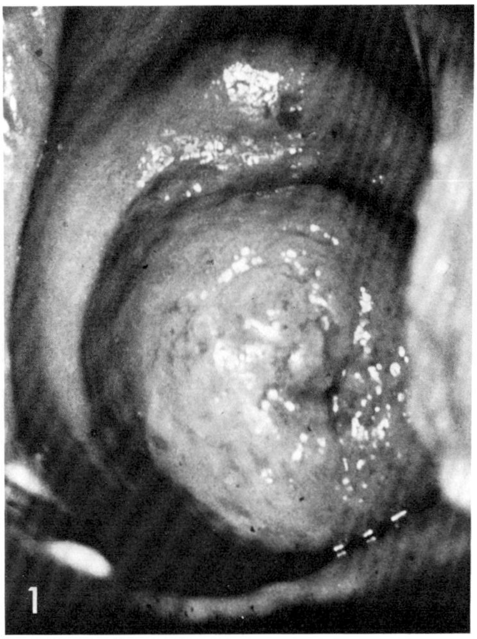
1

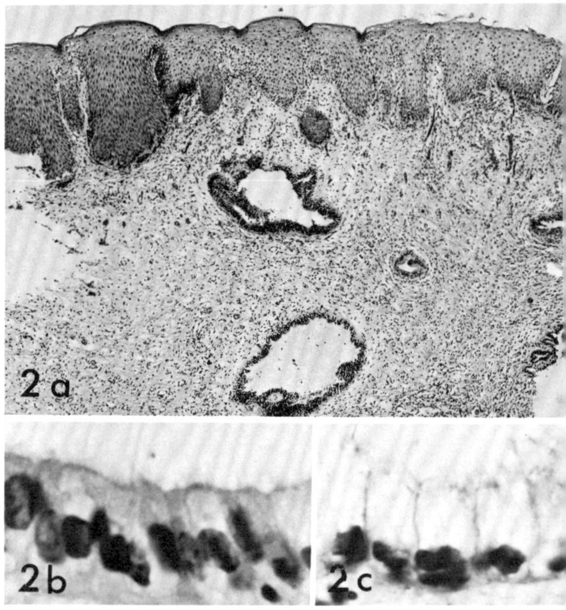
2 a
2 b
2 c

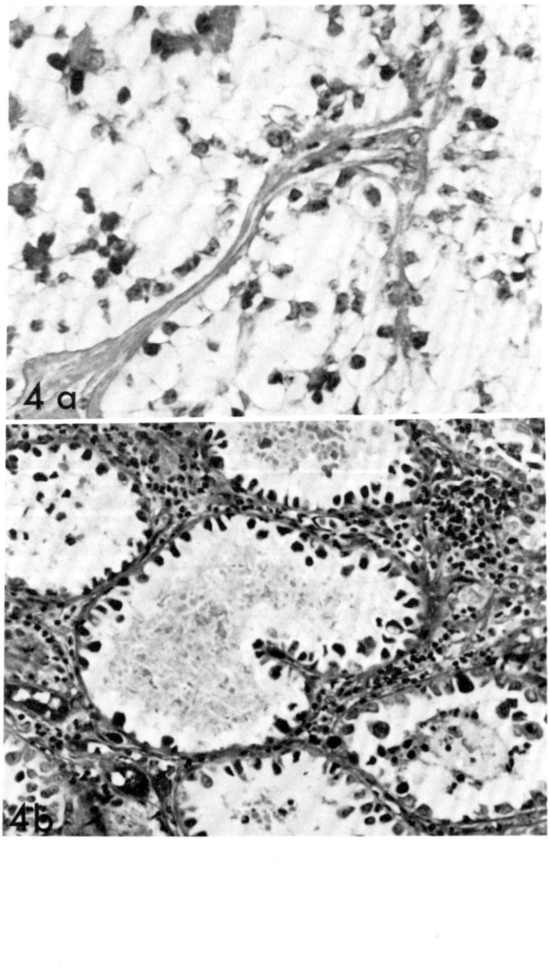
4 a
4 b

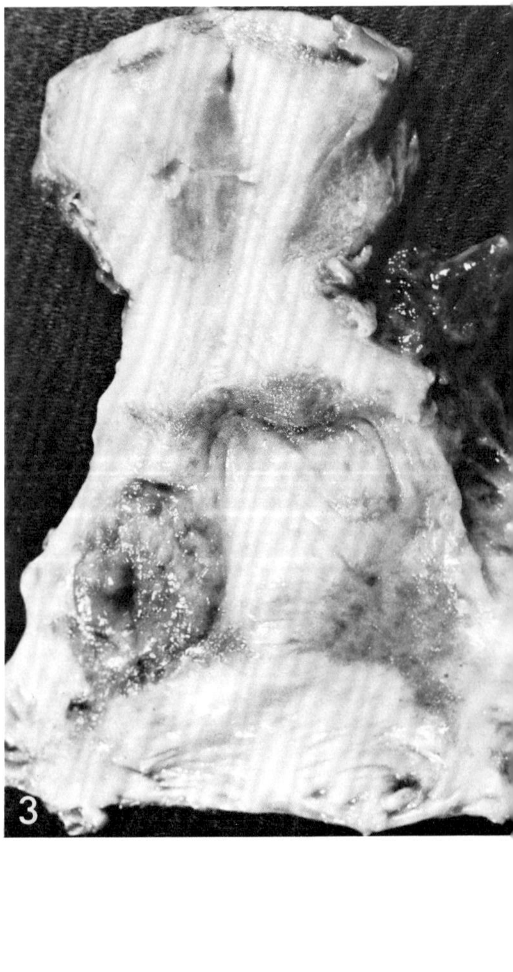
3

of vaginal adenosis fail to stain brown with aqueous iodine solution (Schiller's test). By this means, areas under direct observation that might escape notice can call attention to themselves for mapping and biopsy confirmation. The techniques of colposcopy also lend themselves ideally to repeated visual scrutiny. This is particularly valuable because the women at risk can be clearly selected out of the much larger population pool by the historical fact of stilbestrol exposure.

Biopsy and histological examination quickly identify the cancers, of course. Many cases have come to medical attention through complaints of discharge, particularly when bloody, but screening of asymptomatic women known to have been exposed has disclosed some early lesions and in this group the results of treatment have been most successful.

TREATMENT

There is not enough information to date to permit positive statements regarding the treatment of choice for adenosis. Mechanical excision or destruction of the abnormal areas is followed by clean healing with squamous epithelium, but in many girls the extent and distribution of lesions make this a formidable process. There is good evidence to suggest that gradual replacement of adenosis by squamous metaplasia will occur with the passage of time.

Treatment of cancer, when present, by either surgical or radiotherapeutic methods follows standard oncological procedure. It is notable that spread along lymphatic channels was early and facile, and failure to cure is probably going to be the unfortunate outcome in perhaps 50% of the known cases.

Physicians responsible for the management of individuals exposed to DES in fetal life can keep up to date by following the published results of the DESAD study project. In the female, the risk of benign anomalies, if exposure took place before the 18th week of gestation, is approximately 35%. With this goes a small associated likelihood of problems with fertility and pregnancy and a possibility of adenocarcinoma of the cervix or vagina that is currently estimated at something between one per thousand and one per ten thousand.

Exposure of the male fetus has not been associated with malignant disease in any of the studies reported to date. But the teratogenic potential is expressed also in the development of the masculine genital organs. DES sons have been found to have cysts of the epidydimus, cryptorchidism, hypogonadism, and diminished spermatogenesis in a significantly increased frequency over normal expectations.

Fortunately there is every reason to believe that avoidance of exposure of early developing human fetuses to the stilbene molecule will eliminate these disorders. It is entirely possible that physicians now living will some day look back and note that they observed firsthand the appearance, rise, decline, and disappearance of this phenomenon.

Fig. 1. Speculum view of cervical ridge and pseudo polyp (courtesy of Dr. Duane Townsend; reprinted from J. Reprod. Med., *15:*14, 1975).

Fig. 2. a) Benign adenosis underlying squamous metaplasia. b) High power view, endometrial pattern. c) High power view, endocervical pattern (reprinted from J. Reprod. Med., *15:*15, 1975).

Fig. 3. Clear-cell adenocarcinoma of the vagina (operative specimen; reprinted from Cancer, *25:*175, 1970).

Fig. 4. a) Adenocarcinoma, clear-cell pattern. b) Adenocarcinoma, hobnail-cell pattern (reprinted from J. Reprod. Med., *15:*17, 1975).

BIBLIOGRAPHY

Herbst, A.L., H. Ulfelder, and D.C. Poskanzer (1971) Adenocarcinoma of the vagina. Association of maternal stilbestrol therapy with tumor appearance in young women. N. Eng. J. Med., *284:*878–881.

Herbst, A.L. (1978) Intrauterine exposure to diethylstilbestrol in the human. Proceedings of Symposium on DES, 1977. The American College of Obstetricians and Gynecologists, Chicago.

O'Brien, P.C., K. Noller, S.J. Robboy, A.B. Barnes, R. Kaufman, B. Tilley, and D.E. Townsend (1979) Vaginal epithelial changes in young women enrolled in the national cooperative diethylstilbestrol adenosis (DESAD) project. Obstet. Gynecol., *53:*300–308.

Robboy, S.J., R.H. Kaufman, J. Prat, W.R. Welch, T. Gaffey, R.E. Scully, R. Richart, C.M. Fenoglio, R. Vir-ata, and B.C. Tilley (1979) Pathologic findings in young women enrolled in national cooperative diethylstilbestrol adenosis (DESAD) project. Obstet. Gynecol., *53:*309–317.

Ulfelder, H., and S.J. Robboy (1976) The embryologic development of the human vagina. Am. J. Obstet. Gynecol., *126:*769–776.

Ulfelder, H. (1980) The stilbestrol disorders in historical perspective. Cancer, *45:*3008–3011.

TERATOGEN UPDATE: ENVIRONMENTALLY INDUCED BIRTH DEFECT RISKS, PAGES 23–27 (1986)

Warfarin Embryopathy

JOSEF WARKANY
Children's Hospital Research Foundation, Cincinnati, Ohio 45229

Assigning a teratogenic effect to a drug must be done with caution. Since thalidomide directed general suspicion towards drugs and other chemical compounds a number of products have been accused of teratogenicity without adequate proof. Whereas vigilance and suspicion in this respect are justified and necessary, careful evaluation of useful chemicals is recommended before they are discarded because of unproven accusations. The responsibility of the accusers is considerable because they could deprive patients of the benefits of valuable medication.

RECOGNITION OF A SYNDROME

Ten years ago Di Saia ('66) recorded the pregnancy and delivery by a patient with a Starr-Edwards mitral valve prosthesis. The result was a female infant with hypoplasia of nasal structures, bilateral optic atrophy, blindness, and mental retardation. The history of the case was complex. The mother had been treated a year before the pregnancy for syphilis; during pregnancy she took digitalis, sulfisoxazole, erythromycin, and warfarin (Coumadin); the serological tests remained positive despite repeated courses of treatment. During the 26th week of gestation the mother had an episode considered a pulmonary infarct and she was given i.v. heparin therapy. Although the baby's disease picture was bizarre and it was known that anticoagulant therapy with coumarin derivatives during pregnancy could result in fetal and perinatal death (Mahairas and Weingold, '63; Villasanta, '65) the author limited the publication to the description of the mother and the infant and recommended further studies along these lines.

SUSPICION OF A CAUSE

Two years later Kerber et al. ('68) observed a male infant with a nasal malformation, choanal stenosis, seizures, and mental retardation; this mother also had a complex history. She had a prosthetic mitral valve and was treated with digitalis, penicillin G benzathine, sodium warfarin, and heparin during her pregnancy. The authors pointed out that 2 of 4 reported cases of prosthetic mitral valves in pregnancy had resulted in malformed infants with hypoplastic nasal structures. Common to all 4 cases was warfarin administration and mitral valve disease with a prosthesis. They thought it unlikely that maternal mitral valvular disease influenced the development of the nasal structures of the fetus, and noted that patients with prosthetic aortic valves in pregnancy who had not received anticoagulants during pregnancy had delivered normal infants. Therefore, they considered warfarin the most likely teratogenic agent, particularly when administered in the first 8 weeks of gestation; they called attention to their observation "so that it may be added to the experience of others." A follow-up of Di Saia's patient by Becker et al. ('75) added stippling of bones seen in roentgenograms to the teratologic picture, and in addition they described a premature baby boy (fig. 1) born to a mother with an aortic valve prosthesis and warfarin treatment during pregnancy who had an extremely depressed nasal bridge, deformed extremities, and roentgenograms suggestive of Conradi-Hünermann disease or chondrodysplasia punctata. The cases of Shaul et al. ('75) and of Pettifor and Benson ('75) with comparable congenital malformations were also associated with maternal warfarin use during pregnancy. Shaul et al. ('75) emphasized that the very rare disease picture of chondrodysplasia punctata subsequent to the rare use of warfarin during pregnancy should make one suspect that warfarin during the 1st trimester of pregnancy may have a teratogenic effect and they speculated that the anomalies could be related to bleeding in fetal or embryonic cartilage at an early and critical stage in development. Thus optic atrophy and mental retardation noted in at least 2 of the patients suggested "the possibility that a more generalized insult occurs during organogenesis."

SYMPTOMATOLOGY WIDENS

Later Shaul and Hall ('76) cited 11 cases of similar multiple congenital anomalies asso-

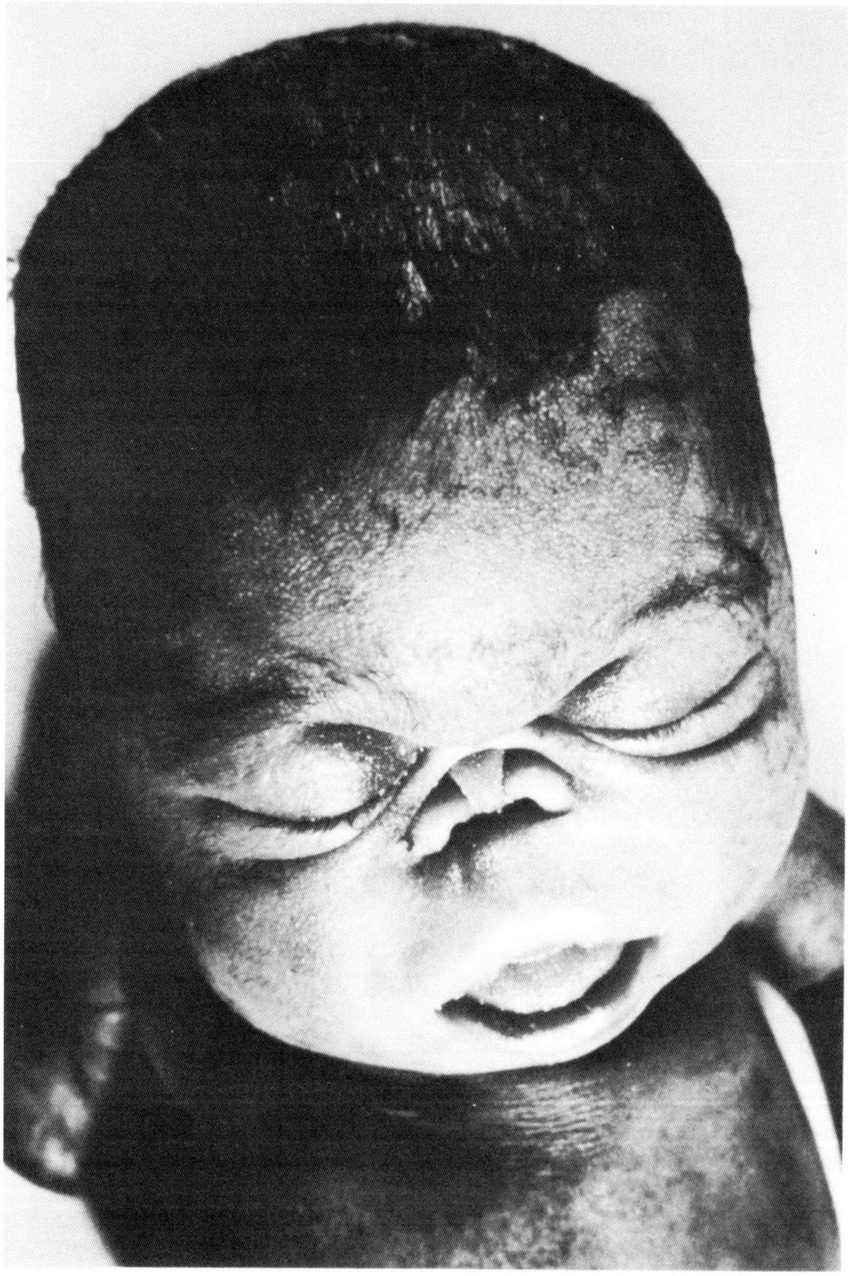

Fig. 1. Face of an infant with extreme hypoplasia of nasal bridge. The child also had opacification of the left optic lens and stippling in cartilaginous areas of epiphyses of extremeties and about spine and pelvis. The mother had been treated with warfarin during pregnancy. Reprinted from Becker et al. ('75; copyright 1975, Am. Med. Ass.) by permission of the author and editor.

ciated with oral anticoagulants. Since bleeding into embryonic or fetal tissues could result in congenital lesions besides chondrodysplasia punctata, nasal deformities, and optic atrophy, a spectrum of anomalies had to be considered. This was discussed by Warkany and Bofinger ('75) who cited von Sydow's ('47) case of a hydrocephalic child possibly damaged in the perinatal period by the mother's treatment with dicoumarin. Quenneville et al. ('59) had mentioned an infant with microcephaly, cerebral agenesis, and optic atrophy born after maternal treatment with a coumarin derivative. Tejani ('73) described a child with hypoplastic nasal bones and cartilages, occipital meningocele, hydrocephaly, microphthalmia, and a persistent truncus arteriosus. In this child of a woman with a mitral valve prosthesis treated with warfarin, the spectrum had spread out to involve many organ systems. Warkany and Bofinger ('75) reported 2 hydrocephalic children, 1 of them with a huge occipital cephalocele and renal malformations; the mothers had been treated with sodium warfarin during pregnancy. In these cases typical chondrodysplasia punctata could not be demonstrated; thus various portions of the spectrum of anomalies may result from maternal anticoagulant treatment. This would be understandable if bleeding into various fetal tissues were the cause of the malformations seen at birth.

In May 1975 Endo Laboratories revised the prescribing information concerning Coumadin (crystalline sodium warfarin) adding a warning about the possibility of fetal malformations related to warfarin therapy during the 1st trimester of pregnancy: "Coumadin should be used in women of childbearing potential only when, in the judgment of the physician, the potential benefits outweigh the possible hazards."

This warning did not end fetal damages by anticoagulant therapy. Holzgreve et al. ('76) reported a boy exposed to warfarin to the twelfth week of gestation. The child appeared normal until 5 months of age when delay in psychomotor development was noted. He had also mild nasal anomalies, pale optic discs, and moderate hypotonia. An E.M.I. scan revealed agenesis of the corpus callosum. In 1979, after review of all published and unpublished cases of warfarin embryopathy, Pauli and Hall ('79) listed 27 cases exposed between the sixth and ninth week of gestation: Seven died in infancy and another six had considerable disability. In individuals exposed in the second or third trimester, central nervous system defects and perinatal hemorrhages occurred.

In a retrospective review of all published cases in which coumarin derivatives were administered during pregnancy, it was found that about one in six of such pregnancies yielded liveborn infants with the warfarin embryopathy, CNS manifestations, or hemorrhage-related abnormalities; about one in six ended in stillbirths or spontaneous abortion so that only two-thirds resulted in apparently normal liveborn infants. Interestingly, a similar literature review of gestational use of heparin showed that pregnancy ended in stillbirths in about one in eight cases and in premature deliveries in one in five (with a third of these prematures dying). A normal outcome was to be expected in only two-thirds of such pregnancies. Thus both coumarin derivatives and heparin carry significant risks to fetuses. Pauli and Hall concluded: "If anticoagulation is necessary, counselling should be given, and if the patient does become pregnant, an offer of therapeutic abortion seems the most prudent course."

Stevenson et al. ('80), writing on hazards of oral anticoagulants during pregnancy, described in detail a female infant born after a 31-week gestation and weighing 1,049 g. The mother, a 23-year-old primigravida, had undergone tricuspid and mitral valve replacement one year before becoming pregnant. She took 5 mg of warfarin sodium each night for anticoagulation. One month before delivery, she experienced hematuria and hemarthrosis of the right knee. At that time the prothrombin time was prolonged to 42 s. At birth the infant's head was large, the optic discs were pale, and the nose was underdeveloped with absence of the nasal bridge and small nares directed forward. There were respiratory difficulties with retractions, cyanosis, acidosis, and depressed muscle tone. Roentgenograms showed stippling of vertebral, femoral, and tarsal epiphyses. At age 16 months length and weight were less than third centile, head size was 50th centile, and there was bilateral optic atrophy; she could not sit alone or pull herself to standing. The authors tabulated features noted in 15 infants exposed to anticoagulation during the first trimester of gestation. The infants' birth weights were graphically presented, which showed that not all of them were reduced. The risk of malformations was 15 to 25%.

After second trimester exposure, intrauterine or parturitional hemorrhages led to impairment of growth, vision, and mental development. Third trimester exposure sometimes resulted in intrauterine bleeding in spite of maintenance of the maternal prothrombine time within safe range. The risk of perinatal hemorrhage from second or third trimester exposure was thought to be 5 to 10%.

Two cases reported by Harrod and Sherrod ('81) are of great interest, since there were three children in a sibship, two with signs of warfarin embryopathy and one entirely normal. The oldest, a normal boy, was born before the mother became sick, whereas two younger children were born after the mother had received warfarin treatment for thrombophlebitis. The second boy had a flattened nose, a high frequency hearing loss, and some delayed language skills. The sister born 3 years later showed marked nasal hypoplasia, a small right opaque cornea, cataract, and widely spaced nipples. Radiologically, stippling of vertebral and calcaneal epiphyses was seen, signs that persisted over 1 year. The reason for continuation of warfarin treatment during the second pregnancy was that the affected boy's signs were not recognized as drug-related.

Baillie et al. ('80) described an eye anomaly attributed to warfarin exposure. The left eye and lacrimal sac were infected with streptococcus viridans, whereas the eye bulbs were normal. There was also a hypoplastic nose due to failure of development of the nasal septum.

Dean et al. ('81) recorded the outcome of three pregnancies of patients with prosthetic valves who were treated with warfarin. One patient, after three abortions, gave birth to a healthy infant and to an infant with complicated cardiovascular anomalies. However, two women with prosthetic valves and warfarin treatment had healthy children.

Kleinebrecht ('82) attempted to explain why some exposed conceptuses are affected while others remain normal. Dosage may play a role. The results of Kort and Cassel ('81) are cited: aiming at a prothrombin level of 40 to 60% of normal seemed to prevent damage. Other decisive factors could be genetic or environmental. Effects of other medications and of nutritional differences could influence the outcome. A long list of drugs is cited that are contraindicated when coumarins are given. Whether coumarins other than warfarin are less teratogenic remains to be seen. Differences in incidence figures can be explained by overreporting of pathologic cases on one hand and underreporting owing to delayed manifestations.

RELATING EFFECTS TO CAUSE

Early incidents illustrated the difficulties of relating a congenital malformation to an environmental cause such as maternal exposure to a drug or chemical (Warkany, '75). Human situations seldom present themselves with the clarity of an experiment. Reports on the mothers' pregnancies contained many factors besides warfarin therapy that had to be considered. All mothers were threatened by some thromboembolic complication for which anticoagulants were prescribed. They had diseases that were treated surgically by valvotomy or with valve prostheses. One mother had a positive serologic reaction to syphilis and another was an alcoholic; and many other drugs were taken besides coumarins. Anticoagulant treatment was recognized as a cause because it was repeatedly mentioned in the pregnancy histories; but also because such drugs are not widely used and nasal deformities with generalized chondrodysplasia punctata are rare malformations. This made the recognition of a causal relation possible. But if a widely used drug caused a common and unspecific malformation, it would be very difficult to prove a causal connection.

Another difficulty arises if a drug or a chemical produces a malformation that can be genetically determined in other instances. Chondrodysplasia punctata induced by warfarin resembles to a certain extent the disease picture known as Conradi-Hünermann disease (Conradi, '14; Hünermann, '31) or chondrodystrophia congenita calcificans which was considered a dominant or a recessive hereditary trait by some authors (Fraser and Scriver, '54; Spranger et al., '71). The warfarin-induced embryopathy would thus represent a "phenocopy" of the hereditary disorder. It is obvious that if dominant and recessive inheritance can be held responsible for a pathologic trait in some patients, it is very difficult to assert that a similar abnormal trait in a sporadic case is due to an environmental teratogenic factor.

Animal experiments have not been very helpful. Kraus et al. ('49) gave bishydroxycoumarin to pregnant rabbits and found that, according to dose, hemorrhagic tendencies or death of the fetuses resulted. Kronic et al. ('74) using sodium warfarin in mice, noted placental hemorrhage, fetal loss, and some minor anomalies, probably signs of delayed maturation and unspecific; but lesions characteristic of chondrodysplasia punctata were not observed.

It must be emphasized that not all children of mothers treated with warfarin and similar anticoagulant drugs were damaged, even when the compounds were given during the 1st trimester of pregnancy. Accessory factors may be involved in the production of the malformations described (Fillmore and McDevith, '70).

PREVENTION

Since physicians have been warned to withhold warfarin from women of childbearing potential it is to be hoped that cases of warfarin embryopathy will not be seen in the future. If this is so, the physicians involved in this preventive research are to be commended for their contributions and the methods employed. They reported their observations objectively in medical journals and expressed suspicions cautiously until the evidence was in. There were no sensational and disquieting reports in the lay press or on television and there was no need for political intervention. The laboratories that distribute the drug alerted physicians of possible dangers to the fetus. The ways used to stop this embryopathy could be used in similar situations without premature involvement of the public which cannot evaluate the risks and benefits of drugs and other chemical compounds.

LITERATURE CITED

Baillie, M., E.D. Allen, and A.R. Elkington (1980) The congenital warfarin syndrome: A case report. Br. J. Ophthalmol., *64:*633–635.

Becker, M.H., N.B. Genieser, M. Finegold, D. Miranda and T. Spackman (1975) Chondrodysplasia punctata: is maternal warfarin therapy a factor? Am. J. Dis. Child., *129:*356–359.

Conradi, E. (1914) Vorzeitiges Auftreten von Knochen- und eigenartigen Verkalkungskernen bei Chondrodystrophia fötalis hypoplastica: Histologische und Röntgenuntersuchungen. Jahrb. Kinderh., *80:*86–97.

Dean, H., S. Berliner, Y. Schoenfeld, and J. Pinkhas (1981) Warfarin treatment during pregnancy in patients with prosthetic mitral valves. Acta Haematol. *66:*65–66.

DiSaia, P.J. (1966) Pregnancy and delivery of a patient with a Starr-Edwards mitral valve prosthesis. Report of a case. Obst. Gyn., *28:*469–472.

Fillmore, S.J., and E. McDevith (1970) Effects of coumarin compounds on the fetus. Ann. Int. Med., *73:*731–735.

Fraser, F.C., and J.B. Scriver (1954) A hereditary factor in chondrodystrophia calcificans congenita. New Eng. J. Med., *250:*272–277.

Harrod, M.J.E. and P.S. Sherrod (1981) Warfarin embryopathy in siblings. Obstet. Gynecol., *57*:673–676.

Hünermann, C. (1931) Chondrodystrophia calcificans congenita als abortive Form der Chondrodystrophie. Z. Kinderh., *51:*1–19.

Holzgreve, W., J.C. Carey, and B.D. Hall (1976) Warfarin-induced fetal abnormalities. Lancet, *2*:914–915

Kerber, I.J., O.S. Warr and C.J. Richardson (1968) Pregnancy in a patient with a prosthetic mitral valve. Associated with a fetal anomaly attributed to warfarin sodium. J. Am. Med. Ass., *203:*223–225.

Kleinebrecht, J. (1982) Zur Teratogenität von Cumarin-Derivaten. Dtch. Med. Woch., *107*:1929–1931.

Kort, H. and G.A. Cassel (1981) An appraisal of warfarin therapy during pregnancy. S. Afr. Med. J., *60*:578–579.

Kraus, A.P., A. Perlow and K. Singer (1949) Danger of dicumarol treatment in pregnancy. J. Am. Med. Ass., *139.*758–762.

Kronick, J., N.E. Phelps, D.J. McCallion and J. Hirsh (1974) Effects of sodium warfarin administered during pregnancy in mice. Am. J. Obst. Gyn., *118:*819–823.

Mahairas, G.H., and A.B. Weingold (1963) Fetal hazard with anticoagulant therapy. Am. J. Obst. Gyn., *85:*234–237.

Pauli, R.M. and J.G. Hall (1979) Warfarin embryopathy. Lancet, *2*:144.

Pettifor, J.M., and R. Benson (1975) Congenital malformations associated with administration of oral anticoagulants during pregnancy. J. Pediat., *86:*459–462.

Quenneville, G., G. Barton, E. McDevitt and I.S. Wright (1959) The use of anticoagulants for thrombophlebitis during pregnancy. Am. J. Obst. Gyn., *77:*1135–1149.

Shaul, W.L., H. Emery and J.G. Hall (1975) Chondrodysplasia punctata and maternal warfarin use during pregnancy. Am. J. Dis. Child., *129:*360–362.

Shaul, W.L., and J.G. Hall Multiple congenital anomalies associated with oral anticoagulants. Am. J. Obst. Gyn., in press.

Spranger, J.W., J.M. Opitz and U. Bidden (1971) Heterogeneity of chondrodysplasia punctata. Humangenetik, *11:*190–212.

Stevenson, R.E., M. Burton, G.J. Ferlauto, and H.A. Taylor (1980) Hazards of oral anticoagulants during pregnancy. JAMA, *243*:1549–1551.

Sydow, G. v. (1947) Hypoprothrombinemia and cerebral injury in infant after dicumarol treatment of mother. Nord. Med., *34:*1171–1172.

Tejani, N. (1973) Anticoagulant therapy with cardiac valve prosthesis during pregnancy. Obst. Gyn., *43:*785–793.

Villasanta, V. (1965) Thrombembolic disease in pregnancy. Am. J. Obst. Gyn., *93:*142.

Warkany, J. (1975) A warfarin embryopathy? Am. J. Dis. Child., *129:*287–288.

Warkany, J., and M. Bofinger (1975) Le rôle de la coumadine dans les malformations congénitales. Méd. Hyg., *33:*1454–1457.

Fetal Hydantoin Effects

JAMES W. HANSON
Division of Medical Genetics, Department of Pediatrics, University of Iowa, College of Medicine, Iowa City, IA 52242

In the more than twenty years since questions have been raised regarding the teratogenicity of anticonvulsant drugs, a substantial body of literature has accumulated, surrounding which there is still debate (Kelly, '84a). Nonetheless, it has become increasingly clear that infants born to mothers with seizure disorders treated with anticonvulsant medications during pregnancy are at an increased risk for congenital defects. Problems including confounding, ascertainment bias, poor statistical power, biologically inappropriate or inconsistent case definition, and present medical seizure disorder management practices, have all plagued epidemiologic studies, rendering firm conclusions problematic.

A comprehensive review of these issues is beyond the scope of this update. However, a variety of lines of human and animal investigation continues to suggest that anticonvulsant medications of the hydantoin group (e.g., phenytoin) have teratogenic effects in at least some exposed fetuses that are not attributable to other concurrently existing prenatal risk factors. When these effects lie near the extreme end of a spectrum of possible outcomes, the resulting pattern of abnormalities has been referred to as the fetal hydantoin syndrome.

MANIFESTATIONS

As originally characterized, the fetal hydantoin syndrome was thought to consist of: 1) abnormalities of growth such as pre- and postnatal growth deficiency and microcephaly; 2) abnormalities of performance such as developmental delay or dull mentality to frank mental deficiency; and 3) dysmorphic craniofacial features commonly including short nose with broad depressed bridge and inner epicanthic folds, mild ocular hypertelorism, ptosis of the eyelid, strabismus, wide mouth, sutural ridging, and short neck with mild webbing; less commonly cleft lip and/or palate (Figs. 1, 2), and limb anomalies including hypoplasia of the nails and distal phalanges with an increased frequency of low arch digital dermal ridge patterns, and fingerlike thumb (Figs. 3–5) (Hanson and Smith, '75).

Less frequently, children displaying these dysmorphic craniofacial and limb features were reported to have major anomalies in other systems, including cardiac anomalies. Concern has also been expressed about an increased incidence of major genitourinary and central nervous system anomalies, more serious limb reduction defects, and diaphragmatic hernia.

Subsequent studies have raised questions about this definition of the syndrome, its components, specificity, and clinical significance (Kelly, '84b; Rating et al., '82; Koch et al., '82). Present information suggests that growth disorders or mental deficiency may indeed be an outcome of prenatal phenytoin exposure (Bjerkedal, '82; Gopfert-Geyer et al., '82; Ogawa et al., '82; Holmes, '85). However, these abnormalities may not necessarily persist in a serious degree in at least some cases (Helge, '82). Furthermore, questions have been raised as to whether or not growth and mental deficiency, as well as major craniofacial or cardiac anomalies, are indeed parts of a comprehensive syndrome or are defects of distinct and separate pathogenesis encountered in this same group of exposed offspring (Kelly et al., '84; Jager-Roman et al., '82). The craniofacial and limb features would appear to be the most consistent markers of the prenatal teratogenic effect of hydantoins.

An additional abnormality, which has now been reported on numerous occasions in children with features of the fetal hydantoin syndrome, is cancer. Phenytoin is oncogenic in adults; developmental arrest types of tumors, especially tumors of neural crest origin such as neuroblastoma, have now been reported in nine infants with features of the syndrome (Allen, '84; Bostrom and Nesbit, '83). These reports suggest a non-random association

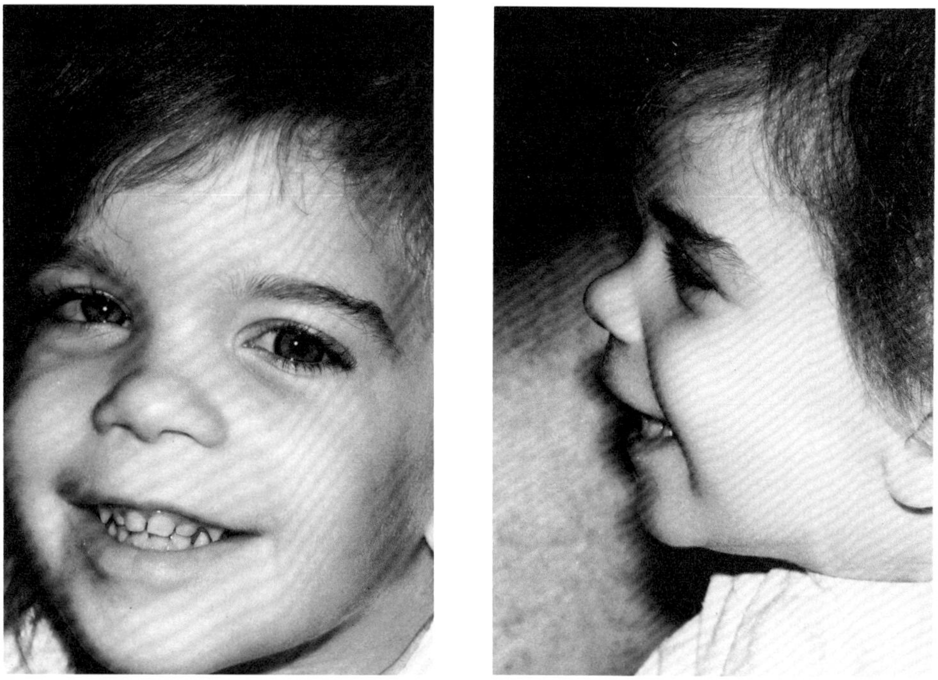

Figs. 1 and 2. Facial features of the fetal hydantoin syndrome—note broad flat nasal bridge with epicanthic folds, mild hypertelorism, strabismus, and wide mouth with prominent upper lip.

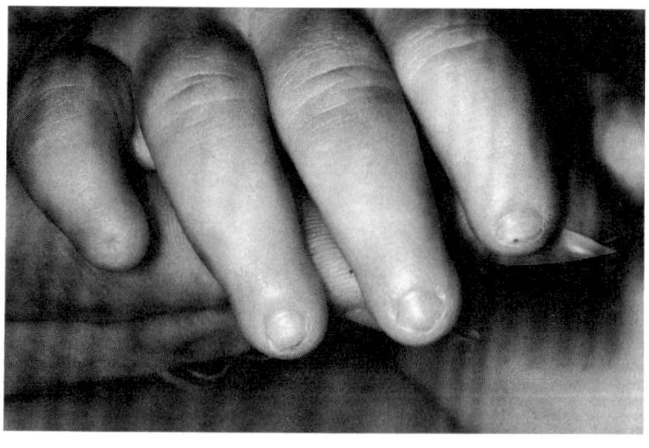

Fig. 3. Hypoplasia of fingernails and distal phalanges.

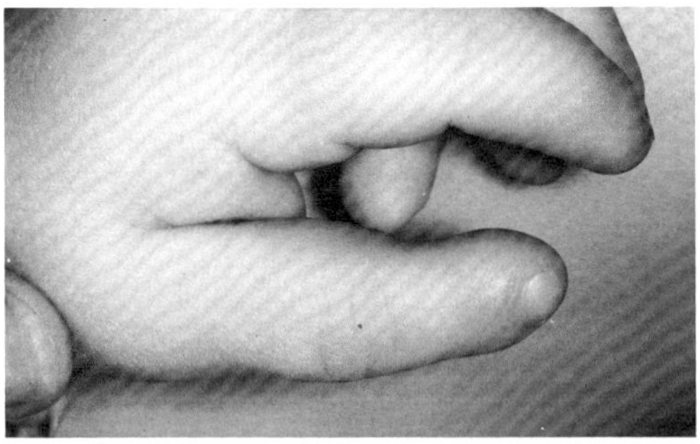

Fig. 4. Finger-like thumb.

reminiscent of the findings among infants exposed prenatally to diethystilbestrol.

DIAGNOSIS

The diagnosis may be considered in any infant exposed prenatally to hydantoin anticonvulsants (diphenylhydantoin, mephenytoin, ethotoin), who also manifests several of the above features. Most affected children manifest only mild craniofacial or limb abnormalities. Mild dysmorphic features such as "short nose with broad bridge," "ocular hypertelorism," "ptosis," or "short neck" are subject to substantial observer variation of interpretation in clinical settings. As a consequence, though careful recent studies (VanLang et al., '84; Holmes, '85) confirm the presence of such abnormalities, diagnosis of

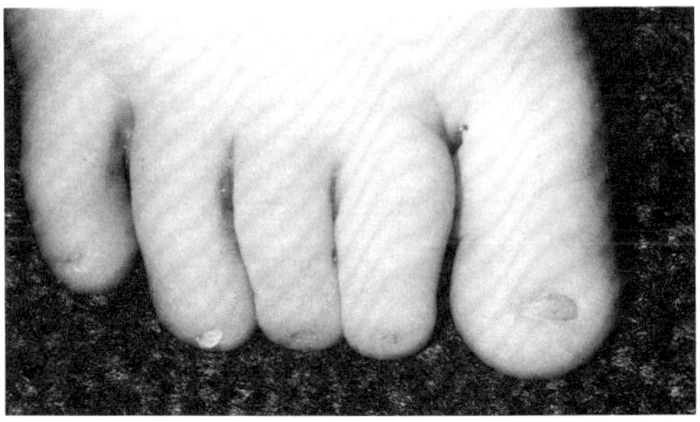

Fig. 5. Hypoplasia of toenails and distal phalanges—note dermal ridges sweeping around nail on dorsum of the great toe.

fetal hydantoin effects is frequently overlooked. Furthermore, these manifestations may be readily confused with the findings in other birth defect patterns. Included among such conditions are the Coffin-Siris, Noonan, Williams, and Aarskog syndromes, neurofibromatosis, and the effects of other teratogenic effects such as alcohol and maternal phenylketonuria. Furthermore, the craniofacial effects of other anticonvulsant drugs such as barbiturates, primidone, and valproic acid may be at least superficially similar (DiLiberti et al., '84; Seip, '76). In many cases, exposures to one or more of these agents may have occurred concomitantly. In such instances it is often difficult or impossible to ascribe observed effects to a single agent. Furthermore, certain genetic conditions that may account for the maternal seizure disorder may likewise be present in the hydantoin-exposed infant. These conditions may themselves produce developmental or growth disturbances.

EPIDEMIOLOGY

A full pattern of abnormalities sufficient to be recognizable as the fetal hydantoin syndrome is probably present in no more than 5 to 10% of exposed infants (Hanson et al., '76). However, careful studies of more subtle indicators of altered growth and morphogenesis, such as radiographic investigations of craniofacial or limb development, or careful clinical investigation for other structural variations, may identify subtle prenatal hydantoin effects in an additional 30% or more of cases (Kelly, '84c; VanLang et al., '84; Holmes, '85). Several authors have suggested that manifestations are likely to be more severe or more frequent in infants exposed to multiple anticonvulsant agents (Koch et al., '82; Holmes, '85). Developmental delay and neurological abnormalities have been suggested to be more frequent in infants whose mothers had seizures during pregnancy despite anticonvulsant therapy (Majewski et al., '81).

The role of genetic factors in predicting fetal outcome remains a source of confusion. Though a number of authors have reported affected siblings (Smith, '80), in some instances the effects among siblings have been dissimilar (Bustamente and Stumpf, '78; Waziri et al., '76). Of particular interest is the observation of heteropaternal twins born to an epileptic mother treated with phenytoin during pregnancy, only one of whom displayed features of the fetal hydantoin syndrome (Phelan et al., '82). Subsequent metabolic studies of these individuals have identified different epoxide hydrolase activities, suggesting that this enzyme may be important in the manifestations of fetal hydantoin effects (Buehler, '85). Further studies will be needed in order to determine whether such pharmacogenetic factors may be important predictive risk factors that could identify a subpopulation of especially susceptible individuals. In this regard Strickler et al. ('85) have recently correlated measurements of an apparently genetic defect in arene oxide detoxification with the presence of more serious malformations (congenital heart disease, cleft lip/palate, microcephaly, limb defects, etc.) in infants exposed prenatally to phenytoin.

Some authors (Shapiro et al., '76) have suggested that paternal epilepsy and/or phenytoin exposure may be a teratogenetic risk factor. The mechanism for such a postulated effect remains unclear, and specific studies to confirm such suggestions are lacking. Nonetheless, it seems unlikely that a consistent phenotype among exposed offspring would be the result of any clastogenic or mutagenic effect of phenytoin during spermatogenesis. Furthermore, the frequency of such effects on the genetic material would be expected to be extremely low. It also seems more likely that paternal disorders of genetic origin resulting in parental epilepsy are themselves the likely risk factors for offspring of epileptic fathers, if such exist.

PATHOGENESIS

At the present time, the pathogenetic mechanisms responsible for fetal hydantoin effects remain uncertain, although it is important to acknowledge that all of the teratogenic or embryopathic observations relate to offspring exposed to chronic anticonvulsant therapy. Few if any of these observations can be utilized to determine results or risks of short term or acute exposure to these agents in pregnancy. A role has been postulated for arene oxide metabolites (Martz et al., '77; Blake and Martz, '80; Holmes, '85). However, other metabolic factors may be important as well (Finnell and Chernoff, '84a). Animal studies reveal not only differences in susceptibility between different species but substantial strain differences as well (Finnell and Chernoff, '84b). A wide variety of teratopathogenic laboratory testing systems, as well as animal models, have been identified for the further investigation of fetal hydantoin effects (Bruckner et al., '83; Finnell, '81; Finnell and Chernoff, '82; Vorhees, '83).

TREATMENT

Surgical correction of major defects may be necessary. In mildly affected children specific treatment may be unnecessary. Effective remedies for more severe deficiencies of growth and performance have not been found. Early childhood stimulation and appropriate educational placement may be of benefit.

PREVENTION

Present preventive measures rely on the exclusion of the teratogen from the prenatal environment. Unfortunately, the safety of alternative drugs remains poorly defined. Barbiturates, primidone, and, most recently, valproic acid have all been implicated as potentially teratogenic agents. Combinations of these medications may be particularly hazardous; thus, monotherapy is a desirable objective wherever possible. The relative contribution of possible genetic and other factors affecting hydantoin metabolism continues to be unclear at the present time. Women with seizure disorders should be informed of the nature and magnitude of risks to the fetus arising from hydantoin therapy prior to considering becoming pregnant. Accurate prenatal diagnostic tests are not currently available for the abnormalities likely to occur.

LITERATURE CITED

Allen, R.W. (1984) Fetal hydantoin syndrome and malignancy. J. Pediatr., *105:4* 681.

Bjerkedal, T. (1982) Outcome of pregnancy in women with epilepsy, Norway, 1967–1978: Gestational age, birth weight, and survival of the newborn. In: Epilepsy, Pregnancy, and the Child. D. Janz et al. eds. Raven Press, New York, pp. 175–178.

Blake, D.A. and F. Martz (1980) Covalent binding of phenytoin metabolites in fetal tissues. In: Phenytoin-Induced Teratology and Gingival Pathology. T.M. Hassell, M.C. Johnston, and K.H. Dudley, eds. Raven Press, New York, pp. 75–83.

Bostrom, Bruce, and M.E. Nesbit, Jr. (1983) Hodgkin disease in a child with fetal alcohol-hydantoin syndrome. J. Pediatr. *103:5* 760–762.

Bruckner, A., Y.J. Lee, K.S. O'Shea, and R.C. Henneberry (1983) Teratogenic effects of valproic acid and diphenylhydantoin on mouse embryos in culture. Teratology, 27:29–42.

Buehler, B.A. (1985) Epoxide hydralase activity: A direct assay for prediction of potential dilantin teratogenesis. Proceedings of the Greenwood Genetic Center, *4:*92–93.

Bustamente, S.A. and L.C. Stumpf (1978) Fetal hydantoin syndrome in triplets. Am. J. Dis. Child., *132:*978–979.

DiLiberti, J.H., P.A. Farndon, N.R. Dennis, and C.J.R. Curry (1984) The fetal valproate syndrome. Am. J. Med. Genet., *19:*473–481.

Finnell, R.H. (1981) Phenytoin-induced teratogenesis: A mouse model. Science, *211:*483–484.

Finnell, R.H., and G.F. Chernoff (1982) Mouse fetal hydantoin syndrome: Effects of maternal seizures. Epilepsia, *23:*423–429.

Finnell, R.H., and G.F. Chernoff (1984a) Editorial Comment: Genetic background: The elusive component in the fetal hydantoin syndrome: Am. J. Med. Genet., *19:*459–462.

Finnell, R.H., and G.F. Chernoff (1984b) Variable patterns of malformation in the mouse fetal hydantoin syndrome. Am. J. Med. Genet., *19:*463–471.

Gopfert-Geyer, I., S. Koch, D. Rating, E. Jager-Roman, A. Hartmann, S. Jacob, G. Offermann, and H. Hedge (1982) Delivery, gestation, data of birth, and neonatal period in children with epileptic mothers. In: Epilepsy, Pregnancy, and the Child. D. Janz et al., eds. Raven Press, New York, pp. 179–187.

Hanson, J.W., and D.W. Smith (1975) The fetal hydantoin syndrome. J. Pediatr., *87(2):*285–290.

Hanson, J.W., N.C. Myrianthopoulos, M.A.S. Harvey, and D.W. Smith (1976) Risks to the offering of women treated with hydantoin anticonvulsants with emphasis on the fetal hydantoin syndrome. J. Pediatr., *89(4):*662–668.

Helge, H. (1982) Physical, mental, social development including diseases: Review of the literature. In: Epilepsy, Pregnancy, and the Child. D. Janz et al., eds. Raven Press, New York, pp. 391–395.

Holmes, L.B. (1985) The effects of exposure to phenytoin in utero. Proceedings of the Greenwood Genetic Center, *4:*92.

Jager-Roman, E., D. Rating, S. Koch, I. Gopfert-Geyer, S. Jacob, and H. Helge (1982) Somatic parameters, diseases and psychomotor development in the offspring of epileptic parents. In: Epilepsy, Pregnancy, and the Child. D. Janz et al., eds. Raven Press, New York, pp. 425–432.

Kelly, T.E. (1984a) Teratogenicity of anticonvulsant drugs: I. Review of the literature. Am. J. Med. Genet., *19:*413–434.

Kelly, T.E. (1984b) Teratogenicity of anticonvulsant drugs: II. A prospective study. Am. J. Med. Genet., *19:*435–443.

Kelly, T.E. (1984c) Teratogenecity of anticonvulsant drugs: III. Radiographic hand analysis of children ex-

posed in utero to diphenylhydantoin. Am. J. Med. Genet., *19:*445–450.
Kelly, T.E., M. Rein, and P. Edwards (1984) Teratogenecity of anticonvulsant drugs: IV. The association of clefting and epilepsy. Am. J. Med. Genet., *19:*451–458.
Koch, S., A. Hartman, E. Jager-Roman, D. Rating, and H. Helge (1982) Major malformations in children of epileptic parents—due to epilepsy or its therapy? In: Epilepsy, Pregnancy, and the Child. D. Janz et al. eds. Raven Press, New York, pp. 313–315.
Majewski, F., M. Steger, B. Richter, J. Gill, and F. Rabe (1981) The teratogeneicity of hydantoins and barbiturates in humans with considerations on the etiology of malformations and cerebral disturbances in the children of epileptic parents. Biol. Res. Preg., *2:1* 37–45.
Martz, F., C. Failinger. and D.A. Blake (1977) Phenytoin teratogenesis: Correlation between embryopathic effect and covalent binding of putative arene oxide metabolite in gestational tissue. J. Pharmacol. Exp. Ther., *203:*231–239.
Ogawa, Y., Y. Nomura, S. Kaneko, K. Suzuki, and T. Sato (1982) Insidious effect of antiepileptic drugs in the perinatal period. In: Epilepsy, Pregnancy, and the Child. D. Janz et al., eds. Raven Press, New York, pp. 197–202.
Phelan, M.C., J.M. Pellock, and W.E. Nance (1982) Discordant expression of fetal hydantoin syndrome in heteropaternal dizygotic twins. New Engl. J. Med., *307:2* 99–101.
Rating, D., E. Jager-Roman, S. Koch, I. Gopfert-Geyer, and H. Helge (1982) Minor anomalies in the offspring of epileptic parents. In: Epilepsy, Pregnancy, and the Child. D. Janz et al., eds. Raven Press, New York, pp. 283–289.
Seip, M. (1976) Growth retardation, dysmorphic facies, and minor malformation following massive exposure to phenobarbital in utero. Acta Paediatr. Scand., *65:*617–621.
Shapiro, S., D. Slone, S.C. Hartz, L. Rosenberg, V. Siskind, R.R. Monson, A.A. Mitchell, O.P. Heinonen, J. Idanpaan-Heikkila, S. Haro, and L. Saxon (1976) Anticonvulsants and parental epilepsy in the development of birth defects. Lancet, *1:*272–275.
Smith, D.W. (1980) Hydantoin effects on the fetus. In: Phenytoin-Induced Teratology and Gingival Pathology. T.M. Hassell, M.C. Johnston, and K.H. Dudley, eds. Raven Press, New York, pp. 35–41.
Strickler, S.M., M.A. Miller, E. Andermann, L.V. Dansky, M.H. Seni, and S. Spielberg (1985) Genetic predisposition to phenytoin-induced birth defects. Lancet, *2:*746–749.
VanLang, Q.N., M.S. Tassinari, D.A. Keith, L.B. Holmes (1984) Effect of in utero exposure to anticonvulsants on craniofacial development and growth. J. Craniofac. Genet. and Dev. Biol., *4:*115–133.
Vorhees, C.V. (1983) Fetal anticonvulsant syndrome in rats: Dose- and period-response relationships of prenatal diphenylhydantoin, trimethadione and phenobarbital exposure on the structural and functional development of the offspring. J. Pharmacol. Exp. Ther., *227:2* 274–287.
Waziri, M., V. Ionasescu, and H. Zellweger (1976) Teratogenic effect of anticonvulsant drugs. Am. J. Dis. Child., *130:*1022–1023.

TERATOGEN UPDATE: ENVIRONMENTALLY INDUCED BIRTH DEFECT RISKS, PAGES 35–38 (1986)

Fetal Trimethadione Syndrome

ALLEN S. GOLDMAN, ELAINE H. ZACKAI, AND SUMNER J. YAFFE
Center for Craniofacial Anomalies and Department of Pediatrics, University of Illinois College of Medicine at Chicago, P.O. Box 6998, 808 South Wood St., Chicago, Illinois 60680 (A.S.G.), Clinical Genetics Center, The Children's Hospital of Philadelphia, and Department of Pediatrics, University of Pennsylvania School of Medicine, Philadelphia, Pennsylvania 19104 (E.H.Z.), and Center for Research for Mothers and Children, National Institute of Child Health and Development, Public Health Service, National Institutes of Health, Bethesda, Maryland 20205 (S.J.Y.)

MANIFESTATIONS

Major features included in the fetal trimethadione (3,5,5-tri-methyloxazolidine-2,4-dione) syndrome are developmental delay, speech difficulty, V-shaped eyebrows, epicanthus, low set ears with anteriorly folded helix, palatal anomaly, and irregular teeth.

Some patients also have intrauterine growth retardation, short stature, microcephaly, cardiac anomaly, ocular anomaly (strabismus, myopia), hypospadias, inguinal hernia, and simian creases (Zackai et al., '75).

Some children exposed to trimethadione in utero have died in the neonatal period with severe anomalies (German and Ehlers '70; Zackai et al., '75; Feldman et al., '77) of the trachea, larynx, and esophagus; of the heart — anomalous right subclavian and left common carotid, patent ductus arteriosus, transposition, hypoplastic heart, valve atresia, and tetralogy of Fallot; of the genitourinary system — absent kidney and ureter, fetal lobulation of kidneys, and hypospadias; of the gastrointestinal tract — omphalocele; and of the skeletal structure — scoliosis, club hand, pterygium colli, and meningomyelocele.

DIAGNOSIS

The diagnosis may be considered in any infant exposed prenatally to trimethadione (or other oxazolidine type anticonvulsant, e.g., paramethadione, 3,4-dimethyl-5-ethyloxazolidine-2,4-dione) who has several of the above features including developmental delay and facial dysmorphia that is apparently specific for trimethadione: broad nasal bridge, V-shaped eyebrows, epicanthal folds, and low set backward sloping ears with anteriorly folded helices (Zackai et al., '75). The diagnosis should be considered in any infant exposed prenatally to trimethadione who has severe anomalies of the trachea, larynx, and esophagus or heart defects (Zackai et al., '75; Feldman et al., '77).

The fetal trimethadione syndrome can be distinguished from the fetal hydantoin syndrome (Hanson, '76; Hanson and Smith, '75) secondary to intrauterine exposure to the hydantoin anticonvulsants that have a similar chemical structure to the oxaxolidines (Fig. 1). The "specific anomalies," i.e., V-shaped eyebrows and low set ears with anteriorly folded helix and lack of phalangeal hypoplasia occur only in the offspring of mothers who have taken trimethadione in the absence of other anticonvulsants. In one child having not only the specific characteristics of the trimethadione syndrome, but also the hypoplasia of nails and distal phalanges characteristic of the fetal hydantoin syndrome, the mother took diphenylhydantoin and trimethadione during the critical period (Zackai et al., '75). The last observation is consistent with the idea that the hypoplasia of nails and distal phalanges is specific for diphenylhydantoin and can be expressed along with the features specific for trimethadione.

The facial dysmorphia characteristic of this syndrome is shown in Figures 2–7.

PROGNOSIS

Data regarding growth and development of children with the fetal trimethadione syndrome who have survived the neonatal period is reported in the literature (German et al., '70; Zackai et al., '84; Rosen and Lightner, '78; Zellweger, '74; Lawrence and Stiles, '75).

Growth

Six of the ten children were small for gestational age. Ten of the ten children were below the 3rd centile for growth. Three young adults (ages ranging from 18.5–22 years) have gone through puberty at the normal time and sexual development is complete in all three. Final adult heights of the two males are 5′2″–5′2.75″ and the female is 4′10″.

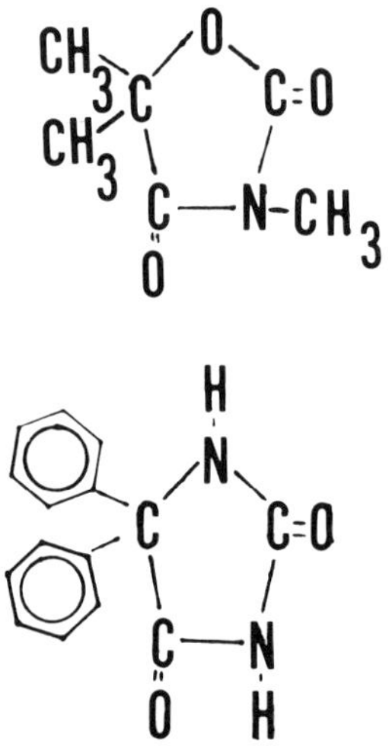

Fig. 1. Chemical structure of trimethadione (above) and diphenylhydantoin (below).

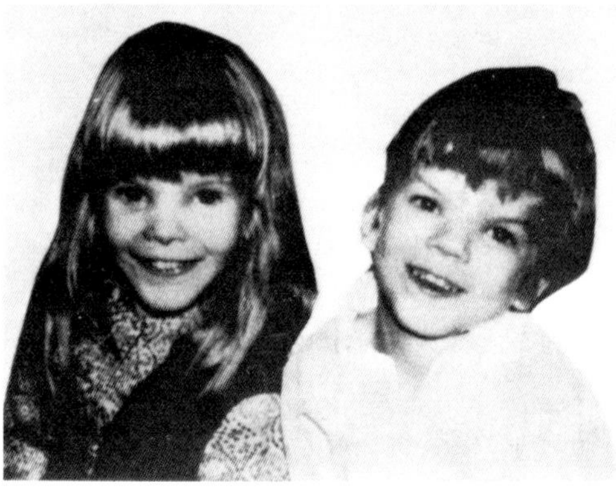

Fig. 2. Patient, age 4¹/₁₂ and sibling, age 5⁶/₁₂. Note broad nasal bridge, epicanthal folds, V-shaped eyebrows.

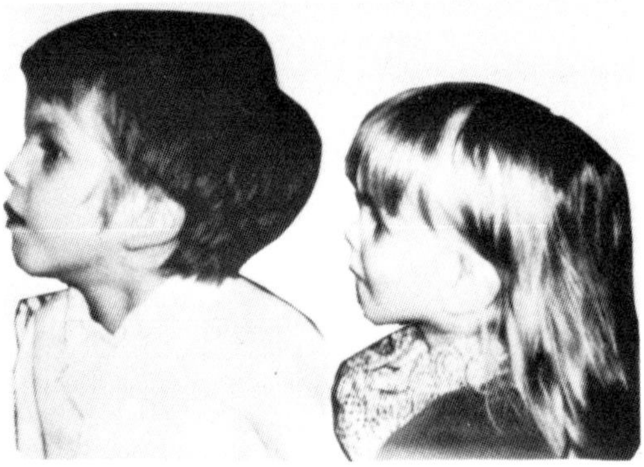

Fig. 3. Patient, age 3⁶/₁₂, and sibling, age 23 months. Note low-set, backward sloped ears with anteriorly folded helices.

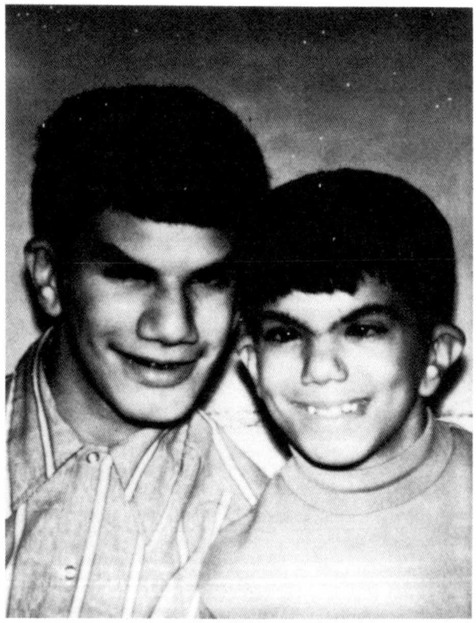

Fig. 4. Patient and sibling. Note broad nasal bridges, epicanthal folds, and V-shaped eyebrows.

Development

One child age 46 months is described as having normal intelligence (Zellweger '74). Two children, ages 2 and 6 years, are described as mentally retarded (Lawrence and Stiles '75). The I.Q. of four children, ages 4 1/12–8 6/12, fell between 80–88 (German and Ehlers, '70; Zackai et al., '75; Rosen and Lightner, '78). One child, age 5 6/12, had an I.Q. of 64 (Zackai et al., '75). The three young adults' I.Q.s were: age 18 1/2, 75; age 19, 85; and age 22, 90 (Zackai et al., '84).

ANIMAL STUDIES

Trimethadione was shown to be highly embryotoxic and teratogenic in the CD-1 mouse, at doses well below those that caused overt maternal toxicity (Brown et al., '79). Malformations were induced in a wide range of visceral organs and in the skeletal system,

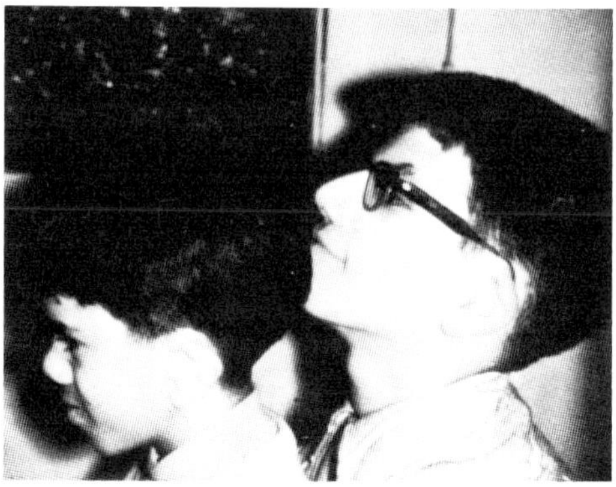

Fig. 5. Two siblings of same family as in Figure 4. Note low-set, backward sloped ears and anteriorly folded helices.

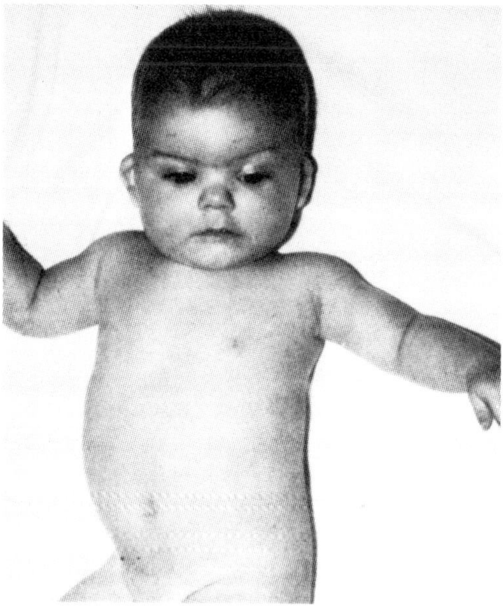

Fig. 6. Patient, D.K. Note broad nasal ridge and V-shaped eyebrows.

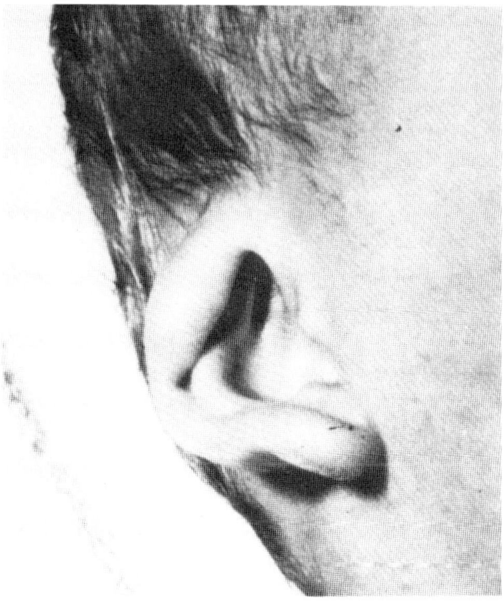

Fig. 7. Patient, D.K. Note small superior aspect of helix and upped and overlapped helix.

the most common defects being of the vertebral column and the aortic arch. Embryos in the late phase of organogenesis (days 11–13) were less sensitive to maternal trimethadione treatment. The tD50 was 5.97 mmol/kg and the maximum levels of embryomortality and congenital malformations were 21 and 74%, respectively, following daily doses of 7.3 mmol/kg. Cleft palate and defects in the great vessels of the heart were the common abnormalities induced during this treatment period.

Studies using the A/J mouse have also supported the above findings (Zackai et al., '84). At maternal doses larger than 200 mg/kg there is a significant production of isolated cleft palate, open eye, and small-for-gestational-age fetuses.

The therapeutic doses in humans that were associated with malformations ranged from 13 to 22 mg/K/d (Zackai et al., '75; Lawrence and Stiles, '75; Rosen and Lightner '78; German and Ehlers '70; Feldman et al., '77). The teratogenic dose range in mice varied from 200 to 1,800 mg kg/d. Thus, the mouse teratogenic range is approximately 10 to 100 times the human therapeutic range.

Since most of the studies dealing with this syndrome have come from the examination of malformed children, the risk of exposure tends to be high. However, we would tend to counsel families that it is probably contraindicated to continue trimethadione therapy in a woman who becomes pregnant.

TREATMENT AND PREVENTION

Surgical correction of major defects may be necessary. The only preventive measures available at the present would be removal of the drug at the critical period of the first trimester. Zarontin is another drug used for petit mal epilepsy, but, unfortunately, the safety of this other oxazolidine during the critical period is not known. Women with seizure disorders of the type requiring trimethadione should be counselled as to the nature and magnitude of the risks to the fetus arising from therapy with this drug prior to consideration of becoming pregnant.

ACKNOWLEDGMENTS

A.S.G. is supported in part by grants DE-4622 and DE-5041 from the National Institutes of Dental Research.

LITERATURE CITED

Brown, N.A., G. Shull, and S. Fabro (1979) Assessment of the teratogenic potential of trimethadione in the CD-1 mouse. Toxicol. Appl. Pharmacol., *51:*56–71.

Feldman, G.L., D.A. Weaver, and E.W. Lovrien (1977) The fetal trimethadione syndrome. Am. J. Dis. Child, *131:*349–354.

German, J., A. Kowal, and K.H. Ehlers (1970) Trimethadione and human teratogenesis. Teratology, *3:*349–354.

Hanson, J.W., and D.W. Smith (1975) The fetal hydantoin syndrome. J. Pediatr., *87:*285–290.

Hanson, J.W. (1976) Teratogen update. Fetal hydantoin syndrome. Teratology, *13:*185–187.

Lawrence, T.Y.K and Q.R. Stiles (1975) Persistent fifth aortic arch in man. Am. J. Dis. Child, *129:*1229–1231.

Rosen, R.C. and E.S. Lightner (1978) Phenotypic malformations in association with maternal trimethadione therapy. J. Pediatr., *92:*240–244.

Zackai, E.H, W.J. Mellman, B. Neiderer, and J.W. Hanson (1975) The fetal trimethadione syndrome. J. Pediatr., *87:*280–284.

Zackai, E.H., D. Cryer, and A.S. Goldman (1986) Long term follow-up of patients with the fetal trimethadione syndrome. J. Craniofac. Genet. Dev. Biol. (in preparation).

Zellweger, H. (1974) Anticonvulsants during pregnancy: A danger to the developing fetus? Clin. Pediatr., *13:*338.

Aminopterin and Methotrexate: Folic Acid Deficiency

JOSEF WARKANY
Children's Hospital Medical Center, University of Cincinnati, Cincinnati, Ohio 45229

Vitamin deficiencies were the first methods successfully used in mammalian experimental teratology. Maternal vitamin A-deficiency (Hale, '33, '37) and riboflavin deficiency (Warkany and Nelson, '40; Warkany and Schraffenberger, '44) produced in pigs and rats ocular and skeletal malformations which were clearly attributable to environmental situations. Subsequently other vitamin deficiencies were employed but all these dietary methods were difficult because embryos with malformations were only born if a borderline deficiency could be attained so that improvement of the vitamin level resulted in the birth of normal young and reduction in early prenatal death of embryos.

Folic acid (pteroylglutamic acid) deficiency was at first not producing congenital malformations in rats since the intestinal flora of pregnant animals can counteract the maternal dietary deficiency. When antibiotics or antimetabolites were added to the deficient diet (Evans et al., '53; Giroud and Lefebvres-Boisselot, '51) depletion was achieved that resulted in congenital malformations. With the help of x-methy-folic acid (Nelson et al., '52) acute folic acid deficiency could be induced which proved promptly teratogenic. Subsequently various antimetabolites became powerful teratogenic tools which made possible conversion of long-term nutritional depletions into short-term chemical experiments. These findings indirectly led to human congenital malformations when the folic acid antagonist aminopterin (4-aminopteroylglutamic acid) was used as an abortifacient. The use was based on observations of fetal death and absorption in rats and mice following injection of small doses of aminopterin during early gestation (Thiersch and Philips, '50). It was thought that the reaction of human embryos to the folic acid antagonist could be tested in women for whom therapeutic abortion was indicated because of tuberculosis, cancer or other illness. Thiersch ('52) gave a total dose of 6-12 mg orally over a period of two to five days to patients less than three months pregnant. The women were closely observed for toxic effects and course of pregnancy. The drug induced fetal death followed by spontaneous abortion of the product of conception in 10 out of 12 cases treated. In two instances in which the dosage of the drug was thought to have been too small for the advanced pregnancies, surgical evacuation of the uterus was carried out; the fetus was hydrocephalic in one, and deformed by cleft lip and palate in the other instance. In one case a spontaneously delivered fetus showed a large meningoencephalocele. Since in three fetuses aminopterin failed to produce immediate death but did induce malformations the dangers of the drug in cases of failed abortion were obvious. In 6 of another 12 patients with cavernous tuberculosis (Thiersch, '56) aminopterin failed to induce abortion and surgical removal of the conceptuses became necessary. In one instance a fetus went to term and the infant that was anencephalic lived for 12 days. After several variations of administration and of drugs, Thiersch ('56) concluded that antimetabolites were too uncertain to induce abortion unless in case of failure surgical intervention could be carried out.

In 1962 Goetsch ('62) reported on 20 abortions attempted with aminopterin of which 15 were for therapeutic reasons and 5 were undertaken with "criminal intent." In five instances no abortion occurred and surgical measures terminated the pregnancy. In one of the resulting fetuses multiple malformations were noted. In the discussion of Goetsch's presentation Alvarez ('62) mentioned two cases in which fetal death or abortion did not occur and the children carried to term were hydrocephalic. Combining the series of Thiersch and Goetsch (Thiersch, '56; Goetsch, '62), one learns that of 44 attempted abortions obstetrically observed, 13 patients (30%) failed to abort so that surgical removal became indicated. With the cases mentioned by Alvarez ('62), seven malformed fetuses were recorded.

As the abortive action of aminopterin became known some pregnant women took the drug without supervision by physicians and a number of these attempts resulted in deformed fetuses or children.

Meltzer in 1956 described a child that had been exposed to aminopterin at 6 to 8 weeks gestation and survived to term. There were anomalies of the occipital bone with lacunae, synostosis of the lambdoid sutures and left talipes equinovarus. A well observed and analyzed case was reported from Cincinnati in 1959 by Warkany et al. ('59). There, a woman who had six normal living children developed signs of folic acid deficiency which could be related to intake of aminopterin tablets purchased from a druggist and used during early pregnancy for attempted abortion. Course of her pregnancy and treatment were described in detail. At the time of expected delivery roentgenograms of the mother's abdomen showed failure of ossification of a large segment of the fetal calvarium. Spontaneous delivery occurred approximately two weeks after the calculated date, but the child had marked intrauterine growth retardation weighing only 1,280 gm. The head was large, the skull was soft and felt like a rubber balloon. Rudimentary, widely separated cranial bones could be felt and the face was relatively small. The eyes were far apart and the ears very low set and deformed; the mandible was small and the posterior palate cleft. The body was small and the extremities assumed abnormal positions (fig. 1). On the second day of life the child died during a period of apnea at 29 hours of age. Autopsy showed a relatively large, non-hydrocephalic brain without gross abnormalities. Although the child's anomalies were thought to be due to exposure to aminopterin in early gestation the authors found it necessary to support this hypothesis by the following arguments: The malformations of the child were compatible with interference with development from the tenth to twelfth week of gestation; the family history was negative for comparable anomalies; and the folic acid antagonists had been found to be teratogenic in man and in animals. In addition, the syndrome presented by the infant was apparently unique and unknown at that time. It was necessary in 1959—the year in which the thalidomide embryopathy was identified—to defend the belief that a drug could produce a syndrome of multiple congenital malformations in man. That the explanation was correct was demonstrated by similar observations which showed a pattern of anomalies characteristic of prenatal aminopterin damage. Emerson ('62) reported a fetus of 24 weeks gestation that had been exposed to aminopterin at six to eight weeks gestational age. Parietal bones

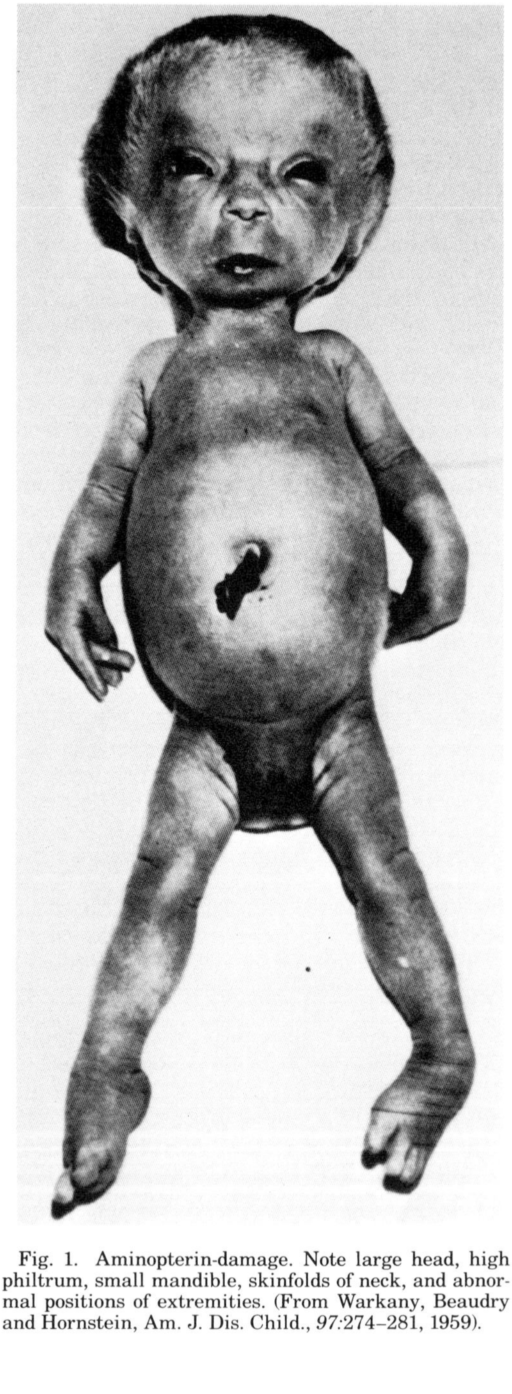

Fig. 1. Aminopterin-damage. Note large head, high philtrum, small mandible, skinfolds of neck, and abnormal positions of extremities. (From Warkany, Beaudry and Hornstein, Am. J. Dis. Child., *97*:274–281, 1959).

were absent, there was hydrocephalus, cerebral hypoplasia, hypertelorism, low set malformed ears, micrognathia, cleft palate and talipes equinovarus. Shaw and Steinbach ('68) described an incident in which aminopterin ingested during early pregnancy for the purpose of abortion produced severe toxic symptoms in the mother and severe damages in the infant who at 39 weeks gestation had marked intrauterine growth retardation and signs similar to those previously described by Warkany et al. ('59). But the girl survived and her development could be observed for many years. Ossification of the skull progressed slowly, developmental quotient at 18 months of age was 75 with good manipulative skills but poor language. Her height and weight remained below the third percentiles and her intelligence at two years of age was considered dull normal. This child was carefully observed during subsequent years (Shaw, '72) during which growth remained retarded and facial appearance peculiar though her social and mental development became eventually normal.

At age 17½ years she was found to be amazingly improved (Shaw and Rees, '80). She was a short, young adult with a normally ossified skull. Her hair was abundant and the eyebrows were present. Micrognathia was still noticeable; her teeth were crowded and protruded. Extremities were normal in length and mobility. Secondary sex characteristics were developed; menstruation had begun at age 11 ½ years and was normal. She seemed well adjusted and did fairly well in school except for arithmetic. Psychometric tests showed her to be within normal limits and she played the organ acceptably.

Another child that survived beyond infancy was described by Brandner and Nusslé ('69). The similarity of the facial features of this boy (fig. 2) with those of the girl (fig. 3) observed by Shaw ('72) is amazing. Brandner and Nusslé ('69) described radiographic details and stressed congenital stenosis of the tubular long bones. Another case of survival has been recently reported by Howard and Rudd ('77).

A methyl derivative of aminopterin, methotrexate, used unsuccessfully as an abortifacient, resulted in congenital malformations with survival of the affected child. Milunsky et al. ('68) observed absence of the frontal bone, synostosis of the lambdoid and coronal sutures, multiple rib anomalies, unusual fa-

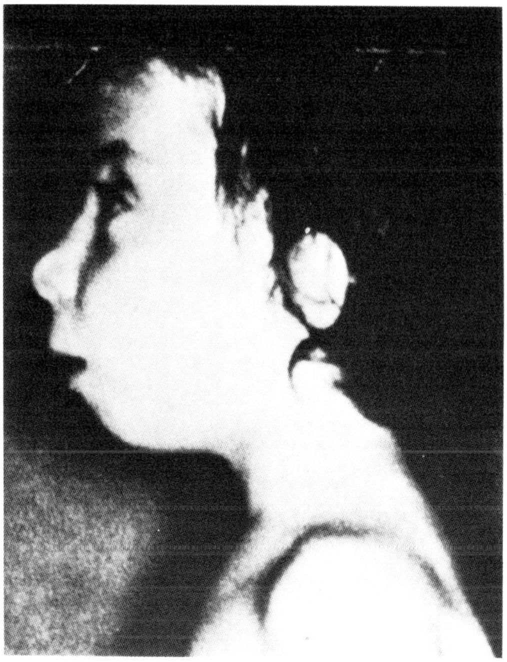

Fig. 2. Aminopterin-damage in a boy at 3 years. (From Brandner M. and D. Nusslé, Ann. de Radiologie, *12:*703–710, 1969).

cies, absence of digits on the left foot and only one digit on the right foot. Growth was markedly retarded at 15 months of age but mental and motor development appeared normal. Another case of methotrexate-induced congenital malformations was reported by Powell and Ekert ('71). The mother had taken large amounts of this drug as treatment for psoriasis. At birth the child showed oxycephaly with fusion of the coronal sutures, wide metopic suture and anterior fontanel, marked hypertelorism, and webbing of the proximal phalanges of the index and middle fingers. At the age of 12 days a left coronal linear cranioplasty was performed and at four months the infant did well and developmental progress was normal.

Reich et al. ('78) wrote about recognition in adult patients of malformations induced by folic acid antagonists. They described in great detail two patients aged 22 and 19 years of age whose mothers reported ingestion of abortifacient drugs during pregnancy. The patients resembled each other and those described before in the literature. The authors tabulated clinical data together with those of

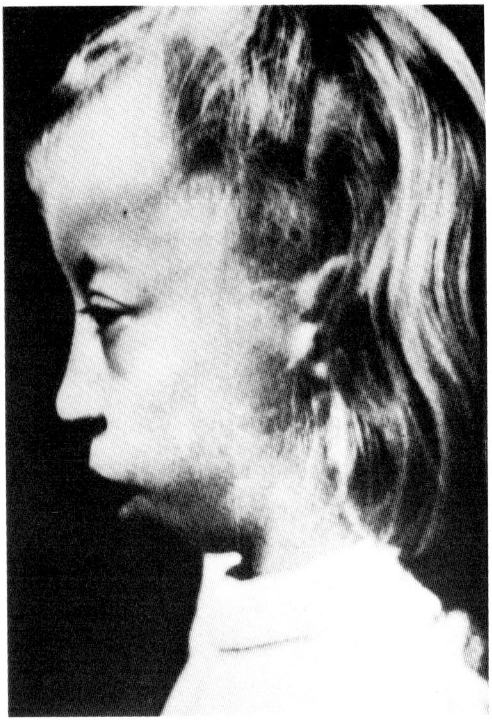

Fig. 3. Aminopterin-damage in a girl at age 9 years. (From Shaw, E.B. Am. J. Dis. Child., *124*:93–94, 1972).

two patients who possibly had been damaged by folic acid deficiency before birth. Thus a syndrome exists now that can be seen in children and adults, which is suggestive of prenatal folic acid deficiency.

In summary, it can be stated that the folic acid antagonists aminopterin and methotrexate administered in early pregnancy have been clearly established as teratogens in human beings. In fact a syndrome of congenital anomalies became apparent, the "aminopterin syndrome" whose most consistent anomaly is cranial dysostosis, i.e., lack of delay of ossification of the bones of the calvarium. This may or may not be associated with hydrocephalus. Hypertelorism, anomalies of the external ears and micrognathia are the rule but posterior palate cleft may be present (Brandner and Nusslé, '69; Emerson '62; Thiersch, '56; Warkany et al., '59) or absent (Shaw and Steinbach, '68). Anomalies of the extremities may be minor or include absence of several digits (Milunsky et al., '68).

The observations of congenital malformations due to folic acid antagonists led to the question of malformations caused by folic acid deficiency of different origins. Vitamin deficiencies can result from inadequate ingestion, absorption or utilization, or from increased requirement or excretion (Waxman et al., '70). Congenital absorption of folate may lead to mental retardation and cerebral calcification in postnatal life (Lanzkowsky et al., '69).

There are some suggestions which link maternal folate deficiency to congenital malformations in the offspring. Hibbard ('64) and Hibbard and Smithells ('65) examined mothers of infants with severe congenital malformations, particularly central nervous system malformations, either prenatally or within two to three days of delivery with the formimoglutamic acid (FIGLU) excretion test to determine their folic acid status. Similar tests were made on matched controls. Mothers of malformed babies had about five times more often positive FIGLU tests than controls. Admittedly these tests done at the end of pregnancy did not show that a deficiency existed during embryogenesis. Subsequently, Smithells et al. ('76) performed a prospective study of vitamins during the first trimester of pregnancy in over 900 cases. In six mothers who gave birth to infants with neural tube defects, first trimester red cell folate and white blood cell vitamin C were significantly lower than in controls. In a study of megaloblastic anemia in pregnancy Fraser and Watt ('64) noted that five malformed babies were born to 17 mothers with such anemias. But Pritchard et al. ('70) investigated the fate of 86 infants of women with folate deficiency so severe as to cause overt megaloblastic anemia. Fetal malformations, birth weight, prematurity, and perinatal mortality were very similar to those of the general obstetric population. Rothman ('70), Scott et al. ('70) and Hall, ('72) found no association between maternal folate deficiency and fetal malformations. Thus it seems doubtful that relatively mild "biochemical" folate deficiencies (Rothman, '70) can be equated with the severe effects of folic acid antimetabolites.

Yet in a study published in 1981 Smithells et al. (1981a,b) wrote about possible prevention of neural tube defects (NTDs) by periconceptional vitamin supplementation. Women who had previously given birth to one or more infants with a NTD were recruited into a trial of periconceptional multivitamin supplementation. One of 178 offspring of fully supplemented mothers (0.6)% had a NTD, compared with 13 of 260 offspring of unsupplemented mothers (5.0%). In an expanded study of the same type, NTD of offspring of fully supplemented mothers were 0.5% and 4% of unsupplemented mothers. If it were correct that NTDs can be prevented or reduced by such simple nutritional supplementation, it would be a great step forward in the prevention of these serious malformations. But the numbers of recruited mothers were small, so that prospective studies on a large scale had to be planned in the UK and the USA. These studies proved to be very difficult because controls can hardly be obtained and the rate of NTDs is generally decreasing in recent years (Editorial, Lancet '82). The usefulness of the recommended method should be proved or disproved within a few years.

LITERATURE CITED

Alvarez, R. de (1962) Discussion of paper: C. Goetsch. Am. J. Obstet. Gynecol., *83:*1474–1477.

Brandner, M., and D. Nusslé (1969) Foetopathie due a l'aminoptérine avec stenose congénitale de l'espace médullaire des os tubulaires longs. Ann. Radiol., *12:*703–710.

Editorial (1982) Vitamins to prevent neural tube defects. Lancet, *2:*255–1256.

Emerson, D.J. (1982) Congenital malformations due to attempted abortion with aminopterin. Am. J. Obstet. Gynecol., *84:*356–357.

Evans, H.M., H.V. Wright, C.W. Asling and M.N. Nelson (1953) Congenital skeletal anomalies resulting from transitory maternal folic acid deficiency. Anat. Rec., *115:*303.

Fraser, J.L., and H.J. Watt (1964) Megaloblastic anemia in pregnancy and the puerperium. Am. J. Obstet. Gynecol., *89:*532–534.

Giroud, A., and J. Lefebvres-Boisselot (1951) Anomalies provoquées chez le foetus en l'absence d'acide folique. Arch. Franç. Pédiat., *8:*648–656.

Goetsch, C. (1962) An evaluation of aminopterin as an abortifacient. Am. J. Obstet. Gynecol., *83:*1474–1477.

Hale, F. (1933) Pigs born without eye balls. J. Hered., *24:*105–106.

Hale, F. (1937) The relation of maternal vitamin A deficiency to microphthalmia in pigs. Texas State J. Med., *33:*228–332.

Hall, M.H. (1972) Folic acid deficiency and congenital malformation. J. Obstet. Gynaecol. Br., *79:*159–161.

Hibbard, B.M. (1964) The role of folic acid in pregnancy. J. Obstet. Gynecol., *71:*529–542.

Hibbard, E.D., and R.W. Smithells (1965) Folic acid metabolism and human embryopathy. Lancet, *1:* 1254.

Howard, N.J., and N.L. Rudd (1977) The natural history of aminopterin-induced embryopathy. Birth Defects: Orig. Art Series, Vol. XIII, No. 3C, pp. 85–93.

Lanzkowsky, P., M.E. Erlandson and A.I. Bezan (1969) Isolated defect of of folic acid absorption associated with mental retardation and cerebral calcification. Blood, *34:*452–465.

Meltzer, H.J. (1956) Congenital anomalies due to attempted abortion with 4-aminopteroglutamic acid. J.A.M.A., *161:*1253.

Milunsky, A., J.W. Graef and M.F. Gaynor (1968) Methotrexate-induced congenital malformations. J. Pediat., *72:*790–795.

Nelson, M.M., C.W. Asling and H.M. Evans (1952) Production of multiple congenital abnormalities in young by maternal pteroylglutamic acid deficiency during gestation. J. Nutr., *48:*61–80.

Powell, H.R., and H. Ekert (1971) Methotrexate-induced congenital malformations, Med. J. Aust., *2:*1076–1077.

Pritchard, J.A., D.E. Scott, P.J. Whalley and R.F. Haling, Jr. (1970) Infants of mothers with megaloblastic anemia due to folate deficiency. J.A.M.A., *211:*1982–1984.

Reich, E.W., R.P. Cox, M.H. Becker, et al. (1978) Recognition in adult patients of malformations induced by folic acid antagonists. Birth Defects, *14:*(6b):139–160.

Rothman, D. (1970) Folic acid in pregnancy. Am. J. Obstet. Gynecol., *108:*149–175.

Scott, D.W., P.J. Whalley and J.A. Pritchard (1970) Maternal folate deficiency and pregnancy wastage. II. Fetal malformation. Obstet. Gynecol., *36:*26–28.

Shaw, E.B., and H.L. Steinbach (1968) Aminopterin-induced fetal malformation. Survival of infant after attempted abortion. Am. J. Dis. Child., *115:*477–482.

Shaw, E.B. (1972) Fetal damage due to maternal aminopterin ingestion. Am. J. Dis. Child., *124:*93–94.

Shaw, E.B. and E.L. Rees (1980) Fetal damage due to aminopterin ingestion: Follow-up at 17½ years of age. Am. J. Dis. Child., *134:*1172–1173.

Smithells R.W., S. Sheppard and C.J. Schorah (1976) Vitamin deficiencies and neural tube defects. Arch. Dis. Child., *51:*944–950.

Smithells, R.W., S. Sheppard, C.J. Schorah, M.J. Seller, N.C. Nevin, R. Harris, A.P. Read, D.W. Fielding, and S. Walker (1981a) Vitamin supplementation and neural tube defects. Lancet, *2:*1425

Smithells, R.W., S. Sheppard, C.J. Schorah, M.J. Seller, N.C. Nevin, R. Harris, A.P. Read, D.W. Fielding, and S. Walker (1981b) Apparent prevention of neural tube defects by periconceptional vitamin supplementation. Arch. Dis. Child., *56:*911–918.

Thiersch, J.B. (1952) Therapeutic abortions with a folic acid antagonist. 4-aminopteroylglutamic acid (4-amino P.G.A.). Am. J. Obstet. Gynecol., *63:*1298–1304.

——— (1956) The control of reproduction in rats with the aid of antimetabolites and early experiences with antimetabolites as abortifacient agents in man. Acta Endocrinol., *28:*37–45.

Thiersch, J.B., and F.S. Philips (1950) Action of 4-aminopteroylglutamic acid on the early pregnancy of rats and mice. Fed. Proc., *9:*346.

Warkany, J., P.H. Beaudry and S. Hornstein (1959) Attempted abortion with aminopterin (4-aminopteroylglutamic acid). Am. J. Dis. Child., *97:*274–281.

Warkany, J., and R.C. Nelson (1940) Appearance of skeletal abnormalities in the offspring of rats reared on a deficient diet. Science, *92:*383–384.

Warkany, J., and E. Schraffenberger (1944) Congenital malformations induced in rats by maternal nutritional deficiency. VI. The preventive factor. J. Nutr., *27:*477–484.

Waxman, S., J.J. Corcino and V. Herbert (1970) Drugs, toxins, and dietary amino acids affecting vitamin B_{12} or folic acid absorption or utilization. Am. J. Med., *48:*599–608.

TERATOGEN UPDATE: ENVIRONMENTALLY INDUCED BIRTH DEFECT RISKS, PAGES 45–49 (1986)

Antituberculous Drugs

JOSEF WARKANY
Children's Hospital Medical Center, University of Cincinnati, Cincinnati, Ohio 45229

When the thalidomide catastrophe proved to the world that drugs taken by pregnant women can endanger their conceptuses it was recommended by some authorities that no drugs at all should be taken during gestation since it was impossible to guarantee harmlessness by testing them in experimental animals and since most of the numerous drugs ingested routinely during prenancy were unnecessary. It is true that many drugs consumed by pregnant women are useless but there are exceptions which present a serious problem to physicians and their patients. Antituberculous drugs are among these exceptions since pregnancy can aggravate active tuberculosis and endanger the mother's life. Streptomycin (SM), dihydrostreptomycin (DHSM), isoniazid (INH), aminosalicylic acid (PAS), rifampicin (RMP), ethionamide (ETA), and ethambutol (ETM) are used for antituberculous treatment and questions about their ototoxic and teratogenic actions are being raised. Many patients taking streptomycin in high doses for a prolonged time experienced labyrinthine and auditory disturbances which soon directed attention to children whose mothers had been treated with that drug during pregnancy.

It has been demonstrated in several studies that SM passes the placental barrier of animals (Heilman et al., '45; Woltz and Wiley, '45; Molitor et al.,'46; Riskaer et al., '52; Podvinec et al., '65) and man (Heilman et al., '45; Woltz and Wiley, '45; Grassot et al., '51; Kreibich, '54). It was shown that the drug concentration in fetal blood was generally lower than in maternal blood but it was also shown that immature rats are more susceptible than adults to the neurotoxic effect of SM (Molitor et al., '46). A report by Filippi and Mela ('57) claimed that congenital malformations of the extremities can be produced by penicillin and SM which led to studies of teratogenicity of antituberculous drugs in man. The observations of ototoxicity of patients treated with SM and observations in animal experiments led to two different questions: 1. Can SM administered to pregnant women damage their fetuses? and 2. Do antituberculous drugs have teratologic effects in man? Attempts will be made to separate the adverse effects of different drugs but often several drugs were used in maternal treatments so that drug specificity could not always be established.

An early report by Watson and Stow ('48) dealt with two women who were treated with 90 or 95 g of SM in pregnancy and developed some loss of vestibular function. Their children were normal and at one year of age there was no evidence of acoustic or vestibular disturbances. In subsequent years a number of similar publications stated that SM was innocuous to the fetus when a daily dose of 1 g or less was used (Sakula, '54), the explanation being that the fetal blood level is lower than the maternal. But by 1976 about 30 cases of hearing or vestibular deficiency had been reported in children of SM and DHSM treated mothers (Schardein, '76; Shepard, '76). Only some of the publications will be mentioned here.

It was apparently Leroux who in 1950 first observed deafness in the infant of a mother who had received only 30 g of SM in daily doses of 1 g during the last month of pregnancy. He published the case in form of a question: Can congenital deafness be acquired through streptomycin? Bolletti and Croatto ('58) observed severe congenital deafness in a 5-year-old girl whose mother had been treated during the last trimester of pregnancy with SM. Rebattu et al. ('60) found high-tone deafness in two children of mothers treated with SM for tuberculous menigitis. The case published by Kern ('62) is of interest since he dealt with a girl who was considered mentally retarded because of unrecognized deafness. The mother had not related the child's handicap to treatment with DHSM received during the first four months of pregnancy. Single case reports of eighth nerve damage by SM or DHSM were not convincing and studies on a larger scale had to be made. Robinson and Cambon ('64) reviewing 200 cases of school children with hearing loss found that none of their mothers had taken SM or DHSM treatment. Among another 100 children with congenital hearing loss there were two whose mothers had received SM during pregnancy. One had been treated early, from the sixth to the fourteenth week of pregnancy, and the other late, during the last four months. Conway and Birt ('65) examined 17 children exposed to SM or DHSM during gestation and eight had minor eighth nerve damage which had not been noticed by the parents. The results of Matsushima ('67) were similar. There was one child with hearing deficit and one with vestibular disturbance among 124 children tested for effects of prenatal chemotherapy. The author found the results inconclusive because they did not differ from a control series. Rasmussen ('69) studied the ototoxic effects of SM and DHSM treatment in 36 children (exposed prenatally) when they were 2 to 15 years old. Only one child had a slight (30 dB) unilateral sensory-neural high tone hearing loss; all had normal vestibular function. Varpela et al. ('69) made a prospective study of 50 children whose mothers had received SM and DHSM at various stages of pregnancy. With exact tests one child was found to have perceptive hearing loss higher than 15 dB and another child had reduced reactivity to water at 30°C. Ganguin and Rempt ('70) examined 44 children older than four years whose mothers had been treated during pregnancy with more than 10 g SM; some had also been given PMS and INH. Histories did not indicate any inner ear damages of the children and social hearing was normal. Yet audiograms showed that five (11.3%) did have perceptive hearing losses with higher frequencies especially affected. There was no relation to total dose but exposure in early pregnancy seemed to have more adverse effects than late exposure. The incidence of hearing loss in 11.3% of the children was higher than that of adults (7.2%) damaged by SM.

This brief presentation of studies of SM and DHSM effects on the unborn child shows that there is no simple answer to the question of risks to fetuses involved with these treatments during pregnancy. Early statements about complete harmlessness were not correct; and other statements about severe and frequent damages were found exaggerated.

There was and is some justification in suspecting single cases of eighth nerve damage in children exposed in utero to SM or DHSM because it was known that these drugs can cause disturbances of hearing and equilibrium in adults treated for tuberculosis. Since on the other hand, congenital deafness can result from many heterogeneous causes a single case could be misinterpreted. Several controlled studies showed that eighth nerve damages of prenatally exposed children were slightly more frequent than in the control groups but most of the exposed fetuses were not affected so that one had to look for accessory injurious factors. High doses and long duration of treatment may be aggravating factors. There were some suggestions that exposure in the first trimester of gestation was more dangerous than later exposures (Ganguin and Rempt, '70) but this was not consistent. The observation that the inner ear reached full adult development by midterm (Robinson and Cambon, '64) does not explain protection since SM and DHSM can damage adult ears too. The fact that transplacental passage reduces drug levels in fetuses probably reduces the danger to the inner ear but increased susceptibility of fetuses to the drugs (Molitor et al.,'46) works in the opposite direction. Since only about 10% of the exposed children suffer eighth nerve damage an individual susceptibility has been invoked (Ganguin and Rempt, '70) to account for this low incidence. Johnsonbaugh et al. ('74) attributed to increased sensibility the hearing loss of a mother and her son after treatment with SM. They quoted also other cases of familial predisposition published before. It should be pointed out that some of the children with hearing loss were so mildly affected that they were not considered hard of hearing by their parents but discovered by audiometric tests.

Aside from eighth nerve damages general teratological effects of tuberculosis and antituberculous drugs were considered by some investigators. Data of McDonald ('61) suggested that children born to women with pulmonary tuberculosis may have an excess of serious congenital malformations. Of 3,295 pregnant women interviewed at their first antenatal visit, 61 gave a history of pulmonary tuberculosis. Two of the tuberculous mothers had anencephalic children, one had a child without kidneys and one a child with a cardiac defect (6.6%). Lowe ('64) in a study of 173 pregnancies in women known to have active tuberculosis (without specific drug treatment) found that seven (4.1%) had infants with congenital defects. Women treated for tuberculosis in early pregnancy with INH, PAS and/or SM in various combinations had 74 children and only two of these (2.7%) had congenital defects. There was nothing to suggest that any of the drugs were teratogenic. Marynowski and Sianožecka ('72) compared the incidences of congenital malformations in infants of 1,619 mothers treated for tuberculosis with those of infants of healthy parturients. In the infants of treated tuberculous women the malformation incidence was 2.34% and in those of healthy women it was 2.56%. Neither the drugs (SM, Hydrazid, PAS) nor the tuberculosis of the mother exerted a teratogenic effect detectable in the neonatal period. The findings of Varpela ('64) were somewhat different. He examined histories of 123 women who had received SM, INH and PAS in various combinations during pregnancy. Malformations of various kinds were observed in 12 children (9.8%), whereas in a control group of 223 mothers only eight (3.6%) of the infants had congenital malformations. Although this looked like a substantial difference the author's conclusions were cautious. He thought that tuberculosis itself could have been responsible; the treated mothers received many drugs other than tuberculostatic; and 6 of the 12 children with malformations had been exposed to antituberculous drugs after the first trimester of gestation. The author stressed the need for additional studies. Marcus ('67) examined 19 children born of mothers treated in the first trimester with antituberculous drugs and found only four minor malformations (umbilical hernias and one undescended testis). He suggested that it is safe, and indeed essential to treat tuberculous women in early pregnancy.

A serious question about brain damage was raised by Monnet et al. ('67) who had observed five children with severe encephalopathies whose mothers had been treated with INH during pregnancy. They knew the INH can have toxic effects on the nervous system and that it can pass the placental barrier. The children had been exposed to INH at different times of gestation: two during the first three months and three after the first trimester. Four children had severe psychomotor retardation and convulsions; the fifth child had a cerebral hemiplegia. The authors discussed that degradation products of INH and hypovitaminosis B_6 could be responsible for these damages. They admitted that such apparent INH injuries must be very rare but they deserve publication since prophylactic administration of vitamin B_6 should be considered for pregnant women who receive INH.

Possible teratogenic effects of ethionamide (ETA) were discussed by Bignall ('65) who cited experiments in rats and rabbits which on high doses had abortions and some malformations. He thought that the drug should not be given to pregnant women although to his knowledge it had not been shown to be teratogenic in man. Reports from Poland were contradictory. Whereas Zierski ('66) by questionnaire failed to obtain reports of malformed children, Potworowska et al. ('66) noted among 23 children exposed to the drug in utero, seven with congenital malformations. Several other studies, representing some 70 cases, found no such relationship to ETA treatment during pregnancy (Schardein, '76).

Ethambutol (ETM) is a useful substance in the treatment of drug-resistant human tuberculosis and Place ('64) reported early that a normal girl was born to a mother with severe tuberculosis treated with this and other antituberculous compoounds before and during pregnancy. Since loss of vision sometimes complicated prolonged treatment with this drug it was stressed that the infant appeared normal on ophthalmological examination. Lewit et al. ('74) examined six human embryos up to age 12 weeks taken from mothers treated during early pregnancy with ETM and found them to be normal. Bobrowitz ('74) observed 38 patients on multidrug therapy who all received ETM through various stages of pregnancy. The children were followed from one to nine years and very thoroughly examined. Eight minor abnormalities were found which did not conform to any pattern and were not more common than in the general children's population. A number of single case reports were also negative for induction of congenital malformations (Schardein, '76).

Rifampicin (RMP) was suspected of teratogenicity and embryotoxicity because of experiments in rodents but there is no proof of damages to children when moderate therapeutic doses are given. Reimers ('71) reported two cases of normal fetal development following RMP treatment in early pregnancy. The treatments were given inadvertently because pregnancy had not been established. One patient had a healthy child and another patient's pregnancy ended in a legalized abortion in the fifth month; the fetus showed no pathological changes. These results and previous reports on 34 similar cases spoke for lack of teratogenicity of RMP in man. Jentgens ('75) describing various combinations of antituberculous drugs (including RMP and ETM) administered to 82 pregnant women observed no increase in malformation rates than generally expected. He was against termination of pregnancy because of antituberculous treatment. But Frahm ('76) observed after treatment with RMP of a 24-year-old woman for pyelonephritis before and during pregnancy, bleeding both in mother and newborn with disturbances in liver function and coagulation. He recommended that RMP be given in pregnancy with caution.

In 1980 Snider et al. published a critical review of tuberculosis treatment during pregnancy. They surveyed the literature on outcomes of 2,787 pregnancies among women who took INH, SM, EMB, and/or RMP during pregnancies. In addition, they added reports on 14 women who inadvertently took antituberculosis drugs while pregnant. They concluded that other than the well known ototoxicity of SM, none of these drugs in normal dosages were proven teratogens to human fetuses. They recommended the use of INH in combination with EMB for a pregnant woman with tuberculosis, if the disease was not extensive. Because of its ototoxicity, SM should not be used, unless RMP is contraindicated or proves unsatisfactory. Routine therapeutic abortion is not medically indicated for a woman who is taking "first-line" antituberculosis drugs.

SM ototoxicity deserves special mention. One in six of the fetuses exposed to this drug developed some hearing loss or suffered deafness severe enough to cause profound social and educational consequences. Streptomycin ototoxicity is independent of the so-called critical period early in embryogenesis and is potentially hazardous throughout gestation. This is not surprising since SM endangers the eighth nerve in postnatal life too. In patients treated with RMP during the first 4 months, there were some elevated rates of congenital malformations that deserved attention, but they were not statistically significantly different from the normal rates.

This review indicates a certain dilemma for physicians faced with a pregnancy in a woman with active tuberculosis. Failure to treat endangers the patient and indirectly her fetus. Treatment with the antituberculous drugs discussed above presents a slight risk of ototoxic and even cerebral damage to the fetus. This risk is probably reduced if treatment is given after the first trimester of pregnancy and doses are kept to a minimum considered effective. But since even adults can suffer damage of the eighth nerve through SM and DHSM one cannot guarantee safety of the fetus at any stage. Treatment with INH should be combined with administration of B_6 (Monnet et al., '67). It has been pointed out that the rarity of ototoxic complications with these powerful drugs can only be explained by unpredictable individual susceptibilities which makes parental counseling very difficult. As in other situations it will be necessary to present to the parents the medical dilemma and then let them decide whether the pregnancy should be continued or not.

LITERATURE CITED

Bignall, J.R., (1965) Study of possible teratogenic effects of ethionamide. Bull. Int. Union Tuberc., *36:*53.

Bobrowitz, I.D. 1974 Ethambutol in pregnancy. Chest, *66:*20–24

Bolletti, M., anbd L. Croatto (1958) Deafness in a five-year-old girl resulting from streptomycin therapy during pregnancy. Acta.Peadiatr. Lat., *11:*1–15.

Conway, N., and B.D. Birt (1965) Streptomycin in pregnancy: effect on the foetal ear. Br. Med. J., *2:*260–263.

Filippi, B., and V. Mela (1957) Malformazioni congenite degli arti ottenute sperimentalmente in embrioni di ratto in seguito a trattamento con penicillina et streptomicina. Minerva Chir., *12:*1047–1052.

Frahm, R. (1976) Zur Problematik der Rifampicin-Behandlung in der Schwangerschaft. Zbl. Gynäk., *98:*1585–1588.

Ganguin, G., and E. Rempt (1970) Streptomycinbehandlung in der Schwangerschaft und ihre Auswirkung auf das Gehör des Kindes. Z. Laryngol. Rhinol. Otol., *49:*496–503.

Grasset, E., H. de Watteville and P. Dossena (1951) Passage de la streptomycine à travers le placenta au cours du développement gravidique. Presse Méd., *59:*1265–1267.

Heilman, D.H., F.R. Heilman, H.C. Hinshaw, D.R. Nichols and W.E. Herrell (1945) Streptomycin: Absorption, diffusion, excretion and toxicity. Am. J. Med Sci., *210:*576–584.

Jentgens, H. (1975) Antituberkulotische Therapie mit Ethambutol und Rifampicin in der Schwangerschaft. Prax. Pneumol., *30:*42–45.

Johnsonbaugh, R.E., H.G. Drexler, I.J. Light and J.M. Sutherland (1974) Familial occurrence of drug-induced hearing loss. Am. J. Dis. Child., *127:*245–247.

Kern, G. (1962) Zur Frage der intrauterinen Streptomycinschädigung. Schweiz. Med. Wochenschr., *92:*77–79.

Kreibich, H. (1954) Sind nach einer Streptomycinbehandlung tuberkulöser Schwangere Schädigungen des Kindes zu erwarten? Dtsch. Gesundh.-Wes., *9:*177–181.

Leroux, M.L. (1950) Existe-t-il une surdité congénitale acquise due à la streptomycine? Ann. Otolaryngol.,

*67:*194–196.
Lewit, T., L. Nebel, S. Terracina and S. Karman (1974) Ethambutol in pregnancy: observations on embryogenesis. Chest, *66:*25–26.
Lowe, C.R. (1964) Congenital defects among children born to women under supervision or treatment for pulmonary tuberculosis. Br. J. Prev. Soc. Med., *18:*14–16.
Marcus, J.C. (1967) Non-teratogenicity of antituberculous drugs. S. Afr. Med. J., *41:*758–759.
Marynowski, A., and E. Sianožecka (1972) Porównanie czestości wystepowania wad wrodzonych u noworodków matek zdrowych i chorych, leczonych z powodu gruźlicy. Ginekol. Pol., *43:*713–715.
Matsushima, M. (1967) A study of pulmonary tuberculosis of pregnant women. Report 7. Effects of chemotherapy during pregnancy on the fetus. Kekkaku, *42:*463–464.
McDonald, A.D. (1961) Maternal health in early pregnancy and congenital defect. Final report on a prospective inquiry. Br. J. Prev. Soc. Med., *15:*154–166.
Molitor, H., O.E. Gresele, S. Kuna, C.W. Mushett and R.H. Silber (1946) Some toxicological and pharmacological properties of streptomycin. J. Pharmacol. Exper. Therap., *86:*151 173.
Monnet, P.,J. Cl. Kalb and M. Pujol (1967) Doit-on craindre une influence tératogène éventuelle de l'isoniazide? Rév. Tubercul (Paris), *31:*845–848.
Place, V.A. (1964) Ethambutol administration during pregnancy: A case report. J. New Drugs, *4:*206–208.
Podvinec, S., B. Mihaljevic, A. Marcetic and M. Simonovic (1965) Schädigungen des foetalen Cortischen Organs durch Streptomycin. Mschr. Ohrenheilk., *99:*20–24.
Potworowska, M., E. Sianožecka and R. Szufladowicz (1966) Leczenic etionamidem a ciaza. Gružlica Choroby Pluc., *34:*341–347.
Rasmussen, F. (1969) The ototoxic effect of steptomycin and dihydrostreptomycin on the foetus. Scand. J. Respir. Dis., *50:*61–67.
Rebattu, J.-P., G. Lesne and M. Megard (1960) Streptomycine, barrière placentaire, troublés cochleovestibulaires. J. Fr. Otorhinolaryngol., *9:*411–420.
Reimers, D. (1971) Missbildungen durch Rifampicin? Bericht über 2 Fälle von normaler fetaler Entwicklung nach Rifampicin-Therapie in der Frühschwangerschaft. Muench. Med. Wochenschr., *113:*1690–1691.
Riskaer, N., E. Christensen and H. Hertz (1952) The toxic effects of streptomycin and dihydrostreptomycin in pregnancy, illustrated experimentally. Acta Tuberc. Pneumol. Scand., *27:*211–212.
Robinson, G.C., and K.G. Cambon (1964) Hearing loss in infants of tuberculous mothers treated with streptomycin during pergnancy. N. Engl. J. Med., *271:*949–951.
Sakula, A. (1954) Streptomycin and the foetus. Br. J. Tuberc., *48:*69–72.
Schardein, J.L. (1976) Drugs as Teratogens. CRC Press, Inc., Cleveland.
Shepard, Th. H. (1976) Catalog of Teratogenic Agents. Second ed. The Johns Hopkins University Press, Baltimore.
Snider, D.E., P.M. Layde, M.W. Johnson, and M.A. Lyle (1980) Treatment of tuberculosis during pregnancy Am. Review Resp. Dis. *122:*65–79.
Varpela, E. (1964) On the effect exerted by first-line tuberculosis medicines on the foetus. Acta. Tuberc. Pneumol. Scand., *35:*53–69.
Varpela, E., J. Hietalahti and M. Aro (1969) Streptomycin and dihydrostreptomycin medication during pregnancy and their effect on the child's inner ear. Scand. J. Respir. Dis., *50:*101–109.
Watson, E.H., and R.M. Stow (1948) Streptomycin therapy-effects on fetus. J. Am. Med. Ass., *137:*1599–1600.
Woltz, J.H.E., and M.M. Wiley (1945) Transmission of streptomycin from maternal blood to the fetal circulation and the amniotic fluid. Proc. Soc., Exp. Biol., *60:*106–107.
Zierski, M. (1966) O wplywie etionamidu na rozwój plodu u ludzi. Gružlica Choroby Pluc., *34:*349–352.

Tetracycline Staining of Teeth

SIDNEY Q. COHLAN
Department of Pediatrics, New York University School of Medicine, New York, New York 10016

The broad spectrum antibiotic tetracycline deposits as a fluorescent compound primarily in calcifying teeth and bones and in growing tumors. Fluorescence in bones probably arises from a complex interfacial interaction presumably involving the 4-ringed naphthacenecarboxamide tetracycline nucleus and calcium, in areas of active mineralization in the organic matrix of newly proliferating bone. This effect of tetracycline has been used to identify both skeletal and gastrointestinal neoplasms, but its most important clinical manifestation is its staining effect on pre- and postnatally developing teeth. The major factors determining tetracycline deposition are dosage, duration of treatment, stage of tooth mineralization, and activity of the mineralization process. As little as 1 g/day tetracycline for 3 days during the 3rd trimester can produce yellow staining of deciduous teeth. Tetracycline-stained teeth may be grey-brown, yellow, or brown. Fluorescence can be elicited by the use of a Wood's lamp. The yellow-stained teeth fluoresce more consistently than the grey-brown or brown. After eruption and exposure to light, yellow-stained teeth gradually darken to brown. The labial surfaces of erupted yellow-stained incisors will darken in time while their palatal aspects and the cheek teeth will remain yellow.

Prenatal

Calcification of deciduous teeth begins at about the end of the 4th month of gestation and ends at about 11–14 months of age. Administration of tetracycline to pregnant women in the 2nd or 3rd trimester of gestation results in staining of the dentine and enamel calcifying at the time of administration. The chronology of deciduous-tooth calcification is well established so that it is possible to predict with reasonable accuracy which areas of which teeth will be affected. Since the permanent teeth begin calcifying after birth they are not affected by prenatal exposure. There is still no consensus as to whether tetracycline deposition in utero predisposes affected teeth to enamel hypoplasia or caries. Some data is available suggesting that high doses of tetracycline given to premature infants may produce enamel hypoplasia.

Postnatal

Calification of the permanent teeth begins at birth and, except for the 3rd molars, is complete by 7–8 years of age. These teeth calcify much more slowly than do deciduous teeth and are therefore less frequently affected. However, long-term therapy during early childhood will affect the permanent dentition. In fact, the original clinical observation of tetracycline-staining of teeth was made by Schwachman and Schuster ('56) in a group of children with cystic fibrosis of the pancreas who were on continuous, long-term tetracycline therapy for control of pulmonary infection.

During 1948–1959 a variety of tetracyclines became clincally available (chlortetracycline, oxytetracycline, tetracycline, and demethyltetracycline). Some data indicate that differences in staining color are a function of the type of tetracycline used and that there are also differences in incidence and intensity. Oxtetracycline is said to have the least staining effect. Since 1963, when the FDA directed manufacturers to include a warning of these side effects in their drug brochures, the incidence of prenatal and postnatal tetracycline tooth staining has sharply declined. The use of tetracyclines during the 2nd and 3rd trimesters of pregnancy and during infancy and early childhood should be restricted to specific indications and where adequate antibiotic alternatives are not available.

LITERATURE CITED

Porter, P.S., E.A. Sweeney, H. Golan and E.H. Kass (1965) Controlled study of the effect of prenatal tetracycline on primary dentition. Proceedings of the 5th Interscience Conference on Antimicrobial Agents and Chemotherapy, pp. 668–671.

Schwachman, H., and A. Schuster (1956) The tetracyclines: applied pharmacology. Ped. Clin. N. Am. *2:*295–303.

Toaff, R., and R. Ravid (1965) Tooth discoloration due to tetracyclines. In: Drug Induced Diseases. Vol. 3. L. Mayler and H.M. Peck, eds. Excerpta Medica, New York, pp. 117–133.

Weyman, J. (1965) The clinical appearances of tetracycline staining of teeth. Br. Dent. J., *118:*289–291.

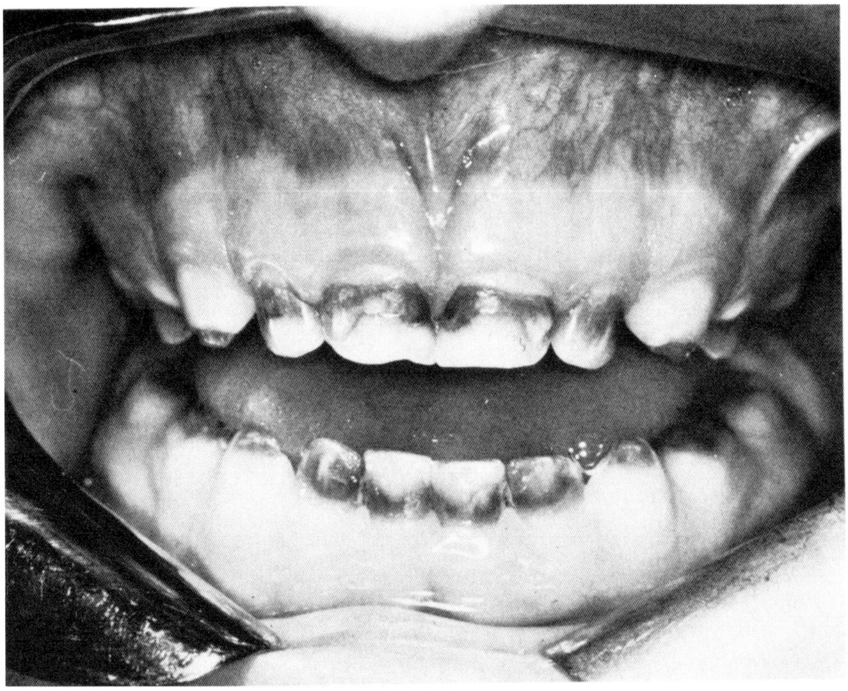

Fig. 1. Yellow-stained hypoplasia of enamel of a 4½-year-old boy who received tetracycline when 2 weeks old.

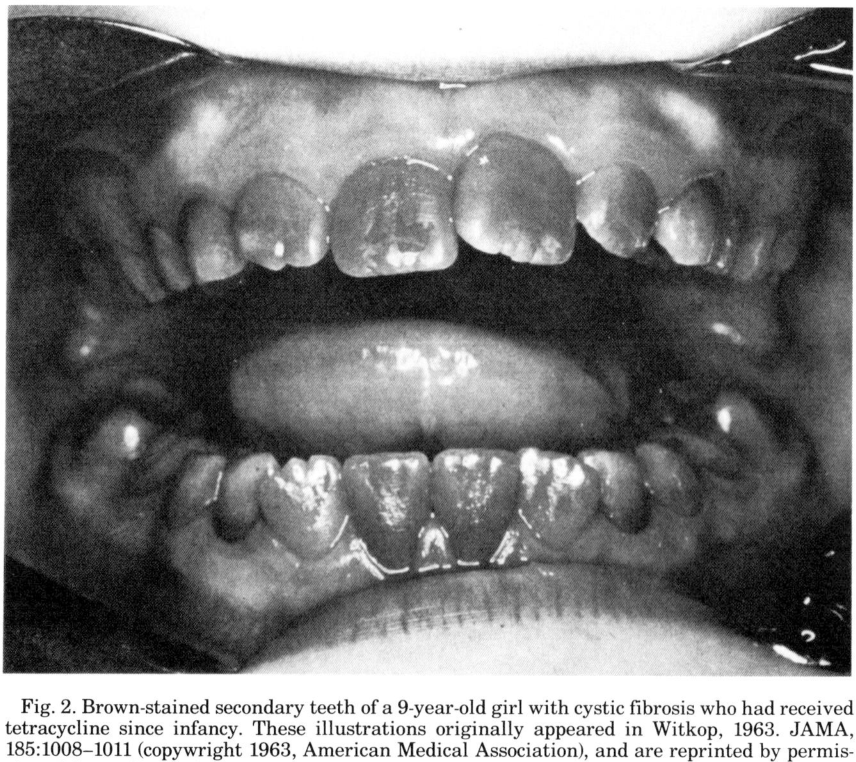

Fig. 2. Brown-stained secondary teeth of a 9-year-old girl with cystic fibrosis who had received tetracycline since infancy. These illustrations originally appeared in Witkop, 1963. JAMA, 185:1008–1011 (copywright 1963, American Medical Association), and are reprinted by permission of the author and editor.

Bendectin

LEWIS B. HOLMES
Embryology-Teratology Unit, Children's Service, Massachusetts General Hospital, Departments of Newborn Medicine and Obstetrics and Gynecology, Brigham and Women's Hospital, and Department of Pediatrics, Harvard Medical School, Boston, Massachusetts 02214

Bendectin has been used widely throughout the world as an agent to treat the nausea and vomiting of early pregnancy for the past 25 years. The drug was first marketed in the United States in 1956 and in Great Britain in 1958. Until 1977 Bendectin (the brand name for the product marketed in the United States; other brand names are Debendox® in Great Britain and Lenotan® in West Germany) contained 10 mg each of doxylamine succinate (an antihistamine with antinausea properties), dicyclomine (an antispasmodic), and pyridoxine (vitamin B_6). Beginning in 1977 Bendectin was reformulated to include only two ingredients, doxylamine and pyridoxine. This change in content was made because new clinical trials, required by 1962 amendments to the Food, Drug and Cosmetic Act, showed that most of the antinausea effect was produced by doxylamine, that pyridoxine added additional effectiveness, and that dicyclomine did not enhance the effectiveness of the other two components.

This review is prompted by the fact that Bendectin was used in the late 1970s by 10–25% of women during pregnancy in the United States and by the fact that there has been extensive debate in the lay press and in the courts as to whether this drug is teratogenic to exposed human fetuses (Brent, '83). This high level of concern is in contrast to the fact that most, but not all, studies (described below) have produced no evidence that exposure to this drug in the first trimester of pregnancy causes an increase in malformations, stillbirths, or growth retardation in the exposed fetuses in comparison to unexposed fetuses.

In 1983 the manufacturer discontinued production of the drug because the cost of insurance against litigation was almost equal to the total revenue from U.S. sales (Wall Street Journal, '83). This decision in effect eliminated the one drug approved by the F.D.A. for use during pregnancy to treat nausea and vomiting. After the high level of publicity in the lay press about the drug and the company's decision in June, 1983, we were impressed with the speed with which pregnant women became unaware of this controversy. In March, 1984, most pregnant women interviewed in a large maternity hospital did not recognize the drug name Bendectin (Holmes, '84). At this time some physicians were recommending that pregnant women with significant nausea and vomiting concoct their own "Bendectin" from medication available without prescription: a portion of a tablet that contains doxylamine and a portion of a tablet of pyridoxine (vitamin B_6). So even if Bendectin is no longer available, exposure of fetuses to the ingredients doxylamine and pyridoxine will continue to occur. As with any exposure that has elicited so much controversy, it will be important to review and to reassess regularly the information available on its effects on the fetus.

ANIMAL STUDIES

Teratologic studies in rabbits and rats treated with Bendectin and two of its components, dicyclomine hydrochloride and doxylamine succinate, have shown no effect on pregnancy maintenance, litter size, fetal weight, and the incidence of malformations (Gibson et al., '68). In these studies the doses of Bendectin used (0, 3, 6, and 30 mg/kg/day) were much greater than the average dosage used in pregnant women (two tablets a day with each containing 10 mg of each ingredient). The period of exposure used for rabbits was days 9–16 (normal gestation is 31 days); the rats studied were exposed daily for 80 days before pregnancy and on each day throughout pregnancy. Controls received an equal volume of the vehicle. The rabbits examined for skeletal malformations were sacrificed on day 28, cleared, and stained with alizarin red S. Among the treated fetuses the frequency of altered manubrium and fused sternebrae was increased in comparison to control fetuses. However, the authors considered these skeletal abnormalities to be minor in nature; they attributed their occurrence to genetic factors in the strain of rabbits that was used.

Hendrickx and his associates ('82,'83) have administered Bendectin to non-human primates for different periods of time. Bendectin was administered at a dose 10 to 20 times the human dose equivalent throughout organogenesis (days 20 to 50 of gestation). Four of seven fetuses delivered at 100 days of gestation had intraventricular septal defects and three more followed postnatally had no clinical signs of heart defects. In a follow-up study 16 rhesus monkeys and eight cynomolgus monkeys were treated with Bendectin at 10 to 40 times the human dose equivalent. Four of 18 exposed fetuses had heart defects—three were muscular ventricular septal defects and one was an atrioventricular septal defect. Three of the four fetuses with heart defects had been exposed to a dose of Bendectin 40 times the human dose equivalent and one fetus was exposed to a dose 10 times the human dose equivalent.

Bendectin was also administered for periods of 4 consecutive days by Hendrickx et al. ('82) at a dose 20 times the human dose equivalent. The gestational days were during organogenesis. Out of eight treated cynomolgus macaque monkeys there was one abortion and seven normal fetuses; the fetuses did not have heart defects.

The study of the effect of Bendectin on non-human primate fetuses is continuing (Kolata, '82).

HUMAN STUDIES

Early studies (General Practitioner Research Group, '63; Yerushalmy and Milkovich, '65) showed no evidence that exposure of the fetus to Bendectin in the first trimester of pregnancy was harmful. However, several case reports were published in which malformed infants were described whose mothers had taken Bendectin during the first trimester (Dickson, '77; Donnai and Harris, '78; Frith, '78; Henderson, '77; Paterson, '77). At about the same time and subsequently the results of several epidemiologic studies, some underway for many years and some conducted because of the renewed concern as to whether Bendectin is teratogenic, have been published (Cordero et al., '81; Eskenazi and Bracken, '82; Fleming et al., '81; Golding et al., '83; Jick et al., '81; Martinez-Frias et al., '84; Michaelis et al., '83; Milkovich and van den Berg, '76; Mitchell et al., '81, '83; Newman et al., '77; Rothman et al., '79; Shapiro et al., '77; Smithells and Sheppard, '78, '80). Both cohort and case-control studies have been carried out. The different study designs and interpretations will be reviewed. Any study with a positive association is included, but all negative studies reported are not included.

Cohort studies

In the cohort studies the prevalence of malformations among the exposed infants was compared to that among the unexposed controls (Table 1). As is reflected in the rate ratio of exposed to control infants, none of these cohort studies showed a significant increase among the exposed infants. One study (Newman et al., '77) actually showed a significant decrease in the rate of malformation, based on the fact that the upper bound of the confidence interval for the rate ratio was less than 1.0 (MacMahon, '81).

Each of these cohort studies had a somewhat different design and thereby inherent strengths and weaknesses. In the National Collaborative Perinatal Project, which was conducted at 12 hospitals throughout the United States between 1959 and 1965, over 50,000 pregnancies were monitored carefully and the infants born were followed for 7 years. Some 1,169 women took doxylamine succinate, one of the ingredients of Bendectin, during the first trimester of pregnancy; in addition, 1,024 of the same women took another ingredient, dicyclomine, during this time period. Comparisons in the prevalence of serious malformations were made between heavily exposed, moderately exposed, and unexposed infants for both drugs. No significant differences were identified. The mean birth weight and perinatal mortality were similar in the exposed infants in comparison to 40,000 unexposed infants. The intelligence scores at age 4 years were comparable in the exposed and over 27,000 unexposed infants.

In 1978 Smithells and Sheppard reported the results of a study using the "prescription technique." They reviewed copies of all prescriptions issued by general practitioners in two cities in Great Britain, Leeds and Liverpool, during a 12-month period in 1974 and 1975. The births of 66.8% of the patients for whom Bendectin was prescribed were traced. The estimated gestational age at which Bendectin was first prescribed was determined by reviewing the mother's maternity record. The outcome of the pregnancy, including abortion, stillbirth, and a liveborn infant with or without malformations, was determined from the same source. There was no difference in the incidence of malformations among the 2,295 Bendectin-exposed infants in Liverpool and Leeds (2.1% and 1.3%, respectively) and the prevalence rate among all infants born in both cities in the same year (2.2% and 1.5%, respectively). No unusual malformations were identified among the exposed infants. There was no difference in the incidence of significant malformations among infants exposed in the first 10 weeks of pregnancy and those exposed later in pregnancy. This paper has been criticized because it assumed all Bendectin would have been obtained by prescription, when in fact it could have been obtained by other means. However, Smithells and Sheppard ('80) found that over-the-counter sales were negligible during this time in the United Kingdom.

Another study using the drug prescriptions to confirm possible exposure was carried out by Golding et al. ('83) on infants born with cleft lip and/or palate in the region of Oxfordshire and West Berkshire, England. Information was obtained about exposure during the first 5 months of pregnancy from general practitioners by questionnaire on both cases and matched controls. Among 240 cases and 480 controls the rate of exposure of Debendox was 6.1% (12 cases) and 2.2% (nine controls) respectively, with a relative risk of 2.88. These differences were significant ($p < 0.02$). The authors noted one limitation of their study was that they ascertained prescriptions, not consumption of Debendox. They noted that "the findings of this study alone do not prove the case against Debendox."

The study reported by Jick and his associates ('81) utilized computerized records of all prescriptions filled by pregnant women in a prepaid health plan. In as much as 98% of the participants reported that they use the pharmacies of the health plan to fill their prescriptions knowledge of drug usage was limited to knowing when the women filled the prescription for Bendectin and when her infants were born. The mothers were not interviewed to determine whether they took Bendectin after they had obtained the drug from the pharmacy. Among the 2,255 exposed infants the rate of malformations was 1.1% in comparison to 1.2% among the 4,582 unexposed controls. There was no increase in the rate of malformations for infants whose

TABLE 1. Cohort studies of malformations among infants exposed to Bendectin (modified from MacMahon, '81)

Study	Number of infants		Rate ratio	90% confidence limits of	
	Exposed	Control		Rate	Ratio
1. (Milkovich and van den Berg, '76) 1959–1966 San Francisco, CA	628	9,577	0.62	0.40	0.96
2. (Newman et al., '77) 1953–1975 New Zealand	1,192	6,741	0.48	0.25	0.96
3. (Smithells and Sheppard, '78) 1974–1975 Leeds and Liverpool, England	2,295	—	1.36	0.71	2.61
4. Heionen (cited by MacMahon, '81) 1959–1965 12 U.S. hospitals	2,193	48,089	1.05	0.83	1.33
5. (Michaelis et al., '83) 1961–1972 Germany	874	874	0.95	0.52	1.73
6. (Fleming et al., '81) mid-1960s Scotland and England	620	22,357	0.65	0.36	1.15
7. (Jick et al., '81) 1977–1979 Seattle, WA	2,255	4,582	0.87	0.58	1.30

mother filled only one prescription. There were more infants with atresia of the intestine among the exposed than the unexposed (four and two, respectively). However, the authors doubted there was any causal association as the 95% lower confidence bound was below unity (0.8) and there was no correlation with the number of prescriptions filled.

Case-control studies

In two of the reported studies the rate of exposure to Bendectin for infants with one type of malformations was compared with the exposure rate among infants with other malformations. By interviewing only mothers who have had infants with malformations there is less likelihood that the mother will be unconcerned, and presumably more forgetful, of exposures in the first trimester, a bias attributed to the mothers of healthy infants. Cordero and his associates ('81) compared the findings in interviews with women in metropolitan Atlanta who had had infants with neural tube defects, cleft lip, cleft palate, all types of intestinal atresia, diaphragmatic hernia, omphalocele, Down Syndrome, and limb reduction defects. These malformations were identified in 1,231 infants between 1970 and 1978, except for those with limb reduction defects. The 115 infants with limb reduction defects, a heterogeneous group that was subdivided into six major categories, were born between 1973 and 1978. These 1,231 infants represent 82.5% of the infants born with selected malformations among 280,000 births. This makes the population base for this case-control study four to 20 times greater than that of the cohort studies summarized above (Table 1).

Of the mothers 9.5% reported first-trimester exposure to Bendectin. No significant differences were found in the exposure of infants with 12 different malformations to this drug. Among all of the types of limb defects exposure to Bendectin was increased significantly only for infants with the amniotic band complex. (The amniotic band complex is a severe and sometimes fatal pattern of malformations of the cranium, face, and extremities that is attributed to entanglement of or adherence of fetal parts to segments of amnion that often disrupts development and produces amputations; Miller et al., '81.) Cordero and his associates ('81) noted that the studies of a large number of infants with the amniotic bands complex have failed to show a significant association with exposure to Bendectin. They concluded there was insufficient evidence to support a causal relationship between amniotic band complex and exposure to Bendectin.

Cordero et al. ('81) stratified their findings to coincide with the period when Bendectin contained two and three ingredients. They found an association between exposure to the two-ingredient Bendectin and encephalocele, but not between the three-ingredient Bendectin and encephalocele. As a strict interpretation of the difference would suggest that the third ingredient, dicyclomine, had a protective effect, they concluded it was unlikely there was any causal relationship between exposure to Bendectin and encephalocele. The same stratification showed an association between three-ingredient Bendectin, but not two-ingredient Bendectin, and esophageal atresia. After reviewing all of these issues, Cordero et al. ('81) concluded: "although we found three weak associations, they do not establish a causal relationship between Bendectin and the birth defects categories we studied." Unfortunately, reporters summarizing the findings in this study have emphasized the associations noted, but neither the qualifying aspects of the study design nor the authors' conclusions.

The second study in which the rate of exposure to Bendectin was evaluated among infants with different types of malformations was by Mitchell and his associates ('81, '83). Study subjects were white, malformed, lived within defined geographic areas (Toronto, Boston, and Philadelphia), and were no more than 6 months of age when the mother was interviewed in her home. The malformed infants were identified on hospital wards or in clinics and office records. In a case-control study of 319 infants with cleft lip and/or cleft palate and 122 infants with heart defects, an increased rate of exposure to Bendectin was not identified among the infants with these malformations.

Two case-control studies of note in which the rate of exposure among malformed infants was compared to health controls were the studies of Rothman and his associates ('79) and Eskenazi and Bracken ('82). Rothman and associates ('79) conducted a case-control study of 390 infants with heart defects who were compared to 1,254 infants who had no malformations. The mothers were asked to complete a questionnaire within a year of the infant's birth. They were asked to list drugs they had taken early in pregnancy. Fifty-four percent of the mothers of infants with heart defects and 41% of the mothers of the controls reported taking drugs. There was a strong association with the use of insulin; this is not surprising as heart defects are more common among infants of diabetic mothers than among infants of nondiabetic women. A small positive association was noted for exposure to exogenous hormones and the occurrence of heart defects. A weak association was found for several common drugs, including aspirin, phenylephrine, and Bendectin. The authors did not consider these weak associations to be significant. They noted that the information was obtained from an open-ended question and was thereby likely to be subject to recall bias. Further evidence of this recall bias was apparent in the case of Bendectin as only 6.6% of the mothers of infants with heart defects and even fewer (3.3%) of the control mothers reported having taken Bendectin. This rate of using Bendectin is contrary to the findings of Mitchell and his associates ('81), who found that 9.5% of the women in the same geographic area reported using Bendectin in the first trimester of pregnancy.

Eskenazi and Bracken ('82) compared the frequency of maternal use of Bendectin in 1974 to 1976 among 1,427 malformed infants, most of whom were newborn infants, and 3,001 unexposed healthy newborn infants. The mothers of 6.3% of the cases and 4.6% of controls reported using Bendectin during the first trimester. Considering infants with all major malformations, the chance of having been exposed to Bendectin in the first trimester was not increased to an extent that was considered significant statistically (odds ratio = 1.40, 95% confidence limits = 0.96, 2.05, p = 0.08). When 16 major malformations were considered, two had statistically significant associations with exposure to Bendectin: six of 35 infants with pyloric stenosis (odds ratio = 4.33, 95% confidence limits = 1.75, 10.75, $p < 0.001$) and four of 32 infants with abnormal heart valves (odds ratio = 2.99, 95% confidence limits = 1.02, 8.74, $p < 0.04$). In an analysis of confounding variables, maternal smoking appeared to increase the risk for pyloric stenosis. The findings in this study by Eskenazi and Bracken ('82) were not confirmed by the work of Mitchell and his associates ('83), whose study of infants with cleft lip and/or cleft palate and heart defects was described earlier. They found that the rate of exposure to Bendectin during pregnancy among 325 infants with pyloric stenosis was not significantly different from the rate of exposure among 3,153 infants with other defects. 17% of the infants with pyloric stenosis were exposed during pregnancy to Bendectin and 20% of the infants with other malformations were exposed; the relative risk was 0.9 (95% confidence interval 0.6–1.2). If the comparison is restricted to infants with pyloric stenosis unassociated with other defects, the relative risk was 0.8 with 95% confidence interval 0.6 to 1.1. In comparing their study to that of Eskenazi and Bracken ('82), Mitchell and his associates ('83) noted that they studied many more exposed cases (56 versus six), which made their findings more powerful in statistical terms. They noted that the lower exposure rate in New Haven, CT (4.6% in comparison to 20% in Mitchell's study in Boston, Philadelphia, and Toronto) made it quite possible that Eskenazi and Bracken did not identify several exposed cases.

As preliminary and unpublished laboratory experiments had suggested a slight incidence of diaphragmatic hernias among rat fetuses exposed to very high doses of Bendectin (Kolata, '81), data on the association between diaphragmatic hernia and exposure to Bendectin collected in the Spanish Collaborative Study of Congenital Malformations was reviewed (Martinez-Frias et al., '84). Between 1976 and 1981, 53 infants with diaphragmatic hernias were identified, five of whom were exposed to Debendox in the first trimester. Exposure among 4,965 malformed controls was 12.7%. The odds ratio was 0.71 with 95% confidence intervals of 0.28 and 1.8, which is not significant statistically. The authors noted that the sample size of their data was large enough for them to have an 82% chance of finding a doubling of the prevalence of a malformation and 100% chance of identifying a three fold increase.

UNCONTROLLED STUDIES

The observation that specific malformations could be caused by exposure to Bendectin has prompted studies of infants with specific malformations. For example, infants with the Poland's anomaly have been reported to have been exposed to Bendectin.

To evaluate the hypothesis that exposure to Debendox caused the Poland anomaly, David ('82) examined 32 individuals with isolated absence of the pectoralis major and 46 individuals with the complete Poland anomaly. Each mother's antenatal drug history was verified by examining her hospital records for that pregnancy and by obtaining records of drugs prescribed by the family doctor. Twenty-six individuals were born before Debendox was introduced into Great Britain, so they could not have been exposed. Exposure was documented for two cases, in one of which the exposure occurred before the critical period of embryogenesis for the pectoralis muscle (estimated to be 43 to 46 days after conception); one occurred after this period. David concluded it was unlikely that exposure to Debendox causes the Poland anomaly.

Robinson and Tross ('84) evaluated seven infants with absence of the external genitals, imperforate anus, and persistence of the cloaca. The history of all environmental exposures and maternal infections was obtained and tabulated for five infants. Three agents, doxylamine succinate, detromethorphan, and acetaminophen, were considered to be potential teratogens, as two or more of the five fetuses had been exposed during the first 12 weeks of pregnancy. Robinson and Tross indicated a reluctance to make "categorical statements about etiology" from only five cases. However, they considered doxylamine succinate (an ingredient of Bendectin as well as several other prescription and nonprescription medications) to be the prime suspect for causing this rare malformation.

PUBLIC AWARENESS

Newspaper reporters and their readers prefer simple statements about whether Bendectin is harmful to the exposed fetus, rather than discussions of risk ratio, confidence intervals, associations that do not reflect causality, etc. Furthermore, it is confusing when respected scientists draw opposing conclusions, as occurred at the public hearings before the Fertility and Maternal Health Advisory Committee of the Food and Drug Administration when it met to review Bendectin in January 1981.

One recurring theme in many newspaper and magazine articles about Bendectin as a possible teratogen is a statement of the similarities to thalidomide, a drug that was also marketed for the treatment of the nausea and vomiting of pregnancy. This analogy recalls to many readers other aspects of the thalidomide tragedy, including the reluctance by the manufacturer to remove the drug from the market. According to Lenz ('79), the newspaper reports were helpful in speeding the process of withdrawing the drug from all pharmacies. Therefore, any comparison of Bendectin to thalidomide conjures up a fear of "cover up" and delay in public recognition that a drug is harmful to the exposed human fetus (Wall Street Journal, '83).

This analogy to thalidomide is unfortunate. The full phenotypic effect of thalidomide is not well known to the public; only the limb deformities have been presented vividly by the lay press. In fact, experience with children with the thalidomide embryopathy showed a wide spectrum of phenotypes, which ranged from the infant with deafness due to an inner ear defect, abducens paralysis, and preauricular tags to the infant with phocomelia with ear and dental anomalies, and intestinal atresia (Lenz, '66). While only a minority of affected children had phocomelia, the opposite seems to be the impression of the public and many physicians. In fact, there seems to be a general tendency to suspect environmental factors as a cause whenever a child has any limb malformation. If one includes all types of limb malformations, such as polydactyly, club foot, and long bone deficiencies, limb malformations are one of the most common and most easily recognized of birth defects. Among 30,000 newborn infants at the Brigham and Women's Hospital in Boston whom we have surveyed, the rate of limb malformations is 7/1,000 (Holmes, '81). By contrast, long bone deficiences, including phocomelia, were rare with a prevalence rate of 0.15/1,000. Because the malformations of nonskeletal structures in the thalidomide embryopathy are not well-known, physicians, parents, and lawyers often consider these infants with absence of a portion of one or more limbs the prototype of the drug-induced birth defect.

Although long bone deficiencies and phocomelia are rare, the high rate of usage of Bendectin (estimated at 10–25% of women in the United States) in the first trimester of pregnancy has meant that many of these malformed infants have been exposed to this drug in the first trimester. When one looks at such an unfortunate infant, it is not surprising that the sympathetic observer turns a deaf ear to the findings of the cohort and case-control studies outlined above.

At least 40% of congenital malformations present in newborn infants remain unexplained. As was noted by the Fertility and Maternal Health Advisory Committee of the FDA in its review of Bendectin, it is difficult, if not impossible, for any study to remove all "residual uncertainty" that an exposure is not harmful.

While we can always wish for more and better studies, two issues must be borne in mind. First, well-designed and extensive epidemiologic studies are expensive. Where will the funds to support these studies come from in this period of limited funding? Second, in view of the extensive data cited above on Bendectin and the limited data available on many other commonly used drugs one can argue that well-designed studies of other drugs would be of greater value to the public at this time.

COUNSELING

Based on the information available in early 1984, parents of exposed fetuses can be told: several epidemiologic studies of infants have failed to show an increased risk of birth defects after exposure to Bendectin or its ingredients during early pregnancy; a few studies have suggested an increased risk for specific abnormalities from exposure, but these observations have not been confirmed by other studies of infants with the same malformations; and animal studies show an increased risk of heart defects after an exposure at a dose that is over ten times higher than the human equivalent and that is given for a much longer time than Bendectin is customarily prescribed.

ACKNOWLEDGMENTS

This work was supported in part by NIH grant HD15241 and contract #HD02839.

LITERATURE CITED

Brent, R.L. (1983) The Bendectin saga: Another American tragedy (Brent, '80). Teratology, *27:*283–286.

Cordero, J.F., G.P. Oakley, F. Greenberg and L.M. James (1981) Is Bendectin a teratogen? JAMA, *245:*2307–2310.

David, T.J. (1982) Debendox does not cause the Poland anomaly. Arch. Dis. Child., *51:*479–480.

Dickson, J.H. (1977) Congenital deformities associated with Bendectin. Can. Med. Assoc. J., *117:*721.

Donnai, D., and R. Harris (1978) Unusual fetal malformations after antiometics in pregnancy. Br. Med. J., *1:*601–602.

Eskenazi, B. and M.B. Bracken (1982) Bendectin (Debendox) as a risk factor for pyloric stenosis. Am. J. Obstet. Gynecol. *144:*919–924.

Fleming, D.M., J.D. Knox, and D.L. Crombie (1981) Debendox in early pregnancy and fotal malformation. Br. Med. J. *283:*99–101.

Frith, K. (1978) Fetal malformation after Debendox treatment in early pregnancy. Br. Med. J. *1:*925.

General Practitioner Research Group (1963) Drugs in Pregnancy Survey. Practitioner, *191:*775–780.

Gibson, J.P., R.E. Staples, E.J. Larson, Wil-Kuhu, D.E. Holtkamp, and J.W. Newberne (1968) Teratology and Reproduction Studies with an Antinauseant. Toxic Appl. Pharmacol., *13:*439–447.

Golding, J., S. Vivian, and J.A. Baldwin (1983) Maternal anti-nauseants and clefts of lip and palate. Hum. Toxicol., *2:*63–73.

Henderson, I.W.D. (1977) Congenital deformities associated with Bendectin. Can. Med. Assoc. J., *117:*721–722.

Hendrickx, A.G., S. Prahalada, G. Janos, T. Nyland, and J. Rowland (1983) Cardiac embryotoxicity studies on Bendectin in macaques. Teratology, *27:*49A.

Hendrickx, A.G., S. Prahalada, and J.M. Rowland (1982) Embryotoxicity studies on Bendectin in cynomolgus monkeys (*Macaca fascicularis*). Teratology, *25:*47A.

Holmes, L.B. (1981) Unpublished data.

Indications for Bendectin Narrowed (1981) FDA Bulletin Vol 11, No. 1, March.

Holmes, L.B. (1984) Unpublished data.

Jick, H., L.B. Holmes, J.R. Hunter, S. Madsen, and A. Stergachis (1981) First trimester drug use and congenital disorders. JAMA, *246:*343–346.

Kolata, G. (1982) FDA to reexamine Bendectin data. Science, *217:*335.

Lenz, W. (1966) Malformations caused by drugs in pregnancy. Am. J. Dis. Child, *112:*99–106.

Lenz, W. (1979) Thalidomide; facts and inferences. Proceedings of the Kyoto International Congress Series NO. 513.

MacMahon, B. (1981) More on Bendectin (Editorial). JAMA, *246:*371–372.

Martinez-Frias, M.L., J. Salvadore, and J.F. Cordero (1984) Debendox and diaphragmatic hernia: No evidence of an association. (unpublished data).

Michaelis, J., H. Michaelis, E. Gluck, and S. Koller (1983) Prospective study of suspected associations between certain drugs administered during early pregnancy and congenital malformations. Teratology, *27:*57–64.

Milkovich, L., and B. van den Berg (1976) An evaluation of the teratogenicity of certain antinauseant drugs. Am. J. Obstet. Gynecol., *125:*244–248.

Miller, M.E., J.M. Graham Jr., and D.W. Smith (1981) Compression-related defects from early amnion rupture: Evidence for mechanical teratogenesis. J. Pediatr., *98:*292–297.

Mitchell, A.A., P.J. Schwingl, L. Rosenberg, C. Louik, and S. Shapiro (1983) Birth defects in relation to Bendectin use in pregnancy II. Pyloric stenosis. Am. J. Obstet. Gynecol. *147:*737–742.

Mitchell, A.M., L. Rosenberg, S. Shapiro, and D. Slone (1981) Birth defects related to Bendectin use in pregnancy. I. Oral clefts and cardiac defects. JAMA, *245:*2311–2314.

Newman, N.M., J.F. Correy, and G.I. Dudgeon (1977) A survey of congenital abnormalities and drugs in a private practice. Aust. N.Z. J. Obstet. Gynecol., *17:*156–159.

Paterson, D.C. (1977) Congenital deformities associated with Bendectin. Can. Med. Assoc. J., *116:*1348.

Robinson, H.B., Jr. and K. Tross (1984) Agenesis of the cloacal membrane: A probable teratogenic anomaly. Perspect. Pediatr. Pathol. *1.*79–90.

Rothman, K.J., D.C. Fyler, A. Goldblatt, and M.B. Kroidberg (1979) Exogenous hormones and other drug exposures of children with congenital heart disease. Am. J. Epidemol. *109:*433–439.

Shapiro, S., O.P. Heinonen, V. Siskind, D.W. Kaufman, R.R. Monson, and D. Stone (1977) Antenatal exposure to doxylamine succinate and dicyclomine hydrochloride (Bendectin) in relation to congenital malformations, perinatal mortality rate, birth weight, and intelligence quotient score. Am. J. Obstet. Gynecol., *128:*480–485.

Smithells, R.W, and S. Sheppard (1978) Teratogenicity testing in humans; a method demonstrating safety of Bendectin. Teratology, *17:*31–36.

Smithells, R.W., and S. Sheppard (1980) Safety of Bendectin. Teratology, *22:*353.

Yerushalmy, J., L. Milkovich (1965) Evaluation of the teratogenic effect of meclizine in man. Am. J. Obstet. Gynecol., *93:*553–562.

—(1983) Defects in the Courtroom. Wall Street Journal, June 15, 1983.

TERATOGEN UPDATE: ENVIRONMENTALLY INDUCED BIRTH DEFECT RISKS, PAGES 61–70 (1986)

Vitamin A Congeners

FRANZ W. ROSA, ANN L. WILK, AND FRANCES O. KELSEY
Center for Drugs and Biologics, Food and Drug Administration, Rockville, MD 20857

ABSTRACT Despite animal vitamin A congener teratogenicity in animal studies since 1954, striking human findings only arose in 1983 following *isotretinoin* (ITR) marketing for oral treatment of severe acne. By November 1985, 44 outcomes with central nervous system (CNS), cardioaortic (CV), microtia, facial palsy, micrognathia, cleft palate, and/or thymic aplasia defects, and 33 spontaneous abortions have been reported. The critical period for exposure appears to be two to five weeks postconception, although this is clinically inexact. ITR half life is less than a day, although a teratogenic metabolite, 4-oxo-isoretinoin, has a half life of several days. Seven defect outcomes and one stillbirth have been reported with another congener, *etretinate* (ETR), used for psoriasis. Three of these had meningomyeloceles. Half life of several months makes levels cumulative. Only one additional defect, which may have occurred by chance, is reported with use stopped before conception (4 months). Other discontinuations 1 to 6 months before conception had 11 normal outcomes and two spontaneous abortions. ITR and ETR dose ranged from 0.5 to 1.5 mg/kg. Normal outcomes are reported both with ITR and ETR, but some of these appear not to have been exposed during the critical period. Less striking defects, abortions, and normal outcomes are less well reported. Because vitamin A analogs are therapeutically important and unplanned outcome not always avoidable, further animal research is needed for better risk/benefits. Megadose *vitamin A (retinol)* use is widespread, but experience poorly observed. Eighteen suspicious birth defect outcomes have been reported from pregnancies with high dose exposure. Twelve had findings similar to those seen in animals and in human retinoid syndromes, e.g., CNS, CV, microtia, and clefts. Epidemiological controls are lacking to establish human teratogenicity, but based on animal studies and experience with ITR and ETR, avoiding long term megadose Vitamin A use in fertile women is warranted.

Vitamin A congeners fall into several categories. Vitamin A is an alcohol form, retinol. It metabolizes to an aldehyde, retinal, and to an acid form, retinoic acid. The naturally occurring form of retinoic acid is all-trans derivative, tretinoin (TR). Isotretinoin (ITR), the 13-cis form, differs only in the direction of the acid tail. All of these analogs are teratogenic in animals. Since the original report of animal teratogenicity with vitamin A by Cohlan ('53), more than a hundred studies have found various analogs teratogenic in numerous species (Shenefelt, '71). However, sporadic reports of possible human teratogenicity did not fit any pattern.

ITR (Accutane® or Roaccutane®), has been marketed since September 1982, as an orally administered agent for treating recalcitrant severe acne. Due to animal teratogenicity, since the onset of marketing, a warning against exposure during pregnancy has been provided, and unavoided pregnancy exposures have been monitored. The first observations of human teratogenicity were communicated by the manufacturer to the FDA and to the public in June 1983 (Roche, '83). An analysis of prospectively and retrospectively reported human pregnancies was initially published in August 1983 (Rosa, '83), with follow ups presented in 1984 and 1985. A detailed review of exposures up to May 1984 was presented by the manufacturer

TABLE 1. Isotretinoin pregnancies with ear, CNS and/or CV defect outcome

	Birth	Isotretinoin exposure[2]	Isotretinoin Mg/d	Defects CNS	Defects Ear	Defects CV	Other
1. P[1]	5/29/83	10 to 33	60	+	+	+	
2. R	6/09/83	−14 to 102	40	+	+		Micrognathia
3. R	6/14/83	−45 to 97	80	+			Stillborn
4. R	6/15/83	26 to 34	40	+	+	+	Hepatic abnormality
5. R	9/29/83	0 to 60	40		+	+	
6. R	6/26/83	−10 to 30	50	+	+		Micrognat., cleft palate, microphthalmia
7. R	7/17/83	−14 to 51	40	+	+	+	Microphalmia
8. P	9/07/83	17 to 22	40	+	+		Blind
9. R	9/19/83	−90 to 35	20	+	+	+	Micrognathia, microphthalmia
10. R	9/25/83	−5 to 44	80		+	+	Micrognathia, cleft
11. R	11/16/83		400	+			Cleft palate
12. P	11/19/83	−90 to 40	80			+	
13. R	11/26/83	to 42	60			+	
14. R	11/29/83	17 to 40	50	+	+		Blind, micrognathia
15. R	12/21/83	to 14		+	+		Midface hypoplasia, strabismus, ptosis
16. R	12/21/83	0 to 126	60	+	+	+	Micrognathia, cleft palate
17. R	1/09/84	−20 to 20	40	+	+	+	
18. R	1/01/84	−300 to 21		+	+		Asymmetry face
19. I	1/12/84	to 56	40	+	+		
20. R	1/22/84	3 to 52	40	+	+		Facial palsy
21. R	2/13/84	−28 to −6?	60	+	+	+	
22. I	3/04/84	−30 to 75	40			+	
23. R	3/14/84	−30 to 35	80	+	+	+	Micrognathia, cleft palate
24.	3/25/84	−60 to 14	80	+	+		Micrognathia
25. R	4/02/84	−120 to −21?	10			+	Miniscule thymus
26. R	4/03/84	−30 to 10	80	+			Spina bifida, nystagmus
27. R	5/08/84	−6 to 73		+	+	+	
28. P	5/14/84	0 to 13	40	+			(not walking age 16 months)
29. R	5/19/84	−30 to 60	tid	+	+	+	Micrognathia
30. R	7/06/84	−120 to 90	40	+			
31. R	8/17/84	0 to 28		+	+	+	Facial dysmorphia
32. R	8/22/84	−6 to 30	80	+	+	+	Micrognathia
33. R	9/24/84	26 to 28	80	+	+	+	SIDS age 4 months
34. R	12/03/84		160	+	+		Hydroureter
35. P	12/03/84	14 to 27	25	+			Micrognathia
36. R	12/ /84	−60 to 30	40	+	+		Micrognathia, cleft palate
37. I	5/02/84	25 to 84		+		+	
38. I	1/18/85	10 to 18		+			
39. R	1/23/85				+		Facial palsy
40. R	2/24/85	−14 to 49	40	+	+	+	Hypoplastic thalamus, T-E and R-V fistula
41. R	2/18/85	7 days 1st mo		+	+	+	
42. P	6/ /85	27 to 39	40	+	+		Micrognathia
43. I	8/ /85			+			Interrupted 13th wk
44. I	1/10/86	0 to 126		+			Interrupted 19th week

TABLE 2. Maternal isotretinoin exposures, summary of main case defect components

CNS	Ear	CV	Cases
+	+	+	15
+	+		13
+		+	1
	+	+	2
+			9
	+		0
		+	4
38	30	22	44

(Roche, '84), and published in detail (Lammer et al., '85a).

Also in 1983, human birth defect outcomes were reported with another retinoic acid congener, etretinate (Tigason®), marketed for treating psoriasis (Sautier, '83). These and other cases were published in 1984 (Happle et al.).

Observation of human teratogenicity with therapeutic vitamin A congeners has reemphasized the potential human teratogenicity of high dose vitamin A (retinol) exposure. Defining, identifying, and quantifying excess vitamin A exposure is difficult. For this and other reasons, adverse outcomes associated with excess exposure are under poor surveillance. Therefore vitamin teratology has been largely dependent on animal studies, ethical pharmaceutical experience, and alert human case reporting of exposures and outcomes.

NATURE OF DEFECTS WITH MATERNAL ISOTRETINOIN EXPOSURE

Forty-four birth defect outcomes involved one or more components of a syndrome of central nervous system (CNS) pathology, small or absent external ears, and/or cardioaortic (CV) defects. The number of infants with each of these components, and the frequency of occurrence of each main component among the total are shown in Tables 1 and 2. External ears and auditory canals are bilaterally low and small or absent. Facial dysmorphia is seen, often with micrognathia and cleft palate. Two infants had midface hypoplasia. Brain defects involve a combination of microcephaly and hydrocephaly, often with posterior fossa cyst and cortical blindness. Three CNS defect reports involved only functional impairment (retardation, and/or blindness), one involved only facial nerve paralysis, and one involved only spina bifida. Three other infants had facial palsy in combination with other defects. Aortic coarctation is prominent among the CV defects. Five infants with one or more of the main defect category components also had thymic hypoplasia.

Nine reports with maternal exposure not during the first trimester of pregnancy and/or defects judged non-teratogenic are not included in the table. These include: 1) McBride's ('85) limb reduction report, judged by Lammer et al. ('85b) to be an amniotic band syndrome; 2) an infant with a club foot with no maternal *isotretinoin* exposure until late pregnancy; 3) an inguinal hernia; 4) an apparently normal infant with sudden unexplained death at age 7 weeks; 5) a markedly premature infant with rotated ears, but without defect at follow up; 6) an infant with congenital cataract, isotretinoin stopped 3 weeks before conception; 7) an infant with spina bifida, *isotretinoin* stopped 7 months before LMP; 8) suspected spina bifida, *isotretinoin* stopped a month before LMP; and 9) Down's syndrome, *isotretinoin* stopped 2 months before LMP. Three uncharacteristic defect outcomes with only the father exposed have been reported. These are an infant with biliary atresia and VSD, another with four limb ectomelia and hydrocephalus, and a third case with anencephaly. Because of the diversity of these outcomes, they probably occurred by chance.

TABLE 3. Prospectively reported maternal isotretinoin exposure outcomes[1]

	Weeks following LMP		
	Before 4th	5th to 7th	Started after 7th
Spontaneous abortions	2	11	
Birth defects	0	4	
Apparently normal	9[2]	10[3]	2
Total	11	25	2

[1]Source: Cohort of exposures provided by Roche Laboratories at FDA Advisory Committee Meeting, May 1984.
[2]Includes case with inguinal hernia only.
[3]Includes one sudden unexplained death at 7 weeks age.

A small *semi-prospective cohort* of 41 exposures reported before outcome was known provided the opportunity to examine the distribution of all outcomes (Roche, '84). An unknown number of spontaneous abortions occur before exposure can be reported. Outcomes of reported exposures differ depending on whether exposure was discontinued by 4 weeks following onset of the last menstrual period (LMP), corresponding approximately to the second week of embryogenesis. Twenty-five prospectively recorded exposures continued beyond the fourth week post LMP include 11 spontaneous abortions, four birth defects, and ten apparently normal births, one of which died from sudden unexplained death at 7 weeks of age. Outcomes of 11 exposures discontinued before the fifth week included nine normal outcomes and two spontaneous abortions (Table 3).

Among 25 reported normal outcomes with maternal exposure information (Roche, '84, Kassis et al., '85), 13 were not exposed beyond the fourth week post LMP, and two were not exposed until after the ninth week (10th and 14th week). Only nine normal outcomes with exposures in the fifth week post LMP (approximately the third and fourth week of embryogenesis), lack possible explanation for the normal outcome. Even some of these might be explained by variation in conception relative to LMP, or inaccuracy in exposure history. Furthermore, follow up is insufficient to rule out functional injury.

Only nine defect cases had exposure reported prospectively, indicating that many exposures have not been recorded or identified. Eight infants thought to be normal at birth were later found to have abnormalities or an adverse experience. These included infants with: 1) small ears later found to have hydrocephalus and blindness; 2) a ventricular septal defect (VSD); 3) cortical blindness and other brain pathology; 4) an apparently normal infant having sudden unexplained death at 7 weeks age; 5) another case with VSD; 6) blindness and deafness; 7) motor retardation (unable to walk at 16 months); and 8) spina bifida and nystagmus. All but two were detected among prospectively reported exposures being followed closely, suggesting less striking injuries, are likely to be missed unless known exposure is being monitored.

DEFECTS WITH MATERNAL ETRETINATE EXPOSURE

Although ITR is marketed in other countries, no malformation has been reported with this exposure outside of the United States and Canada. However, Sautier Laboratories in Geneva, which markets another orally administered retinoid, *etretinate* (ETR), Tigason®, outside the United States, communicated to physicians in July 1983 that four birth defect outcomes had been observed among 14 maternal exposures to that agent. Two additional defect outcomes were included in a publication by Happle et al. ('84), and another reported by Roche Laboratories ('85). Three of the seven had meningomyeloceles (two spina bifida, and one encephalocele), three had craniofacial and skeletal abnormalities, and the seventh a severe brain defect with anopthalmia. One had low set ears, but microtia was not described in any, nor were there any cardio-aortic defects. Ten normal outcomes have also been reported with exposures during pregnancy. However, because of long half life (in contrast to ITR), ETR carries a warning to avoid pregnancy within 6 months of use. To date, all but one of eight defect outcomes with ETR occurred with exposures past the missed menstrual period. The exception was a unilateral lower leg hypoplasia, occurring with exposure stopped 4 months before conception (Grote, et al., '85). This malformation is uncharacteristic, and may not have been due to the exposure. Three normal outcomes have been reported with exposure stopped during the month before conception, and three other normal outcomes with exposures discontinued 2 to 4 months before conception. A spontaneous abortion occurred with exposure stopped in the second month before conception and another with discontinuation in the third month. (Roche Laboratories, '85). Abortion reports are difficult to utilize in establishing risks because of the commonness of spontaneous abortions.

BIRTH DEFECTS WITH MATERNAL VITAMIN A (RETINOL) EXPOSURE

Prior to 1984, the FDA had received only two reports of birth defects with excessive maternal *vitamin A exposure.* One infant with a maternal exposure of 40,000 units daily throughout pregnancy had facial anomalies, extremely small ear canals with a false fibrous eardrum in front of one normal ear drum, and a high arched palate without cleft. The other exposed to 60,000 units daily, had absence of the right ear, cleft palate and hare lip. Microtia is the most unique finding with *isotretinoin* exposure. Both of these reports

TABLE 4. Human birth defect reports with high maternal vitamin A exposure

Defects	Daily units vitamin A	Source
1. Tiny ear canals, facial dysmorphy, high palate	40,000 before and throughout pregnancy	MD report to FDA
2. Absent right ear, cleft palate/lip	60,000 before and throughout pregnancy	MD report to FDA
3. Bilateral cleft lip	50,000 3rd to 9th week	MD report to FDA
4. Microcephalus	27,000+ before and throughout pregnancy	NY State Birth Defect Registry[1]
5. Absent right ear and canal	25,000− before and throughout pregnancy	NY State BDR[1]
6. Absent left auditory canal, "Vater's syndrome"	25,000+ before and throughout pregnancy	NY State BDR[1]
7. Hypoplastic left ear	25,000− throughout	NY State BDR[1]
8. Low "deformed" ears, micrognathia, microphthalmia	18,000+ throughout	NY State BDR[1]
9. Transposition	33,000+ throughout	NY State BDR[1]
10. Hyp. left ventricle, ectopic neurones	100,000 vit A/50,000 vit D, before and throughout (induced 18th week abortion)	MD report to FDA
11. Cleft lip/palate/cheek/ jaw/left eye (absent)	50,000	Danish National Health Service
12. Heart defect, cleft palate		Morris and Thomson, 1974
13. Bilateral hydroureter	25,000–50,000 throughout	Bernhardt and Dorsey, 1979 and Scorta
14. Bilateral hydroureter	40,000	Pilotti, 1965
15. Facial palsy, hemifacial atrophy, epibulbar dermoid, micrognathia, bilateral oculomotor palsy, left preauricular appendices (Goldenhar syndrome)	500,000 × 1, 2nd month	Mounoud, et al., 1975
16. Microhydrocephaly, hypoplastic kidney and adrenals	150,000 19 to 40th day	Strange et al., 1978
17. Partial sirenomelia, low ears, pt colli	150,000 A/ 210 mg E/d −14 to 21st day	Von Lennep et al., 1985
18. Micrognathia, low ears, lumbar hemivertibrae, narrow sacrum, slender ilea, femoral hypoplasia, tibial diathesis, dislocated radii, contracture elbows, club feet	25,000	MD report to FDA

[1] Vallet et al., 1985.

were received before the reports of microtia with human exposure to *isotretinoin.* Since 1984, ten more unpublished case reports have been obtained with possible human vitamin A teratogenesis. These are listed, together with six published case reports, in Table 4. Because of the long half life, vitamin A levels are cumulative, and depend greatly on the duration of use. All but one of the 18 birth defects reported with high dosage of vitamin A occurred with long term exposure continuing past conception. The single exception was a massive "accidental" exposure occurring in the first month of pregnancy (Mounoud et al., '75). Some of the exposures are in combination with high dosages of other vitamins. For example, the case report of left ventricular hypertrophy was also exposed to 50,000 units of vitamin D daily. This finding is consistent with subaortic stenosis previously reported with maternal vitamin D excess (although stenosis was not detectable in the

TABLE 5. Comparison of teratogenicity of retinoids in small animals: lowest dose found teratogenic (mg/kg/day)[1]

Type	Rat	Mouse	Rabbit	Hamster
Vitamin A (palmitate)	90	50	5	
Tretinoin	6	3	6	7
Isotretinoin	150		10	
Etretinate	8	4	2	

[1]Adapted from Kamm (1981), Shenefelt (1971), and Kochhar et al., (1983).

18 week abortus).

Marketing data in the United States show widespread high dose vitamin A utilization. In 1983 marketing to pharmacies (IMS America, '84) was as follows.

25,000 unit:	107,500,000 pills
50,000 unit:	11,400,000 pills
100,000 unit:	4,900,000 pills

The amount sold through nutrition stores, supermarkets, and other channels is unknown but extensive. Enthusiasts take multiples of over-the-counter 25,000 unit vitamin A pills and/or multivitamin capsules containing up to 20,000 units each. In a telephone survey conducted in 1980 by the FDA Center for Food Safety and Applied Nutrition (Stewart et al, '85), covering 1080 female respondents aged 16 to 64, 314 (29.1%) were using vitamin supplements including vitamin A (not including maternal supplements). Fifteen (1.4%) were supplementing with 15,000 units daily or more.

High vitamin exposures and their outcomes are both poorly defined and observed. None of the 18 reports of suspected vitamin A teratogenesis have been provided through a manufacturer. (In contrast, for prescription therapy, the FDA receives 80% of suspected adverse drug reaction reports from ethical pharmaceutical manufacturers). Although hypervitaminosis A from dietary sources is well known, no birth defect case reports have been reported, perhaps due to lack of recognition or exposures. FDA is anxious to receive additional reports of excess periconceptional vitamin A exposures (preferably prospectively) and the nature of the conceptus.

Six of the listed case reports are from an exposure survey of selected defect categories in the New York State Birth Defect Registry (Vallet et al, '85). A comparison exposure survey on controls has not yet been completed. At this time no denominators exist for developing control rates. Thus the evidence for human vitamin A teratogenicity is limited to animal studies, the teratogenicity of therapeutically proscribed ITR and ETR, and the characteristics of uncontrolled case reports.

COMPARISON OF HUMAN OBSERVATIONS WITH NON-HUMAN STUDIES

Table 5 compares teratogenic potential of vitamin A analogs in small animals. The underlined numbers indicate the *lowest no-effect dose* for teratogeneses. This suggests ITR teratogenicity is less than other retinoids in the rat and mouse although similar in the rabbit.

Wilson ('71) felt that TR was less teratogenic in primates than in rodents, in that he was unable to find primate teratogenicity at the 10 mg/kg dosage, which is teratogenic in rats. However, among six Rhesus exposed to 30 mg/kg or higher doses for three days, four aborted, one produced a fetus with microtia, hydrocephaly, and facial dysmorphy with micrognathia, and another fetus had growth retardation. Fantel et al. ('77) were able to find a high frequency of craniofacial and musculoskeletal defects in the Pigtail Rhesus at a TR dosage of 7.5 to 10 mg per kg from day 20 to 24. Table 6 shows teratogenic findings by system, comparing TR in hamsters and monkeys with ITR in humans. The hamster observations are from Shenefelt's extensive study reported in 1972. Some 40 types of defects produced were analyzed by dose and time of exposure. The spectrum is remarkably similar to that found in the human with ITR.

Table 7 compares the spectrum of outcomes in experimental and prospective observations in primates. Although monkeys had some abortions, no exposures earlier than 17 days were tested, to see when the risk starts. However it is clear in Shenefelt's hamster studies that even high doses of TR had no abortifacient effect until after the fifth day. This supports the human prospective findings that ITR exposures discontinued prior to the 14th day were less likely to cause

TABLE 6. Comparison of retinoic acid teratogenicity

Golden Hamster tretinoin[1]	Rhesus tretinoin[2]	Human isotretinoin
	Nervous system	
Microcephaly	Microcephaly	Hydrocephaly
Spina bifida	Vermus abnormality	Microcephaly
Encephalocele	Hydrocephalus	Posterior fossa cyst
Exencephaly		Cortical blindness
		Facial nerve palsy
		Spina bifida
	Cranio-facial and oral	
Cranial abnormalities	Cranial abnormities	Micrognathia
Maxillary hypoplasia	Maxillary hypoplasia	Cleft palate
Mandibular hypoplasia	Mandibular hypoplasia	Mandibular hypoplasia
Cleft palate, lip	Cleft palate	Maxillary hypoplasia
	Ear	
Absent, deformed	Deformed/micro	Micro ears/canals
Middle/inner ear abnormality	Low set	Low set
	Eye	
Exophthalmus	Exophthalmus	Microphthalmia
Microphthalmus	Coloboma	
Coloboma		
	Cardio-vascular	
Transposition	Transposition	Transposition
Hypoplastic aorta		Hypoplastic aorta
VSD		VSD
	Extremities	
Short	Ectrodactyly	
Ectrodactyly	Syndactyly	
	Other defects	
Anal atresia	Anal atresia	Esophageal atresia
Uterus	Amastia	
Thymic hypoplasia	Thymic hypoplasia	Thymic hypoplasia
Kidney	Kidney	Kidney
Umbilical artery		Umbilical artery
Thyroid		
Olfactory bulbs		
Omphalocele		
Pituitary		
Absent gall bladder		
Situs inversus	Dextrocardia	

[1]Schenefelt (1971).
[2]Wilson (1971), Fantel (1977), Newell-Morris et al., (1980), Hendrickx et al., (1980).

TABLE 7. Comparison of primate observations (unduplicated cases)

	Rhesus (tretinoin)			Human (isotretinoin)
	Wilson	Fantel	Hendrickx	prospective
Dose mg/kg/day	30+	10	20–40	0.5–1.5
On days	23–25	20–44	19–44	14–49
Number of outcomes	6	19	15	25
Spontaneous abortion only	4	7	1	11
Syndrome	1	11	8	4
Single other outcome	retardation	0	amastia	SIDS
Apparently normal	0	1	4	9

TABLE 8. Primate defects with maternal retinoid exposure

	Rhesus tretinoin[1]	Human		
		Isotretinoin	Etretinate	Retinol
Dose mg/kg/d:	7.5–40	0.4–1.5	0.4–1.5	0.2–1.5
Defect cases:	21	44	7	18
Microtia	12	32	1	4
Craniofacial	19	16	3	4
Brain	4	30	1	4
Facial palsy	1	5		1
Micro/anophalmia	2	3	1	2
Facial clefts	2	7		4
Meningomyelocele		1	3	
Cardio-aortic	1	21	0	2
Limb reduction	7	1	2	4
Thymic hypoplasia	1	5		
GI atresia	1	1		1
Urinary				4
Amastia	1			

[1]Wilson et al., (1971); Fantel et al., (1977), Newell-Morris et al., (1980), Hendrickx et al., (1980).

abortion (two out of 11) compared to exposures continuing past the 14th day (11 of 25 aborted). No non-human primate data is available on ITR. Because of small numbers, no effect dose has been determined. However, the teratogenic dose of ITR in the human, 0.4 to 1.5 mg/kg/day, is lower than with TR in monkeys (7.5–40 mg/kg/day).

Table 8 compares defects in Rhesus TR exposures with human exposures to ITR and ETR. Strongest correspondence is in the ear, facial, and oral findings. Cranial defects seen in monkeys were lacking in humans, except secondary to brain defects. Brain pathology was reported in only three monkeys and heart defect in only one. Limb and vertebral defects, which were prominent in the monkeys, were also lacking in the human ITR exposures. However, two of eight defect cases with ETR had cranial synostoses, three had meningomyeloceles, and two syndactylies. This suggests difference in findings is due to agent rather than species.

Geelen (1979) extensively reviewed animal studies of hypervitaminosis A. The spectrum of defects is similar to that with retinoic acid, including malformations of the nervous system, spina bifida, ear aplasia, cranio-facial defects, ocular defects, cleft palate, cardiovascular defects, intestinal atresias, urogenital, and skeletal defects. However, the dosage tested was generally far in excess of likely human exposures. Dosage comparisons are complicated by the long time required for peak levels to accumulate.

NEED FOR FURTHER STUDIES

Although there is similarity in teratogenic findings between species with different retinoids, differences are apparent. ITR, which appeared to be less teratogenic than TR in rats and mice, is teratogenic at very low doses in humans. The dose and distribution of defects with TR in the hamster, more closely predicts the human teratogenicity with ITR, than the Rhesus findings. The hamsters' lowest teratogenic dose, 7 mg/kg in a single dose, is close to human dosage allowing for 5-day accumulation of the teratogenic metabolite, 4-oxo-ITR (Webster, '85). In the hamster studies it was also possible to examine differences depending on the timing of exposure, showing exposures discontinued early do not cause abortion or defects. This also appears to support the human observations. In contrast, higher dosages of TR were required to cause defects in monkeys.

Human teratogenicity with less than 1 mg/kg/day ITR and ETR therapeutic exposures is characteristic and strong. With this recognition, defect reports are increasingly appearing with high vitamin A exposures. The possibility can be considered that in contrast to rodents, primates are less susceptible to vitamin A forms other than ITR and ETR. Variability of exposure levels, or more generally, the inability to define a denominator for teratogenic exposure levels has hampered terato-epidemiology of non therapeutic excess vitamin A exposure. Monkey studies so far have been limited to TR, suggesting this is less teratogenic than ITR and ETR. Comparative experimental monkey studies are desirable to compare the teratogenicity of retinol, as well as ITR and ETR, to clarify relative teratogenicity between vitamin A congeners, and to clarify whether observed differences are due to species or agent.

CONCLUSIONS

1. Although teratogenic findings with different vitamin A congeners in various species have similarities, differences are apparent.
2. ITR appears less teratogenic than TR in rats and mice, but is teratogenic at very low doses in humans.
3. The dose and distribution of defects with TR in *hamsters*, more closely predicts the human teratogenicity with ITR than the *monkey* findings. The lowest teratogenic dose, a single dose of 7 mg/kg, is close to the repeated human dosage when allowing for cumulation of the 4-oxo-ITR metabolite. The scope of hamster studies allows examining differences depending on the timing of exposure, showing TR exposures discontinued early do not cause abortion or defects. This also supports human ITR experience.
4. ETR has been associated with three meningomyeloceles, among a total of eight defect outcomes. Although this was seen in hamsters with TR, only one human case has been reported with ITR.
5. The dearth of human epidemiology for vitamin A is subject to difficulty in defining an exposure denominator, and poor observation of outcomes. Although suggestive case reports have been accumulated, confirmation of human teratogenicity requires comparison of dose exposures in controls with those in selected defect categories, or of defect outcomes in high dose exposed, compared with non-exposed. Vitamin A is a valuable nutrient and necessary during pregnancy. However the recommended daily amount, 5,000 units, can be met easily from dietary sources. Although the data so far do not provide human dose/risk estimates, findings in laboratory studies and human experience with other vitamin A analogs provide reason for cautioning against long term exposures of 25,000 units per day or more in women who may become pregnant.
6. Study of retinol and ITR in non-human primates for comparison with TR findings might strengthen our knowledge, and is desirable because of the epidemiologic difficulties.

ACKNOWLEDGMENTS

Acknowledgement is made for providing case information to: 1) reporting physicians; 2) The Roche Laboratories, Nutley N.J.; and 3) Edward J. Lammer of the Birth Defects Branch, Centers for Disease Control, now with the Embryology-Teratology Unit, Massachusetts General Hospital.

This report is not an official statement of the Food and Drug Administration.

LITERATURE CITED

Bernhardt, I.B., D.J. Dorsey (1979) Hypervitaminosis A and congenital renal anomalies in a human infant. Obstet. Gynecol.,*45:*7505.

Cohlan, S.Q. (1953) Excessive intake of vitamin A as a cause of congenital anomalies in the rat. Science, *117:*535.

Fantel, A.G., T.H. Shepard, L. Laura, et al. (1977) Teratogenic effects of retinoic acid in pigtail monkeys. 1. General features, Teratology, *15:*65–72.

Geelan, J.A.G. (1979) Hypervitaminosis A induced teratogenesis. CRC Crit. Rev. Toxico., *November 1979.*351–375.

Grote, W., D. Harms, U. Janig, et al. (1985) Malformation of fetus conceived four months after termination of maternal etretinate treatment. Lancet, *1:*1276.

Happle, R., T. Traupe, T. Bounameaux, T. Fisch (1984) Teratogene warkung von etretinat beim menschen. Deutsche Med Wochensch, *1984:*39.

Hendrickx, A.G., S. Silverman, M. Pellegrini, and A.J. Steffek (1980) Teratological and radiocephalometric analysis of craniofacial malformations induced with retinoic acid in Rhesus monkeys (Macaca mulatta). Teratology, *22:*13–22.

IMS America, Ltd. (1983), Ambler, PA.

Kamm, J.J. (1981) Toxicology, carcinogenicity and teratogenicity of some orally administered retinoids. J. Am. Acad. Dermatol., *6(4)Suppl:*652–9.

Kassis, I., S. Sunderji, R. Abdul-Karim (1985) Isotretinoin and pregnancy. Teratology, *32:*145–6.

Kochhar, D.M., P.A. Kuczynski-Brown, and C.I. Tellone (1983) Comparative teratogenicity of all-trans- and 13-cis-retinoic acid in mice as studied by in vivo and in vitro methods. Teratology, *27:*58A.

Lammer, E.J., D.T. Chen, R.M. Hoar et al. (1985a) Retinoic acid embryopathy. N. Eng. :J. Med., *313:*837–841.

Lammer, E.J., D.B. Flannery, M. Barr (1985b) Does isotretinoin cause limb reduction defects? Lancet, *8450 ii:*328.

McBride, W.G. (1985) Limb reduction deformities in child exposed to isotretinoin in utero on gestation days 26–40 only. Lancet, *1:*1276.

Morris, G.M., A.D. Thomson (1974) Vitamin A and rat embryos. Lancet *2:*899.

Mounoud, R.L., D. Klein, F. Weber (1975) A propos d'un cas de syndrome de Goldenhar: Intoxication aigue à la vitamine A chez la mere pendant la grossesse. J. Genet. Hum., *23(2):*135–154.

Newell-Morris, L., J. Sirianni, T. Shepard, et al. (1980) Teratogenic effects of retinoic acid in pigtail monkeys (Macaca nemestrina). II Craniofacial features. Teratology, *22:*87–101.

Pilotti G., A. Scorta (1965) Ipervitaminosi A gravidica e malformazioni neonatali dell' appatato urinario. Minerva Ginecol, *17:*1103–1108.

Roche Laboratories, July 1983. Letter to physicians.

Roche Laboratories, May 1984. Presentation to FDA advisory committee.

Roche Laboratories, June 1985. Presentation to FDA advisory committee and public hearing on etretinate safety.
Rosa, F.W. (1983) Teratogenicity of isotretinoin. Lancet, *2:*513.
Sautier, Laboratories, Geneva, letter to physicians dated 27 July 1983. Bilan des effets tertogenes du Tigason et du Roaccutane.
Shenefelt, R.E. (1971) Morphogenesis of malformations in hamsters caused by retinoic acid: Relation to dose and stage at treatment. Teratology, *5:*103–118.
Stange, L., K. Carlstom, M. Eriksson (1978) Hypervitaminosis in early human pregnancy and malformations of the central nervous system. Act. Obstet. Gynecol. Scand., *57:*289–291.
Stewart, M.L., J.T. McDonald, A.S. Levy, R.E. Schucker, and D.P. Henderson (1985). Vitamin/mineral supplement use: A telephone survey of U.S. adults. J. Am. Diet. Assoc., *85(12):*1475.
Vallet, H.L., A.D. Stark, K. Costas, S. Thompson, R. Davis, and N. Teresi (1985) Isotretinoin (Accutane®), vitamin A, and human teratogenicity. Presentation American Public Health Association meeting, Washington, D.C., November 20, 1985.
Von Lennep, E., N. El Khazen, G. De Pierreux G et al. (1985) A case of partial sirenomelia and possible vitamin A teratogenesis. Prenat Diagn, *5(1):*35–40.
Webster, W.S. (1985) Isotretinoin embryopathy: Effects of isotretinoin and 4-oxo-isotretinoin on postimplantation rat embryos in vitro. Teratology, *31(3):*59A.
Wilson, J.G. (1971) Abnormalities of intrauterine development in non-human primates. Acta Endocrinol. Sci., *166*:261–292.

TERATOGEN UPDATE: ENVIRONMENTALLY INDUCED BIRTH DEFECT RISKS, PAGES 71–75 (1986)

Penicillamine

FRANZ W. ROSA
Epidemiology Branch, Center for Drugs and Biologics, Food and Drug Admnistration, Rockville, Maryland 20857

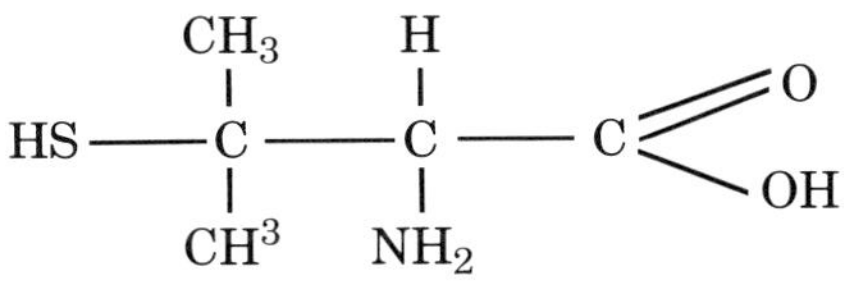

Penicillamine (3 mercaptovaline) is a heavy metal chelator, and has been used since 1956 to manage Wilson's disease, a genetic disorder characterized by high tissue copper (Walshe, '56). Its chelating function also has been employed in mercury, cadmium, and lead toxicity problems (Lyle, '81). Because it can substitute a sulfhydryl radical in amino acids, and thus solubilizes cystine, it is used in cystinuria (Crawhill, '81). It has been increasingly employed for rheumatoid arthritis, scleroderma (Multicentre Trial Group, '73), and autoimmune diseases (Harris and Sjordsma, '66), because of an immune suppressant and/or direct tissue function in these conditions. Penicillamine also has been used experimentally as an antineoplastic (Littman, '63). The dextro-isomer, D-penicillamine (Cupramine^R or Depen^R) is used clinically.

A total of 35,000 "mentions" of use in women age 15 to 44 in 1983 were projected from the IMS America National Disease and Therapeutic Index ongoing interview of a representative sample of office-based physicians. This includes repeat prescriptions and therefore exceeds the number of users. Because use is often long-term, the chances of exposure coinciding with pregnancy are increased. Of total mentions, 82% were for arthritis, 4% for Raynaud's disease, 5% for other cardiovascular problems, 3% for heavy metal poisoning, 2% for scleroderma, and only 2% for metabolic conditions (Wilson's disease and cystinuria).

Observations on penicillamine teratogenicity are desirable for therapeutic guidance with that agent, to elucidate possible heavy metal deficiency pregnancy problems in the human (which have been observed in other animals), to identify possible teratogenicity of structurally related agents such as captopril (an agent used for managing hypertension, and now also being tried for rheumatoid arthritis), and to elucidate teratogenic mechanisms.

HUMAN BIRTH DEFECT CASE REPORTS WITH CUTIS LAXA

1) The report raising the question of human teratogenicity was by Mjolnerod ('71). The mother had been taking penicillamine, 2,000 mg daily, throughout pregnancy for cystinuria. The infant was born with connective tissue defects including lax skin, fragility of veins, and hyperflexibility of the joints. The appearance resembled Ehlers-Danlos syndrome (dermatorrhexis cutis hyperelastica). The infant died at age 7 months following abdominal surgery for an undisclosed reason.

2) A second case (Solomon et al., '77) had growth retardation, flat face, low ears, flexion contractures, inguinal hernia, and lax skin. The infant died on the third day of life following surgery for an undiagnosed acute abdominal condition. The mother had taken 900 mg penicillamine for rheumatoid arthritis daily for the first 16 weeks and later resumed in the last trimester of pregnancy. The authors speculated that the coincidence of the two cases of cutis laxa from penicillamine-treated women who did not have Wilson's disease and the absence of any such outcomes from women with Wilson's disease could be due to a protective effect of the high copper levels in the latter mothers.

3) A third case reported by Linares et al. ('79) had transient cutis laxa. Punch biopsy at age one month showed a decrease of elastic fibers. The mother had received 1500 mg

D-penicillamine daily throughout pregnancy for Wilson's disease. This was the first observation of this type of defect in a mother being treated for Wilson's disease, despite observation of at least 29 pregnancy completions on penicillamine therapy (Scheinberg and Sternlieb, '75; Walshe, '77).

4) A fourth case was described by Beck et al. ('81). The mother had been exposed to D-penicillamine, 2,000 mg daily, throughout pregnancy for cystinuria. The 3-kg newborn had a syndrome manifested by "bloodhound" facies, with dysplastic ears and micrognathia, and generalized cutaneous laxity. In addition there were an interrupted aortic arch and hypoplastic left ventricle, leading to death on the fifth day. Thymic hypoplasia and absent parathyroids were disclosed at autopsy. The combinations of aortic arch defect, ear dysplasia, micrognathia, thymic, and parathyroid dysplasia are characteristic of DiGeorge's syndrome (Lapoint and Pawa, '79). Dermal punch biopsies from this infant were studied by electron microscope and fibroblast culture. Collagen bundles were normal, but no elastic fibers were seen, other than an amorphous component without integration. These findings were said to be similar to those seen in infants with genetic (recessive) cutis laxa.

5) A fifth case was decribed by Harpey et al. ('83). The mother had been treated for Wilson's disease with daily doses of 1,200 mg D-penicillamine and 250 mg pyridoxine throughout pregnancy. The 3-kg infant had micrognathia, low set ears, inguinal hernia, loose folds of skin in the neck and axillae, and abnormally lax skin in other areas of the body. Joint mobility was described as normal. At birth the infant had a serum zinc of 85 μg/dl (normal 110–130), and serum copper of 80 μg/dl (normal 20–50). The mothers serum copper was 19.7 μg/dl (normal 212–368), and her ceruloplasmin was 10 μg/dl (normal 80–120). From day 15 to day 30 the infant was given zinc supplementation. At 4 months of age the infant's skin appeared normal.

OTHER HUMAN BIRTH DEFECT CASE REPORTS

Four other birth defects with maternal penicillamine exposure have been reported to the Food and Drug Administration. Cutis laxa was not described in any of these cases. Only the third case has been previously published.

1) One of these patients was born in 1966 and had hydrocephalus, which was responsive to placement of a ventricular catheter. No other defects were described. The mother had been taking penicillamine for cystinuria throughout pregnancy, "in reduced dosage."

2) An infant born in 1982 had cerebral palsy with blindness at birth and bilateral club feet. He died of "crib death" in the fourth month. The mother was treated for Wilson's disease with 1,000 mg D-penicillamine daily. She also had an unidentified viremia at 7 weeks of pregnancy.

3) A 2.4-kg girl born in 1983 was described to have arthrogryposis multipex manifested by flexion deformities of the wrists, hands, fingers, and lower extremities (Gal and Ravenel, '84). Both hips were dislocated. CT scan and ultrasound demonstrated marked hydrocephalus with intraventricular hemorrhage. Death occurred at 18 hours. Autopsy documented the brain and external findings. No other internal abnormalities were found. D-penicillamine, 750 mg daily throughout pregnancy, maintained good control of the mother's Wilson's disease. The pregnancy had been complicated by a ruptured splenic artery aneurysm requiring emergency surgery at 24 weeks gestation. There was marked polyhydramnios at birth.

4) The last case, also born in 1983, had webbing between the fingers of the left hand and between two toes on each foot, and an extra left thumb. The mother was treated for scleroderma with D-penicillamine (dosage not stated) and ColBenemid®, both discontinued five weeks following her last menstrual period.

ANIMAL STUDIES

Penicillamine interferes with condensation of both collagen and elastin crosslinks by compressing free lysine-derived aldehydes. Abnormalities in dermal collagen have been induced in weanling rats by penicillamine, but not by Cu deficiency; nor did Cu prevent the penicillamine action. (Jaffe, '68).

The University of California (Davis) Department of Nutrition group has reviewed possible relationships of penicillamine and heavy metal deficiency teratogenesis and studied this in rats (Hurley and Keen '79; Keen et al., '82). Cu deficiency is known to cause enzootic ataxia in newborn lambs, characterized by spastic paralysis and incoordination, apparently due to reduced CNS myelination and poorly developed, light, brittle, fracture-prone bones. Cu-deficiency teratogenicity has also been shown experimentally. Guinea pigs fed Cu-deficient diets during pregnancy and lactation had pups with CNS abnormalities similar to those in lambs. Rats had pups which were hyperirritable and whose brains had areas of pallor, edema, and necrosis but, unlike lambs, lacked nerve fiber degeneration. Young dogs and swine fed Cu-deficient diets had deformed leg bones apparently associated with impairment of osteogenesis. Amine oxidase and cytochrome oxidase were low. There was a high ratio of soluble-to-insoluble collagen which could have reduced crosslinkages necessary for the formation of normal bone matrix (Rucker and Tinker, '77).

D-penicillamine was teratogenic in rats causing cutis laxis, abdominal herniations, incomplete diaphragms, and reduced ossification of phalanges and tail vertebrae. These were associated with dose-related reductions in maternal Cu levels (Keen et al., '83). The lowest dose-causing-defect dosage, 25 mg/kg/day, is similar to the therapeutic dose in the human, 20–30 mg/kg/day. Supplementation with Cu, 50–100 mg/kg, prevented malformations and resorptions (Mark-Savage et al., '81). Rat maternal Cu deficiency produced by another Cu chelator, triethylenetetramine (TETA), resulted in resorptions and fetal hemorrhage and edema (Keen et al., '83). Skeletal defects were not consistently noted. This again was preventable by Cu supplementation (Cohen et al., '83).

Steffek et al. ('74) found 400 mg of penicillamine daily for 8 days starting on the tenth day caused resorptions in rats; 360–400 mg daily from day 10 to day 15 caused 40–80% cleft palates. Lower doses did not cause either resorptions or deformities.

Tracheobronchomegaly has also been produced in rats by Kilburn and Hess ('82), with D-penicillamine added to low-copper diet. They also extended the above reported rat findings of cleft palates and observed gibbous vertebral deformities. They provide a review penicillamine embryotoxicity.

DISCUSSION

Penicillamine teratogenicity is evidenced by both human and animal observations. The most striking observation is the finding of cutis laxa in five infants. The fact that the mothers of the first two cases with this finding were treated for indications other than Wilson's disease suggested that the high copper levels in the Wilson's disease cases might be protective. However, subsequently two cases of cutis laxa have been associated with maternal penicillamine for Wilson's disease. The numbers of observations are insufficient to clarify a dose relationship. The small amount of copper in the body, even in Wilson's disease cases, would appear to be insufficient to inactivate the amount of penicillamine administered.

Rat experimental studies support the human findings although the dosage and defect findings vary. Although Cu deficiency was associated with penicillamine teratogenesis, and Cu supplementation was preventive, the defects in rats with Cu deficiency induced without penicillamine did not show the cutis laxa characteristic of penicillamine exposure. Furthermore, defects seen in other animals with maternal Cu deficiency have not shown cutis laxa. The protective effect of Cu added to the diet might be due to chelation inactivation of penicillamine rather than correction of a teratogenic copper deficiency.

The disappearance of cutis laxa in the two surviving cases indicates that a continuing interference with collagen is required to maintain this defect. However, one of the infants had a full-blown DiGeorge's syndrome and two others had manifestations, micrognathia and ear defects, suggesting interference with neural crest migration in early embryogenesis. The mechanism responsible for this may differ from that causing the cutis laxa. The possibility of penicillamine sulfhydryl radical substitution in nucleic acids (Tisman et al., '72) or some other mechanism of interference with early embryonic cellular reproduction should be considered. Cu may be protective for one mechanism, but not for another.

The four birth defect cases without cutis laxa outcomes are less distinctive. Three of these apparently had intrapartum brain damage. This has been observed in animals with maternal Cu deficiency. Unfortunately copper levels were not available in any of these cases, two of which occurred with penicillamine for indications other than Wilson's disease. The fourth birth defect with syndactyly and an extra thumb is unrelated to any other human or animal observations, and probably is a chance observation.

Copper is a key component of at least seven important proteins, including ceruloplasmin, erythrocuprein, hepatocuprein, cerebrocuprein, cytochome-C oxidase, tyrosinase, and monoamine oxidase. Copper deficiency produced by penicillamine could be expected to have broad developmental effects. Walshe ('82) has provided a preliminary report of nonteratogenicity with TETA management of Wilson's disease pregnancies.

Most pregnancies exposed to penicillamine have normal outcomes. Endres ('81) extended the earlier reviews previously cited; 85 pregnancies with exposure to D-penicillamine and normal outcomes were tabulated. In 44 of these the therapy had been continued throughout pregnancy. The latter included six in which the indication was cystinuria, four with a rheumatoid arthritis indication, and 32 with Wilson's disease. At that time the authors were aware of only the two birth defect outcomes with penicillamine therapy (the first two in the preceding section on birth defect outcomes): one with rheumatoid arthritis and the other with cystinuria. No birth defect outcomes were observed when the penicillamine had been discontinued in early pregnancy. More recently, Gregory and Mansell ('83) reported that seven maternal exposures to D-penicillamine (500–1,500 mg/day) for cystinuria, discontinued between 6 and 20 weeks of pregnancy, had six normal outcomes and one miscarriage. Normal outcomes are likely to be less reported than abnormal.

Heavy metal supplementation might be protective but might interfere with penicillamine function (Keiser et al., '68).

CONCLUSION

Embryotoxicity of maternal penicillamine exposure found in animal studies is evidenced by reports of five human births with cutis laxa. Three other human pregnancy outcomes with intrauterine brain injury are less characteristic. Most pregnancy outcomes have been normal.

Unless a safer therapy can be confirmed, penicillamine management of women with Wilson's disease should be continued throughout pregnancy, since the benefits of continuation outweigh risks. However, the available evidence suggests that a prudent course for conditions for which there are safer alternatives would be to discontinue penicillamine during pregnancy. Although cutis laxa appears to depend on continued exposure, the DiGeorge's syndrome case and micrognathia in other cases suggest risk in very early pregnancy, warranting caution in employing penicillamine in women who may become pregnant.

TERMINAL NOTES

The views expressed in this review do not necessarily represent an official position by the Food and Drug Administration.

Extensive reference material for this report by Drs. C.L. Keen and Lucille Hurley and their group at the University of California, Davis, Department of Nutrition, is gratefully acknowledged.

LITERATURE CITED

Beck, R.B., K.N. Rosenbaum, P.H. Byers, K.A. Holbrook, L.W. Perry (1981) Ultrastructural Findings in Fetal Penicillamine Syndrome. Presentation and abstract March of Dimes 14th Annual Birth Defects Conference, San Diego, CA 6/16/1981.

Cohen, N.L., C.L. Keen, B. Lonnerdal, L.S. Hurley (1983) The effect of copper supplementation on the teratogenic effects of triethylenetetramine in rats. Drug-Nutrient Interac., *2:*203–210.

Crawhall, J.C. (1981) Experience with penicillamine in the treatment of cystinuria. J. Rheumatol. (Suppl. 7), *8:*100–102.

Endres, W. (1981) D-penicillamine in pregnancy—to ban or not to ban? Klin Wochenshr *59:*535–7.

Gal, P., S.D. Ravenel (1984) Congenital contractures and hydrocephalus with penicillamine and maternal hypotension. J. Clin. Dysmorphol., *2(2):*9–12.

Gregory, M.C., M.A. Mansell (1983) Pregnancy and cystinuria. Lancet, *ii:*1158–60.

Harpey, J.P., M.C. Jaudon, J.P. Clavel et al. (1983) Cutis laxa and low serum zinc after antenatal exposure to penicillamine. Lancet, *ii:*858.

Harris, E.D., Jr, A. Sjordsma (1966) Collagen profile in various clinical conditions. Lancet, *ii:*101–711.

Hurley, L.S., C.L. Keen (1979) *Copper in the Environment, Part II Health Effects.* Nriagu J.O., ed. John Wiley and Sons, New York, p. 33.

IMS America (1983) *National Disease and Therapeutic Index.* Ambler, Pa.

Jaffe I.A., P. Merriman, D. Jacobus (1968) Copper relation to penicillamine induced defect in collagen. Science, *161:*1016–1017.

Keen, C.L., B. Lonnerdal, L.S. Hurley (1982) Teratogenic effects of copper deficiency and excess. In *Inflammatory Diseases and Copper.* J.R.J. Sorenson, ed. Humana Press, Clifton, NJ pp. 109–121.

Keen, C.L., N.L. Cohen, B. Lonnerdal, L.S. Hurley (1983a) Teratogenesis and low copper status resulting from triethylenetetramine in rats. Proc. Soc. Exp. Biol. Med., *173:*598–605.

Keen, C.L., P. Mark-Savage, B. Lonnerdal, L.S. Hurley (1983b) Teratogenic effects of D-Penicillamine in rats: Reaction to copper deficiency. Drug-Nutrient Interact. *2:*17–34.

Keiser, H.R., R.I. Henkin, M. Kare (1968) Reversal by copper of the lathyrogenic action of D-penicillamine. Proc. Soc. Exp. Biol. Med., *129:*516–522.

Kilburn, K.H., and R.A. Hare (1982) Neonatal deaths and pulmonary dysplasia due to D-penicillamine in the rat. Teratology, *26:*1–9.

Lapointe, N., S. Pahwa (1979) Thymic agenesis. Item 943. In *Birth Defects Compendium,* 2nd Ed. Bergsma D, ed. A.R. Liss, New York.

Linares, A., J.J. Zarranz, J. Rodriguez-Alarcon, J.L. Diaz-Perez (1979) Reversible cutis laxa due to maternal D-penicillamine treatment. Lancet, *ii:*43.

Littman, M.L., T. Taguchi, Y. Shimizu (1963) Acceleration of growth of sarcoma 180 with pyridoxamine and retardation with penicillamine. Proc. Soc. Exp. Biol. Med., *113:*667–674.

Lyle, W.H. (1981) Penicillamine in metal poisoning. J. Rheumatol. (Suppl. 7), *8:*96–99.

Mark-Savage, P., C.L. Keen, L.S. Hurley (1981) Reduction by copper supplementation of teratogenic effects of D-penicillamine. Presentation at Teratology Society

Annual Meeting. June 1981. Teratology, *25 (2):*50A (Abstract).
Mjolnerod, O.K., K. Rasmussen, S.A. Dommerud, S.T. Gjeuldsen (1977) Congenital connective tissue defect probably due to D-penicillamine treatment during pregnancy. Lancet, *i:*673–675.
Multicentre Trial Group (1973) Controlled trial of D-penicillamine in severe rheumatoid arthritis. Lancet *i:*275–280.
Rucker, R.B., D. Tinker (1977) Structure and metabolism of arterial elastin. Int. Rev. Exp. Pathol., *17:*1
Scheinberg, I.H., I. Stenlieb (1975) Pregnancy in penicillamine treated patients with Wilson's disease. N. Engl. J. Med., *293:*1300–2.
Solomon L., G. Abrams, M. Dinner, L. Berman (1977) Neonatal abnormalities associated with D-penicillamine during pregnancy. N. Engl. J. Med., *296:*54–55.
Steffek, A.J., A.C. Verrusio, and C.A. Watkins (1974) Cleft palate in rodents after maternal treatment with various lathyrogenic agents. Teratology, *5:*33–40.
Tisman, G., V. Herbert, L.T. Go, L. Brenner (1972) Inhibition by penicillamine of DNA and protein synthesis by human bone marrow. Proc. Soc. Exp. Biol. Med., *139:*355–363.
Walshe, J.M. (1956) Wilson's disease: New oral therapy. Lancet, *i:*25–26.
Walshe, J.M. (1977) Pregnancy in Wilson's disease. Q.U. Med., *46:*73–83.
Walshe, J.M. (1982) Treatment of Wilson's disease with trentine (triethylenetetramine). Lancet, *i:*643–6.

Congenital Rubella—An Encapsulated Review

SHELDON B. KORONES
Departments of Pediatrics and Obstetrics and Gynecology, University of Tennessee, Center for the Health Sciences, and the Newborn Center, E. H. Crump Women's Hospital and Perinatal Center, Memphis, Tennessee 38163

Rubella is a worldwide disease characterized by an apparent low attack rate in open populations, and by a considerably higher one in closed populations. Accurate estimates of attack rates vary widely because of the frequency of asymptomatic infection. Serologic data suggest that for every clinically recognized infection there are one or two asymptomatic ones. In northern temperate zones, the peak incidence of disease occurs during March, April, and May. Notable epidemics seem to occur every 6 to 9 years throughout the world. Rubella infection is quite infrequent during infancy, rising considerably between ages 5 to 14 and gradually reaching a peak at about 35 years of age. In the United States, this pattern has been altered considerably by ongoing massive immunization programs that attempt to vaccinate all children before school entry. Of the 2,000 cases of rubella that were reported in the United States in 1982, 62% of the affected individuals were over 15 years of age. Compared to the era before vaccination, overall incidence of the disease has declined by more than 90%. Although the incidence of rubella in women of childbearing ages has declined to that extent, 10 to 15% of these women are still susceptible to infection (1,2).

The overriding concern with postnatal rubella has been its occurrence in pregnant women and its transmission to the fetus. Epidemics of postnatal infection are associated with a high incidence of tragic fetal involvement. Postnatal rubella is generally mild and self-limited, but the fetal infection, particularly during the earlier months of gestation, is often devastating. Fetal disease is associated with major anomalies, with destruction of normal tissue, and with chronic infection that persists for months or years after birth. The aftermath of the most recent epidemic in the United States, which occurred in the middle 1960s, was an estimated 11,000 wasted pregnancies and approximately 20,000 children with congenital malformations that were severe and multiple in most instances (3). The virus has been recovered from the abortus, the placenta, amniotic fluid, and from the throat, urine, meconium, conjunctival and cerebrospinal fluids of liveborn infants. At necropsy, the virus has been grown from virtually every organ of the body. It has also been cultured from a surgically extirpated ductus arteriosus, from a cataractous lens, and from liver tissue obtained by biopsy (4). The earliest of fetal infections are associated with greater severity and a higher incidence of disease. If fetal infection occurs during the first 8 weeks, up to 85% of those affected will be left with some defect that is identifiable within the first 4 years of life. Between the ninth and twelfth gestational weeks, 52% are similarly involved; between the thirteenth and twentieth weeks the incidence declines to 16%. Thus, multiple organ involvement is more likely to occur in the earliest fetal infections (1).

One of the hallmarks of congenital infection is chronicity and a protracted period of virus shedding. At 1 month of age virus has been recovered from the throats of approximately 85% of infected babies; at 5 to 8 months of age the incidence of positive cultures is 33%. Virus shedding is rare beyond these ages, but it has been recovered from the urine and from an extirpated lens past 2 1/2 years of age. The shedding of virus by chronically infected infants is probably one of several factors that maintain a residuum of virus and a source of contagion in the community. As an example, small outbreaks among personnel have occurred sporadically during the hospitalization of chronically infected infants (1).

CLINICAL MANIFESTATIONS

The clinical manifestations are as widespread as the infection itself. They have been noted in the cardiovascular and central nervous systems, eyes, ears, blood, liver, and bones. In severe disease hypoplastic intrauterine growth retardation is almost the rule; in most organs there are in fact fewer cells than normal.

Cataracts, patency of the ductus arteriosus, and deafness were regularly described in earlier literature as the collective hallmark of congenital rubella. This classic clinical triad was first perceived in 1941 by the Australian ophthalmologist Sir Normal Gregg. Lundstrom's milestone epidemiologic study during the 1950s (reported in 1962) unearthed a variety of additional abnormalities, some of which had been previously reported by others in case reports (5). Then, during the pandemic of 1964, when isolation of the virus became feasible, most of these signs could be clearly attributed to maternal infection during pregnancy. Sever et al., in 1969, labeled the broader and newly appreciated clinical entity the "expanded rubella syndrome" (3).

Cardiovascular abnormalities

Except for infrequent involvement of the myocardium, the malformations attributed to fetal rubella seem to involve changes in the caliber of various blood vessels that are in turn due to damage in vessel walls, particularly in the endothelium. The resultant vascular changes are seen most often in patency of the ductus arteriosus and stenosis of the peripheral branches of the pulmonary artery. The coexistence of both these lesions is quite frequent. Stenosis also occurs in the main pulmonary artery and its principal branches, and it may be unilateral or bilateral. Pulmonic valve stenosis may exist alone or in combination with patent ductus arteriosus and peripheral pulmonary artery stenosis. The same pattern is evident in coarctation of the aorta, and stenosis of the renal artery. The cardiovascular malformations associated with fetal rubella infection do not involve changes in gross cardiac structure. Thus, malformations such as truncus arteriosus, transposition of the great vessels, and common atrioventricular canal are not considered to be results of fetal infection. Severe myocardial necrosis, with or without an inflammatory response, has occurred in a number of infants whose congestive failure, often refractory to treatment, may be present at birth or shortly thereafter. Electrocardiograms resemble those of adults with myocardial infarction (6).

Eye defects

Ocular abnormalities have been identified in 30 to 70% of infected infants. The most common lesions are cataracts, corneal opacities, microphthalmia, and pigmentary retinopathy. Cataracts have been identified in approximately half of all infants with rubella, affecting both eyes in 75% of them. They are usually identified at birth or soon thereafter, but occasionally they are not discernible until several weeks later. Opacities of the cornea may result from congenital glaucoma due to rubella, or to delayed maturation of Descemet's membrane. In instances of delayed maturation, corneal clouding eventually disappears as maturation of Descemet's membrane proceeds. Microphthalmia, unilateral or bilateral, occurs in 20% of infected infants. If only one eye is microphthalmic it is cataractous, while pigmentary retinopathy is identifiable in the eye of normal size. So-called "salt and pepper" retinopathy is a pigmentary lesion that has no regular pattern of distribution. It is characterized by alternating areas of hypertrophy and atrophy of the retinal pigmentary epithelial cells. Although this retinopathy has not been thought to cause functional impairment, recent reports have described delayed appearance of visual impairment as a consequence of subretinal neovascularization (7,8).

Neurologic abnormalities

Signs of central nervous system involvement are evident in approximately 25% of infected neonates. In some infants central nervous system infection is indicated by a full anterior fontanelle at birth, hypotonia, and lethargy, which are soon followed by irritability, disturbed sleep, and intermittent opisthotonic posture. In others, pronounced undergrowth is associated with severely delayed motor performance and development, hyporeactivity, and hypotonia. Yet another group of infants may present with an abrupt onset of the signs of acute meningitis, including seizures. Some neonates are asymptomatic even in the presence of high CSF protein and pleocytosis. In consonance with the chronicity of rubella infection, abnormalities of central nervous function are often progressive during the first months or years of life. Microcephaly may develop gradually, becoming apparent within the first 6 to 12 months of age. A number of the abnormalities produced by fetal infection are often undetectable until the second year of life or even later. These include hearing defects (peripheral and central), delayed language development, delayed motor, intellectual, and behavioral development, deficient educability, autism, and subacute progressive panencephalitis (9,10).

Skin lesions

Cutaneous abnormalities are common and varied. The best known of these are the "blueberry muffin" lesions, which are commonly evident at birth. Their distribution is generalized; they may involve the palms and soles, but are most often situated on the face, neck, and upper trunk. Many are raised and infiltrated; others are macular. Their color varies from deep blue to gray to purple, and individually they range from 2 to 8 mm in diameter. The "blueberry muffin" lesion is a localized area of erythropoiesis in the upper dermis. Petechiae and ecchymoses associated with thrombocytopenia are also quite common. Occasionally red macular lesions, similar to the rash of postnatal rubella, are present at birth or later during the neonatal period (7).

Other abnormal signs

Thrombocytopenia has been reported in 40 to 80% of affected infants. Hepatosplenomegaly is virtually the rule in congenital rubella infection. Hepatitis is not unusual. The histologic appearance is characterized by giant cell transformation, persistent foci of erythropoiesis, bile duct proliferation, and focal inflammatory response. These morphologic changes and abnormalities of liver function tests (obstructive jaundice and elevated enzymes) are not unique to congenital rubella infection (6,7).

Interstitial pneumonitis has been noted at birth. Alternatively, it may first appear a few weeks later. The pneumonitis is occasionally fulminating, but in most instances it clears in several days or weeks (6).

Skeletal changes have been observed radiologically in over half of infected infants. Longitudinal radiolucent streaks (celery stalks) are most often in the metaphases; at the knee these radiolucencies may be particularly pronounced. The bones are generally osteoporotic; spontaneous fractures may occur. "Celery stalk" lesions usually disappear by 3 to 6 months of age but they occasionally persist or worsen, particularly in severely affected infants (11).

DIAGNOSIS

Neonatal disease can be anticipated when maternal infection has been documented. Documentation of maternal infection after reported exposure requires a rising antibody titer (usually HI) in paired sera. Maternal disease and exposure to infection is more readily identifiable during epidemics, but sporadic maternal disease is difficult to identify. Approximately half of infected mothers are asymptomatic and totally unaware of infection or of an exposure. In the neonate, isolation of the virus is the most certain diagnostic modality. Cultures should be taken as soon after birth as is feasible; virus shedding diminishes or disappears with relative rapidity. The pharynx, conjunctiva, cerebral spinal fluid, and urine are most likely to yield virus. In the absence of cultures, demonstration of rubella IgM antibody is reliable. Short of these data, increased concentrations of total serum IgM in an infant with a combination of clinical signs attributable to intrauterine rubella are probably diagnostic. Since maternal IgG antibodies are passively acquired by the fetus, their presence in neonatal serum is of no diagnostic value. However, persistence of the neonatal titer to approximately 6 to 12 months of age, particularly in an infant with telltale clinical signs, is probably sufficient to establish the diagnosis.

PREVENTION

The goal of rubella vaccination is the prevention of fetal infection. Immunization is accomplished by the administration of a live attenuated human diploid cell vaccine which, compared to other vaccine preparations, apparently produces higher antibody titers, a wider range of serologic responses, and resembles the natural infection more closely in that IgA secretory antibody in the oral pharynx are produced.

In the United States, active immunization of children at 15 months of age is recommended. The vaccination program in this country is aimed at herd immunity among children, who are the major source of infection in pregnant women. Immunization is also recommended for susceptible non-pregnant women who must therefore avoid pregnancy for three months following their vaccination. Vaccine cannot be given during pregnancy, in individuals who are allergic to neomycin, or to those who are acutely febrile. Vaccine viruses can infect the fetus and produce fetal damage as well. Although fetal involvement is extremely uncommon, its possibility requires that vaccination and pregnancy are not concurrent.

REFERENCES

1. Alford, C. A. and P. D. Griffiths [1983] Rubella. In: Infectious Diseases of the Fetus and Newborn Infant. J. S. Remington and J.O. Klein, eds. W. B. Saunders Co., Philadelphia, pp. 69–103.
2. Hanshaw, J. B. and J. A. Dugeon [1978] Rubella. In: Viral Diseases of the Fetus and Newborn. W. B. Saunders Co., Philadelphia.
3. Sever, J. L., J. B. Hardy, K. B. Nelson, M. R. Gilkeson, [1969] Rubella in the collaborative perinatal research study. II. Clinical and laboratory findings in children through 3 years of age. Am. J. Dis. Child. *118:*123–132.

4. Monif, G. R., G. B. Avery, S. B. Korones, and J. L. Sever [1965] Postmortem isolation of rubella virus from three children with rubella syndrome defects. Lancet, *1:*723–724.
5. Lundstrom, R. [1962] Rubella during pregnancy: A follow-up study of children born after an epidemic of rubella in Sweden, 1951, with additional investigation on prophylaxis and treatment of maternal rubella. Acta Paediat. Supp., *133:*1–110.
6. Korones, S. B., L. E. Ainger, G. R. G. Monif, J. Roane, J. L. Sever, and F. Fuste [1965] Congenital rubella syndrome: Study of 22 infants. Myocardial damage and other new clinical aspects. Am. J. Dis. Child., *110:*434–440.
7. Cooper, L. Z., P. R. Ziring, A. B. Ockerse, B. A. Fedun, B. Keily, and S. Krugman [1969] Rubella: Clinical manifestations and management. Am. J. Dis. Child., *118:*18–29.
8. Schaffer, D. B. [1981] Eye findings in intrauterine infections. Clin. Perinatol. *8(3):*415–443.
9. Desmond, M. M., G. S. Wilson, J. L. Melnick, D.B. Singer, T. E. Zion, A. J. Rudolph, R. G. Pineda, Z. Mir-Hashen, and R. J. Blattner [1967] Congenital rubella encephalitis. J. Pediatr., *71:*311–331.
10. Monif, G. R. G. and J. L. Sever [1966] Chronic infection of the central nervous system with rubella virus. Neurology, *16:*111–112.
11. Rudolph, A.J., E. B. Singleton, H. S. Rosenberg, D. B. Singer, and C. A. Phillips [1965] Osseous manifestations of the congenital rubella syndrome. Am. J. Dis. Child. *110:*428–433.

The Congenital Rubella Syndrome

MARY ANN SOUTH AND JOHN L. SEVER
National Institute of Neurological and Communicative Disorders and Stroke, National Institutes of Health, Bethesda, Maryland 20205

Gregg's classic descriptions (Gregg, '41,'44) of the association between maternal rubella and defective offspring were published 40 years ago. Those first descriptions included not only this ophthalmologist's observations on the peculiar cataracts, but also the cardiac malformations, hearing loss, and mental retardation that together constitute the major manifestations of the congenital rubella syndrome. For 20 years thereafter, these original descriptions were refined in great detail, statistics were gathered regarding the frequency of each finding in relation to the others, and many less frequently associated findings were described. However, the next breakthrough in this field was not possible until the techniques for viral isolation in tissue culture were developed. The rubella virus was first isolated in 1962 (Parkman et al., '62; Weller and Neva, '62) thus setting the stage for the recognition in 1964 that the congenital rubella syndrome is associated with a chronic viral infection of the fetus (Alford et al., '64; Heggie and Weir '64). This discovery was accompanied by the definition of the "expanded" or "acute" rubella syndrome, a constellation of symptoms accompanying other chronic congenital infections (Rudolph et al., '65a) (Fig. 1). Directly following the 1964 rubella pandemic, extensive and highly detailed studies of the effects of intrauterine rubella infections were begun. Fortunately, the development of rubella vaccines has prevented further large epidemics in the United States, but new cases of congenital rubella are still reported. Interest has been renewed by the finding of late-occurring effects of congenital rubella infection.

This report will update the newer findings in congenital rubella syndrome, as well as summarize some new analyses of the studies following the 1964 epidemic. The term "congenital rubella syndrome" (CRS) will be used to denote any combination of the findings now known to result from gestational rubella. "CRS infant" or "CRS child," or "CRS adult" will be used to designate any person who experienced intrauterine infection with the rubella virus, regardless of resultant abnormality. "Rubella associated defect" refers to any defect now known to occur in increased frequency in CRS offspring, particularly those of cardiac malformations, hearing loss, mental retardation, and the ophthalmologic findings of cataract, glaucoma, microphthalmia, and resulting blindness.

VIROLOGY AND IMMUNOLOGY

The virologic finding of chronic fetal infection, with continuing virus excretion for months or years after birth, was the key to understanding the devastating effects of intrauterine infection with the rubella virus. A review of the literature revealed scattered descriptions of each of the components of the "expanded" rubella syndrome (except the osseous lesions, Rudolph et al., '65b) long before the virologic discovery was made. However, there was no unifying concept until after the continuing fetal infection was found. Now comparisons could be made with the other known chronic intrauterine infections: syphilis, cytomegalovirus, herpes II, and toxoplasmosis. The rubella studies provided insight into all intrauterine infectious processes, and widened the whole field of teratogenesis by infectious agents. The immunologic studies of the chronically infected CRS infants furnished data key to the definitions of the ontogeny of the immune system, which were just beginning to blossom at the time of the 1964 rubella epidemic. Advances were necessary in the methodology for provision of medical care, rehabilitation, and education for multiply handicapped children who were infectious. Thus, the increase in knowledge resulting from this virologic finding was very extensive, reaching far outside the field of virology.

The duration of virus excretion in CRS has not been finally determined. Although most survivors become intermittent virus excretors during the first few months of life (Sever

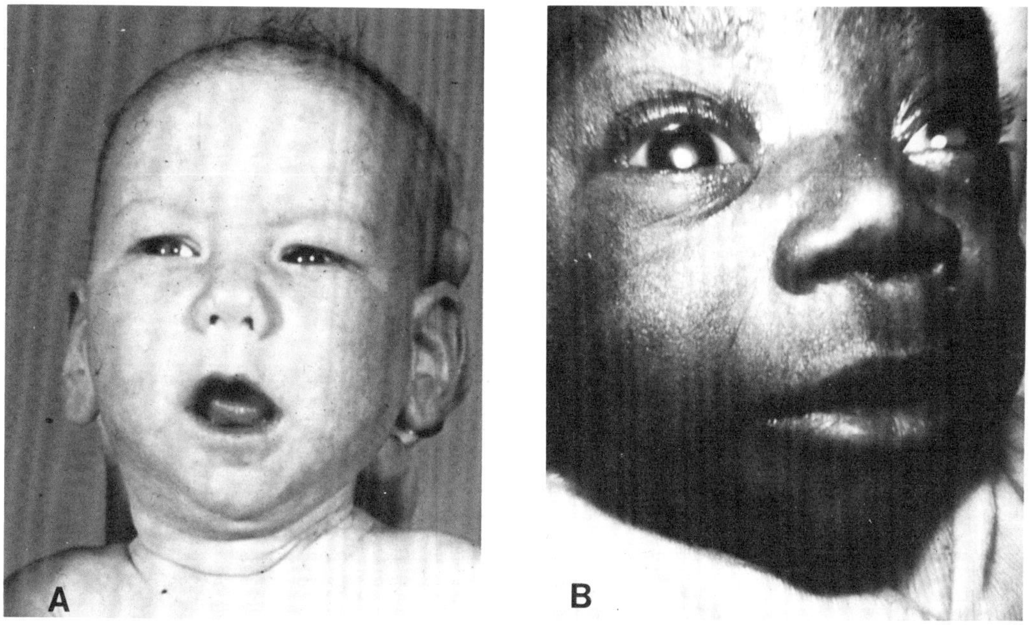

Fig. 1. A. Child with the "expanded" or "acute" congenital rubella syndrome who had hepatosplenomegaly, thrombocytopenia, cataracts, deafness, congenital heart disease, and mental retardation. In addition this patient had cutis marmorata, a peculiar mottling common in infants and young children with the congenital rubella syndrome. B. CRS patient, showing cataracts.

and Monif, '65), a few continue to have virus regularly recoverable for more than 2 years after birth (Rawls et al., '67; Michaels and Kenny, '69). Rubella may cause a chronic encephalitis (Desmond et al., '67, '78), producing viral excretion into the cerebrospinal fluid even when mucosal sites have been cleared. Rubella virus has been detected in the brain in progressive rubella panencephalitis (Weil et al., '75; Wolinsky, '78), which develops decades after the prenatal infection. The virus has also been recovered from other immunologically privileged sites, such as in cataractous lenses removed at surgery (Menser et al., '67a).

Mucosal excretion of rubella virus has been detected in a 4 1/2-year-old boy with CRS who was not ill at the time (Shewman et al., '82). Also, a 29-year-old survivor of Gregg's CRS group in Australia was found to be excreting rubella virus during an attack of a flu-like illness (Menser et al., '71). All these cases, considered together, suggest that the rubella virus may be harbored in a secluded site and persist in a form that can be occasionally activated throughout the lifetime of the person who has experienced congenital rubella infection.

The incidence of fetal infection following maternal rubella at various stages of gestation has recently been determined (Miller et al., '82). The study included all pregnant women in England and Wales, January 1976 to September 1978. More than 1,000 women had serologically confirmed rubella. Infection of the products of conception could be studied in 269 cases, either by virus isolation or by persistence of rubella antibody in survivors. The frequency of congenital infection after maternal rubella with rash (258 women) was more than 80% in first trimester, 54% at 13–14 weeks, 25% at the end of the second trimester, and 100% after 36 weeks. No congenital infection was found in 11 children whose mothers had asymptomatic rubella. These figures agree generally with other smaller prospective studies. For example, Rawls et al. ('68) in a study of first trimester rubella, found 11 of 14 (79%) with fetal infection.

The devastating effects of the 1964 pandemic might be explained by three mechanisms: (1) increased virulence of the epidemic strain of rubella virus; (2) increased infectivity of the virus, leading to an increased incidence of transplacental infection; (3) sheer number of rubella cases with increased exposure of pregnant women combined with a very large number of susceptible women of childbearing age. There is insufficient evidence to support any one of these explanations, and no apparent opportunity to gain further information on this point.

The 1964 discovery of the chronic excretion of rubella virus in the CRS infants created a great stir in immunologic circles. Was this a human model for tolerance? The idea that a fetus has capacity for immune responsiveness was brand-new in 1964. IgM or "19S" had been defined as the "early response" immunoglobulin, with IgG as the later and more permanent one and the one to undergo placental transfer. IgA had just been found to be concentrated in the mucosal secretions; IgE had not yet been discovered. It was in the late fall of 1964 that the lymphoid cell system was first proved to be divided into the T and B cell components. The in vitro techniques to measure the proliferative response of lymphoid cells to mitogens such as phytohemagglutinin (PHA) were being worked out. Rubella antibody could be measured by complement fixation or the laborious neutralization techniques. Hemagglutination inhibition and radioimmunoassay techniques had not been applied to rubella, and enzyme-linked immunosorbent assay (ELISA) was not yet invented. So at the time of presentation of the CRS infants during the 1964 epidemic, concepts had been formed, but the methodology for asking crucial immunologic questions was primitive at best. Nevertheless, the question of tolerance was quite thoroughly explored. Classic tolerance was ruled out immediately, when antibody of fetal origin was found. Then a concept of "split" tolerance in the T cell, but not the B cell, system was put forward, but there were no tools to measure this kind of reactivity. In this search, many immune defects were found in the CRS infants (Fuccillo et al., '74; South and Alford, '80). However, none of them explained the chronic viral excretion, for this excretion was present in the infants with no definable immune defects just as it was in the small minority of patients who had a deficient immune response. Besides, the immune defects were mostly temporary, and the virus excretion went on for months or years after they had reversed to normal; the permanent defects persisted even after virus excretion had ceased.

Thus, congenital rubella infection joined the group of human viral infections known to be chronically active despite immune responsiveness. The questions of tolerance remain unanswered even until now.

OCCURRENCE OF ANOMALIES IN CRS

The 1964 rubella epidemic resulted in more than 1,800,000 cases of rubella in the United States. By the best estimates available, 20,000–30,000 infants were damaged by in utero rubella infection during this epidemic (Cooper, '75). A large proportion of these infants were multiply handicapped with various combinations of severe abnormalities of heart, eye, hearing, and central nervous system function. Many excellent studies of these very damaged infants were reported. However, the incidence of damaged offspring of women having rubella could not be estimated from these retrospective studies. One prospective study, the Collaborative Perinatal Research Study (Sever et al., '65, '69) was in progress during 1964–65. The only other large prospective study, the British study of the 1978 epidemic (Miller et al., '82) does not offer an opportunity to estimate incidence of anomalies, since 60% of the pregnancies were aborted and no assessment of embryonic anomalies could be made. However, this study does provide the only prospectively derived data for fetal infection following maternal rubella. A correlation of the two studies produces the best estimates of incidence of anomalies following fetal infection that are (or indeed are ever likely to be) available.

Findings in the Collaborative Perinatal Research Study are presented in Figure 2. Among infants whose mothers had rubella during the first month of gestation, 70% had one or more severe rubella-associated anomalies. If the rate of fetal infection from the 1978 British epidemic (80% in the first trimester) is applied to these figures from the 1964 epidemic, it is reasonable to conclude that very nearly every fetus infected with rubella during the first month of gestation develops in an abnormal manner. The fetal infection rate drops to 54% by 13–14 weeks of gestation, and the Collaborative Study data show an incidence of 40% affected children in this period. The anomalies are different, and there are fewer multiply handicapped children at this stage, yet the effect of the rubella infection can be clearly dis-

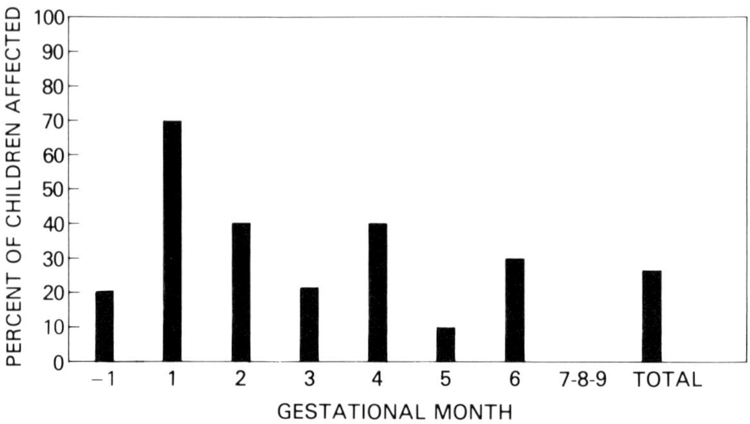

Fig. 2. Children in the Collaborative Study, 1964 rubella epidemic, analyzed for frequency of rubella associated defects by gestational month of maternal rubella.

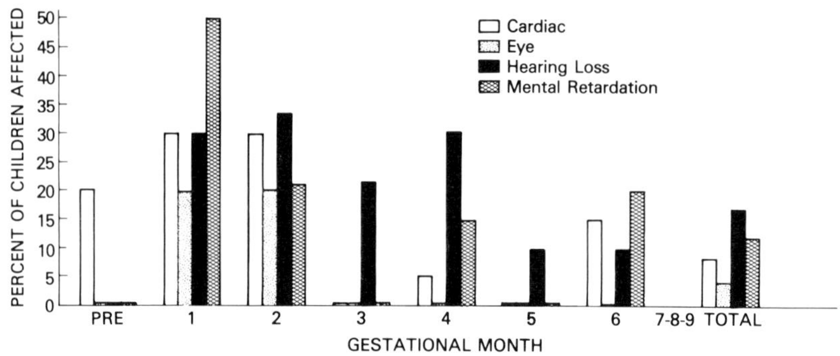

Fig. 3. Children in the Collaborative Study, 1964 rubella epidemic, analyzed for the four major rubella associated defects by gestational month of maternal rubella.

cerned in a great majority of all children infected by rubella even into this second trimester of gestation. After the end of the second trimester's gestation, rubella causes disability rarely, even though the fetal infection rate rises from 25% to 100% during the third trimester. It is impossible at this time to rule out subtle or late effects of rubella, but there is no evidence for fetal damage due to infection at this stage.

Figure 3 shows the distribution of CRS defects found in the Collaborative Study. These data are in general agreement with other studies (Cooper, '75; Dudgeon, '75). Hearing loss is the most common of all the rubella associated defects. Mental retardation (IQ score below 70) is next most frequent; there has not been an assessment of the prevalence of children who have specific learning disabilities, minor motor abnormalities, or simply a decreased intellectual capacity from "what might have been." Cardiac anomalies are third most frequent. These are probably underestimated since the diagnosis of isolated peripheral pulmonary artery stenosis can easily be missed. The eye defects of cataract, glaucoma, or microphthalmia occur least frequently of these four major manifestations of CRS.

Grouping of the four major defects in the CRS children from the Collaborative Study is summarized in Table 1. Eye defects (cata-

TABLE 1. Grouping of four CRS related defects: Collaborative perinatal research study[1]

	No. of children
Children with multiple handicaps	
Hearing, MR, cardiac, eye	4
Hearing, MR, cardiac	1
Hearing, MR	5
Total	10
Children with single handicaps	
Hearing loss	8
Mental retardation	6
Cardiac	4
Eye	0
Total	18

[1]Hearing = hearing loss; MR = mental retardation (IQ less than 70); cardiac = cardiovascular malformation; eye = cataract, glaucoma, microphthalmia (does not include chorioretinitis).

ract, glaucoma) occurred only in combination with defects of other systems. At the opposite extreme, hearing loss was the most common defect, occurring most frequently among the isolated defects and in all the multiply handicapped children. Mental retardation also occurred in each of the multiply handicapped children and was second most frequent among the single handicaps. There was a normal sex distribution among the offspring of the women who had rubella during pregnancy; however, there were twice as many males as females among the handicapped offspring (19 males and 9 females). Among the multiply handicapped children there were seven males and three females, and all of the children who had a combination of all four defects were males.

The occurrence of immune deficiency in CRS was not studied prospectively during and after the 1964 epidemic period. Studies of a few of these CRS infants, utilizing the relatively poor laboratory methods of that time, revealed some defect of immune function in a large majority. Manifestations included decreased proliferative response to mitogens, dysgammaglobulinemia, hypogammaglobulinemia, selective IgA deficiency, and anergy upon skin testing for delayed hypersensitivity. All these defects were transient except the IgA deficiency, which did not correlate with clinical susceptibility to infection in the older CRS child. However, many of the patients in these studies died, and the continued effect of their immune defect could not be assessed (South and Alford, '80).

Vaccine strains of rubella can cross the placenta and infect the fetus. However no anomalies have been associated with any of the attenuated strains (Preblud et al., '81; Centers for Disease Control, '81, '83a).

GESTATIONAL TIMING OF MATERNAL RUBELLA

Assessment of gestational age at the time of rubella infection necessarily involves several inaccuracies. First, the exact date of either ovulation or fertilization is rarely known. The date of the first day of the mother's last menstrual period (LMP) is generally used as a practical marker of these dates. Second, the exact time during the pregnancy at which fetal infection takes place can only be estimated. The incubation period for the infection must be taken into account. It is not known whether the virus can cross the placental barrier during the initial incubation period, or whether rubella may even infect the unfertilized ovum. Evidently it can be harbored somewhere in an infectious state for many days after the mother's illness is over, since there have been well-documented cases of infected infants from women who had rubella several weeks before the LMP. In addition, it is not known whether the fetus undergoes an incubation period similar in length to the mother's. Third, it is not known how long it takes after introduction for the virus to infect a significant number of embryonic cells. Therefore the assignment of age at rubella infection is a gross estimate at best.

A most important consideration in the pathogenesis of the disease is the continuance of fetal infection. Once the virus attacks the fetus, it remains throughout gestational life and may continue the destructive activity begun when infection first occurred, and the effects of this destruction accumulate throughout the period of active infection.

Two types of fetal damage can be recognized: those occurring as disturbances of organogenesis and those resulting from tissue destruction and scarring (Rosenberg et al., '81). Many of the cardiac and eye defects are of the first type. Hearing loss, brain damage, cataracts, chorioretinopathy, and peripheral pulmonary artery stenosis (PPS) are reasonably classified as the second type. The occurrence of the first type is necessarily confined to those children contracting rubella during organogenesis, but these same infants, as well as those infected later in gestation, demonstrate the second type of damage as a cumulative effect of their continuing fetal rubella infection. Table 2 summarizes from

TABLE 2. Last gestational week in which maternal rubella resulted in congenital defects

	Heart disease (PPS)[1]	Cataracts/ glaucoma	Deafness
108 Cases from literature (Dekaban et al., '58)	14	10	20
England (Peckham, '72)	8	8	24
Johns Hopkins (Hardy, '73)	12 (20)	12	21
Japan and Seattle (Ueda et al., '79)	13	8	19
England and Wales (Miller et al., '82)	<11	<11	16
U.S. (Shaver, '83)	12	12	28
Collaborative study	8 (22)	8	21

[1]Numbers in parentheses refer to last gestational week in which peripheral pulmonic stenosis was reported.

seven studies the latest gestational age at which rubella infection resulted in particular defects. Cataracts and cardiac malformations occurred through 12 weeks, with PPS through 24 weeks, and deafness through 28 weeks. In Figure 3, an analysis is made from the Collaborative Study of times in gestation for the most frequent occurrence of these defects. Eye malformations were confined to early gestational rubella, as were cardiac malformations with the exception of PPS. On the other hand, deafness and mental retardation occurred into the sixth month, with little decrease after the end of the first month. None of these defects occurred in third trimester gestational rubella.

Although rubella virus is present in neural tissue of the infected fetus, developmental malformations of the brain are uncommon even in early gestational rubella (Griffith, '77). Most of the CNS damage occurs because of encephalitis associated with cerebral vasculitis (Rorke, '73). Since the encephalitis, once established, can continue for years (Desmond et al., '78) cumulative damage can be expected.

In the Collaborative Study, no child with a history of maternal rubella in the last trimester had an IQ score below 70, and the number with borderline scores (70–80) was not significantly different from matched controls. Probably the development of the elements of the blood-brain barrier protects the CNS from infection with rubella virus during this late gestational period, or the more mature cells do not support the growth of the virus.

Late manifestations cannot yet be accurately related to gestational age at maternal rubella. Late onset hearing loss seems to occur in the same gestational time frame as that of hearing presenting earlier in life. Shaver ('83) found defects of carbohydrate metabolism in individuals contracting rubella as late as the fifth gestational month, and autoantibodies were found through the sixth gestational month. Progressive rubella panencephalitis, since it can also occur following postnatal rubella, cannot be limited to any gestational age group.

LATE MANIFESTATIONS OF CRS

Disabilities due to congenital rubella infections that first make their appearance years after birth are designated "late manifestations." Three of these will be discussed in some detail: deafness, endocrinopathies, and progressive rubella panencephalitis (PRP). Other defects that may also be regarded as late manifestations are subretinal neovascularization following rubella chorioretinopathy (Frank and Purnell, '78; Deutman and Grizzard, '78) and late vascular effects of fibromuscular proliferation in pulmonary and systemic arteries (Forrest et al., '69a). The result of the chronic rubella encephalitis beginning in utero, although producing new disabilities in the child as he grows older, is best regarded as a continuing rather than a late manifestation.

The profound bilateral sensorineural hearing loss characteristic of CRS usually reveals itself in the early weeks of life. However, there are numerous reports of CRS children who had good evidence of hearing ability and who then became deaf. The most extreme example of this late onset deafness was in a CRS child who had numerous normal audiograms, developed normal speech patterns, and attended to everyday activities adequately until age 10 when he first began to display signs of progressive deafness. At age 11 he was diagnosed as having profound bilateral sensorineural hearing loss (Desmond et al., '78, personal communication). Thus deafness must be regarded, in some cases, as a late manifestation of CRS. The mechanism for this type of late onset hearing loss is not known. Its onset does not seem to correlate with progressive damage of any other system.

The first reported CRS associated endocrinopathy was insulin dependent diabetes mellitus (Menser et al., '67b), an association noted in one 24-year-old CRS adult from the 1940 Australian epidemic. The same group (Forrest et al., '69b) then reported this and four additional cases. Soon reports of diabetes in CRS children surviving the 1964 epidemic appeared (Plotkin and Kaye, '70; Johnson and Tudor, '70). An expanded study of 50 older subjects revealed a 20% incidence of overt or latent diabetes (Forrest et al., '71). All these diabetic patients had a prenatal history of rubella before the 16th week of gestation, all were deaf, and most had other rubella associated defects of eyes and heart. All had diagnosis of diabetes before the age of 30. On continued follow-up (Menser et al., '74), 40% of these CRS subjects had developed overt or latent diabetes.

All these reports suggest that diabetes is by far the most common endocrinopathy in CRS survivors. However, other endocrine disorders have been seen in small numbers of CRS persons, sometimes in combination with diabetes. Hypothyroidism (Ziring et al., '75, '77; Hanid, '76; Comas, '76), hyperthyroidism (Floret et al., '80) and hypoadrenalism (Ziring et al., '77) have been reported as well as two cases of growth hormone deficiency (Preece et al., '77). Thus the endocrinopathies are emerging as common late disabilities in CRS.

Progressive rubella panencephalitis (PRP) is in many ways analogous to subacute sclerosing panencephalitis (SSPE). PRP is the "slow virus" manifestation of rubella encephalitis as SSPE is of measles. Like SSPE, PRP begins insidiously, 10 or more years after the primary infection. There is progressive deterioration of intellectual and motor function, with dementia near the end of the invariably fatal course. Evidence for rubella virus as the basis for this condition is very well established. There is an intense immune response against rubella antigens, with high titers of antibody measurable in both serum and CSF, which can be absorbed out with rubella-infected cells. There has been identification of viral antigen in brain tissue by immunofluorescent techniques, and in immune complexes found in CSF and serum as well as by elution from brain tissue. The virus has been recovered from one brain specimen by a "rescue" technique of tissue culture (Wolinski, '78).

The pathologic morphology of PRP (Rosenberg et al., '81) resembles SSPE without inclusions and with perivascular deposits. Both cerebrum and cerebellum are involved, and the lesions do not conform to a vascular distribution, distinguishing it from a simple continuation of neonatal rubella encephalitis. The inflamatory process consists of a meningeal and perivascular lymphocytic and plasmacytic infiltrate with focal and nodular gliosis. It is diffuse but predominates in white matter, most actively in hippocampus and brain stem.

PRP has now been described in 12 cases, (including 2 cases with postnatal rubella infection) (Lebon and Lyon, '74; Weil et al., '75; Townsend et al., '75, '76; Wolinsky, '78). All reported cases are in males. There is so far no recognizable correlation with presence of rubella associated defects or with severity of neonatal symptoms, and no risk factors can be ascertained. As in SSPE, precipitating events remain completely mysterious.

PATHOGENESIS

Pathogenetic mechanisms in congenital rubella are of two types: direct viral effect and effects due to the immune response (Naeye and Blanc, '65; Rosenberg et al., '81). The direct effect of rubella virus is confined almost entirely to inhibition of cell replication (Rawls and Melnick, '66), since this virus is generally not cytopathogenic for human cells. The marked slowing of cell doubling time at critical points in organogenesis prohibits accumulation of sufficient cell mass to shape the embryonic parts normally. Also, the early embryonic cells may require a certain minimum number of replicative cycles as a part of their differentiative activity. By this mechanism, many of the major permanent defects as well as the low birth weight characteristic of CRS can be understood. Also, temporary and permanent effects on the immune system can be explained by inhibition of cell replication. The immunocytes are the cells with the greatest proliferative potential of any in the body; therefore, inhibition of proliferation produces most profound effects on the development of the immune system. When proliferation of immunocytes is limited, cells cannot be generated to function in bringing the infection under control. Thus a vicious cycle is set up. An immune response is mounted only after a population of immunocytes can escape this cycle. Most fetuses with congenital rubella who survive to term will have accomplished this escape and begun to limit the infection, perhaps with the aid of transplacentally transmitted antibody. The evidence of this immune response is in precocious architectural development of lymphoid tissues, lymphoid hyperplasia, inflammatory lesions of various infected tissues, and immunologic activity measurable in the laboratory. However, a few infants at birth will still be caught in a state of "immune paralysis." If they are able to emerge from this state, they may be left with evidence of permanent immune damage (absence of IgA). A few will not be able to escape, and will remain in a state of immune deficiency with regard to all antigens, not just rubella virus (Singer et al., '69). Survival in this state is limited, therefore few of these infants have been studied (South and Alford, '80).

Once the immune response has developed, permanent damage can be inflicted by inflammatory mechanisms. Immune cytolysis, interruption of blood supply by inflammation of vascular walls, and subsequent scarring all contribute to permanent damage in the developing child (Rosenberg et al., '81).

The immune apparatus is finally able to limit the infection but cannot immediately rid the body of the infectious agent. The rubella virus was able to enter cells in the embryonic state and to persist in the progeny of infected cells without being exposed to the neutralizing antibody in the extracellular fluids. The only method for elimination of the virus is by immune elimination of all the infected cells. The mechanisms for immune modulation prohibit this "self-destruct" method from operating in an organism in which a large percentage of all cells are infected. Evidence for this concept comes from the finding that lymphocyte mediated cytotoxicity against rubella-infected cells is absent in CRS subjects (Fuccillo et al., '74).Therefore the virus is allowed to persist. Uninfected cells will eventually "outgrow" the infected cells with their limited proliferative capacity. Then the infected cells may be eliminated one by one.

All CRS children who have been examined lack lymphocyte mediated cytotoxicity for rubella. In addition, some children with congenital rubella will lose their rubella antibody and become susceptible to reinfection (Kenrick et al., '68; Hardy et al., '69; Cooper et al., '71; Peckham, '72; South and Alford, '80), unlike normal individuals experiencing rubella infection postnatally. These may be the children whose defense mechanisms are most "successful" in entirely eliminating the virus, not leaving even enough viral antigen to maintain lasting immunity. They have a perfectly normal course and a primary immune response, both cellular and humoral, when challenged with a wild or vaccine rubella strain.

In other children with CRS the rubella virus certainly has the capacity to avoid even this slow elimination process and to persist, probably in a latent phase, and especially in the central nervous system, in the presence of high titers of antibody. This capacity is demonstrated many years later in the development of PRP. The other late lesions may be due either to persistent viral infection or to the developmental effects of earlier inflammation and scarring. Autoimmune mechanisms may play a very significant role in the evolution of these late manifestations. Also, genetic factors must be important, especially in the endocrinopathies, as suggested by studies of HLA markers (Menseret al., '74; Rubinstein et al., '82; Shaver et al., '84).

RUBELLA VACCINE AS A CONTROL MEASURE FOR CONGENITAL RUBELLA SYNDROME

Rubella vaccine was developed through an intensive effort following the isolation of the rubella virus in tissue culture. The first vaccine was licensed in the United States in 1969. The HPV-77 and Cendehill strains were used first, and subsequently various vaccines were tested. The presently used vaccine, Wistar RA 27/3 (Ingalls et al., '70) was licensed in 1979. These vaccines are efficacious in inducing immunity in 95% or more of vaccinees. Side effects of rash and lymphadenapathy in children, and of arthralgia in adults, are frequent but not disabling. Frank arthritis is reported in less than 1% of vaccinees, peripheral neuritic symptoms are rare. There is no increased risk of these reactions for persons who are already immune when vaccinated; therefore, the vaccine is recommended for adminstration without prior serologic testing (Centers for Disease Control, '81). Rubella vaccine virus is able to traverse

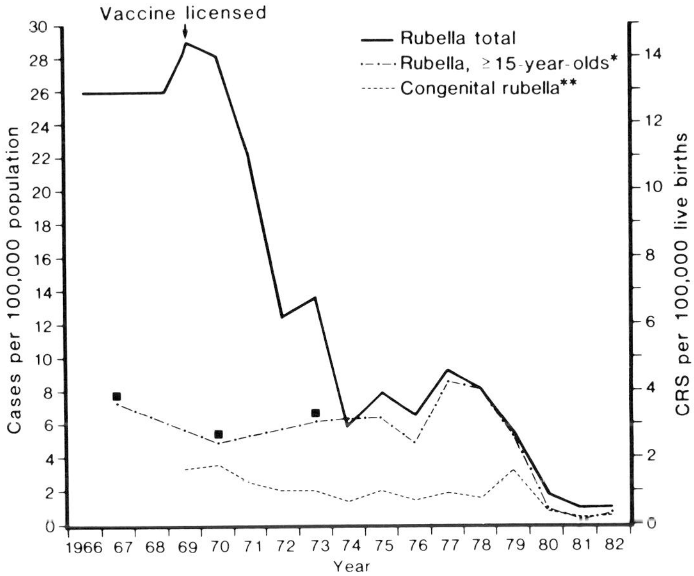

Fig. 4. Incidence rate of reported rubella and congenital rubella cases, United States, 1966–1982. *Includes proration of ≥15-year-olds with unknown ages. **Rate per 100,000 births of confirmed and compatible cases of congenital rubella syndrome (CRS), by year of birth. Reporting for recent years is provisional, as cases may not be diagnosed until later in childhood. ■, average annual U.S. estimate of rubella incidence in ≥15-year-olds, based on data from Illinois, Massachusetts, and New York City for the 3-year periods 1966–1968, 1969–1971, and 1972–1974. Age-specific data were not available for U.S. totals until 1975. (Reproduced from the Centers for Disease Control Morbidity and Mortality Weekly Report, Volume 32, pp. 505–510 (1983)).

the placenta and infect the fetus. Therefore, although there has been no demonstration of teratogenicity from attenuated strains, the vaccine is not recommended for pregnant women (Centers for Disease Control, '81, '83a).

In the 10 years following the introduction of vaccine in the United States, the overall incidence of reported rubella decreased about 70% (Center for Disease Control, '78), and reported CRS decreased from 2.7/100,000 live births in 1969 to 0.9/100,000 live births in 1977 (Sordula et al., '79; Preblud et al., '80; Center for Disease Control, '83b) (Fig. 4). Despite these improvements in statistics, the levels of rubella susceptibility in young adults remained at 10–20%, similar to the seronegativity rate among adults before vaccine became available. This was due largely to the age gap between the group in which the vaccine had so far been used, and the women who remained in their childbearing years. Consequently, the "epidemic" year 1978 produced an increase in CRS cases both in the United States (Lamprect et al., '82; Orenstein and Greaves, '82) and the United Kingdom (Miller et al., '82). In the United States, vaccine programs had concentrated on the infant and preschool child, the most important reservoir for contagion, while in the United Kingdom, the target for immunization programs had been the pre-adolescent female approaching her childbearing years. Modifications have now been made in both programs, utilizing wider distributions of vaccine. There has now been a further decrease in both rubella and congenital rubella, so that in 1982 only nine cases of congenital rubella were reported in the United States (Centers for Disease Control, '83b) (Fig. 4). If enough "herd immunity" effect can be generated through vaccine programs, epidemics can be prevented, with a reduction to near zero of exposure of persons who have not yet been immunized or did not respond to their immunization.

Since the only reservoir of rubella virus is the human host, it is possible to imagine that rubella, like smallpox, may someday be eliminated from the earth. However, in order to achieve this state, all CRS persons will have had to live out their life spans, for each person who became chronically infected in utero is at least theoretically a life-long virus carrier and potential source of contagion (Menser et al., '71). Further, it is possible that a CRS woman can transmit rubella virus to her offspring in utero (Menser et al., '68). Finally, reinfection is possible especially after vaccine-induced immunity; therefore CRS in the offspring of a seropositive woman is possible and has been well documented in several cases (Bott and Eizenberg, '82). Thus many generations of strictly successful rubella prevention would be necessary to achieve a status in which total rubella eradication could become theoretically possible.

LITERATURE CITED

Alford, C.A., F.A. Neva, and T.H. Weller (1964) Virologic and serologic studies on human products of conception after maternal rubella. N. Engl. J. Med., *271:*1275–1281.

Bott, L.M., and D.H. Eizenberg (1982) Congenital rubella after successful vaccination. Med. J. Aust., *1:*514–515.

Centers for Disease Control (1978) Rubella and Congenital rubella, United States, 1977–78. MMWR, *27:*495.

Centers for Disease Control (1981) Rubella prevention. MMWR, *30:*37–47.

Centers for Disease Control (1983a) Rubella vaccination during pregnancy—United States, 1971–1982. MMWR, *32:*430–432.

Centers for Disease Control (1983b) Rubella and congenital rubella—United States, 1980–83. MMWR, *32:*505–510.

Comas, A.P. (1976) Congenital rubella and acquired hypothyroidism secondary to Hashimoto thyroiditis. J. Pediatr., *88:*1065–1066.

Cooper, L.Z. (1975) Congenital rubella in the United States. In: Infections of the Fetus and the Newborn Infant. Progress in Clinical and Biological Research. S. Krugman and A.E. Gershon, eds. Alan R. Liss, New York, Vol. 3, pp. 1–22.

Cooper, L.Z., A.L. Florman, P.R. Ziring, and S. Krugman (1971) Loss of rubella hemagglutination inhibition antibody in congenital rubella. Am. J. Dis. Child.,*122:*397–403.

Dekabon, A.S., J.O. O'Rourke, and T. Cornman (1958) Abnormalities in offspring related to maternal rubella during pregnancy. Neurology (Minneapolis), *8:*387–392.

Desmond, M.M., G.S. Wilson, J.L. Melnick, D.B. Singer, T.E. Zion, A.J. Rudolph, R.G. Pineda, M.-H. Ziai, and R.J. Blattner (1967) Congenital rubella encephalitis. Course and early sequelae. J. Pediatr., *71:*311–331.

Desmond, M.M., E.S. Fisher, A.L. Vorderman, H.G. Schaffer, L.P. Andrew, T.E. Zion, and F.I. Catlin (1978) The longitudinal course of congenital rubella encephalitis in non-retarded children. J. Pediatr., *93:*584–591.

Deutman, A.F., and W.S. Grizzard (1978) Rubella retinopathy and subretinal neovascularization. Am. J. Ophthalmol., *85:*82–87.

Dudgeon, J.A. (1975) Congenital rubella in the United Kingdom of Great Britain. In: Infections of the Fetus and the Newborn Infant. Progress in Clinical and Biological Research. S. Krugman and A.E. Gershon, eds. Alan R. Liss, New York, Vol. 3, pp. 22–34.

Floret, D., D. Rosenberg, G.N. Hage, and P. Monnet (1980) Case report: Hyperthyroidism, diabetes mellitus and the congenital rubella syndrome. Acta Paediatr. Scand., *69:*250–261.

Forrest, J.M., M.A. Menser, and R.D.K. Reye (1969a) Obstructive arterial lesions in rubella. Lancet, *1:*1263–1264.

Forrest, J.M., M.A. Menser, and J.D. Harley (1969b) Diabetes mellitus and congenital rubella. Pediatrics, *44:*445–447.

Forrest, J.M., M.A.Menser, and J.A. Burgess (1971) High frequency of diabetes mellitus in young adults with congenital rubella. Lancet, *1:*332–334.

Frank, K.E., and E.W. Purnell (1978) Subretinal neovascularization following rubella retinopathy. Am. J. Ophthalmol., *86:*462–466.

Fuccillo, D.A., R.W. Steele, S.A. Henson, M.M. Vincent, J.B. Hardy, and J.A. Bellanti (1974) Impaired cellular immunity to rubella virus in congenital rubella. Infect. Immun., *9:*81–84.

Gregg, N.M. (1941) Congenital cataract following German measles in the mother. Trans. Ophthalmol. Soc. Aust., *3:*35–45.

Gregg, N.M. (1944) Further observations on congenital defects in infants following maternal rubella. Trans. Ophthalmol. Soc. Aust., *4:*119–131.

Griffith, J.F. (1977) Non-bacterial infections of the fetus and newborn. Clin. Perinatol., *4:*117–130.

Hanid, T.K. (1976) Hypothyroidism in congenital rubella. Lancet, *2:*854.

Hardy, J.B. (1973) Clinical and developmental aspects of congenital rubella. Arch. Otolaryngol., *98:*230–236.

Hardy, J.B., J.L. Sever, and M.R. Gilkeson (1969) Declining antibody titers in children with congenital rubella. J. Pediatr., *75:*213–220.

Heggie, A.D., and W.C. Weir (1964) Isolation of rubella virus from a mother and fetus. Pediatrics. *34:*278–280.

Ingalls, T.H., S.A. Plotkin, F.R. Philbrook, and R.F. Thompson (1970) Immunization of school children with rubella (RA 27/3) vaccine. Lancet, *1:*99–101.

Johnson, G.M., and R.B. Tudor (1970) Diabetes mellitus and congenital rubella infection. Am. J. Dis. Child., *120:*453–455.

Kenrick, K.G., R.F. Slinn, D.C. Dorman, and M.A. Menser (1968) Immunoglobulins and rubella-virus antibodies in adults with congenital rubella. Lancet, *1:*548–551.

Lamprecht, C., V. Schauf, D. Warren, K. Nelson, R. Northrop, and M. Christiansen (1982) An outbreak of congenital rubella in Chicago, JAMA, *247:*1129–1133.

Lebon, P., and G. Lyon (1974) Non-congenital rubella encephalitis (letter). Lancet, *2:*468.

Menser, M.A., J.D. Harley, R. Hertzberg, D.C. Dorman, and A.M. Murphy (1967a) Persistence of virus in lens for three years after prenatal rubella. Lancet, *2:*387–388.

Menser, M.A., L. Dods, and J.D. Harley (1967b) A twenty-five year follow-up of congenital rubella. Lancet, *2:*1347–1350.

Menser, M.A., R.F. Slinn, L. Dods, R. Hertzberg, and J.D. Harley (1968) Congenital rubella in a mother and son. Aust. Paediatr. J., *4:*200–202.

Menser, M.A., R.F. Slinn, J.M. Forrest, M.J. Nowak, and D.C. Dorman (1971) Rubella viruria in a 29-year-old woman with congenital rubella. Lancet, *2:*797–798.

Menser, M.A., J.M. Forrest, M.C. Honeyman, and J.A. Burgess (1974) Diabetes HLA antigens, and congenital rubella. Lancet, *2:*1058–1059.

Michaels, R.H., and F.M. Kenny (1969) Postnatal growth retardation in congenital rubella. Pediatrics, *43:*251–259.

Miller, E., I.E. Cradock-Watson, and T.M. Pollock (1982) Consequences of confirmed maternal rubella at successive stages of pregnancy. Lancet, *2:*781–784.

Naeye, R.L., and W. Blanc (1965) Pathogenesis of congenital rubella. JAMA, *194:*1277–1283.

Orenstein, W.A., and W.L. Graves (1982) Congenital rubella syndrome: A continuing problem. JAMA, *247:*1174–1175.

Parkman, P.D., E.L. Buescher, and M.A. Artenstein (1962) Recovery of rubella virus from army recruits. Proc. Soc. Exp. Biol. Med., *111:*225–230.

Peckham, C.S. (1972) Clinical and laboratory study of children exposed in utero to maternal rubella. Arch. Dis. Child., *47:*571–577.

Plotkin, S.A., and R. Kaye (1970) Diabetes mellitus and congenital rubella. Pediatrics, *46:*650–651.

Preblud, S.R., M.K. Serdula, J.A. Frank, Jr., and A.R. Hinman (1980) Current status of rubella in the United States, 1969–1979. Institutional reports from the Center for Disease Control. J. Infect. Dis., *142:*776–779.

Preblud, S.R., H.C. Harrison, J.A. Frank, Jr., W.L. Graves, A.R. Hinman, and K.L. Herrmann (1981) Fetal risk associated with rubella vaccine. JAMA, *246:*1413–1417.

Preece, M.A., P.J. Kearney, and W.C. Marshall (1977) Growth-hormone deficiency in congenital rubella. Lancet, *2:*842–844.

Rawls, W.E., and J.L. Melnick (1966) Rubella virus carrier cultures derived from congenitally infected infants. J. Exp. Med., *123:*795–816.

Rawls, W.E., C.A. Phillips, J.L. Melnick, and M.M. Desmond (1967) Persistent virus infection in congenital rubella. Arch. Opthalmol., *77:*430–443.

Rawls. W.E., J. Desmyter, and J.L. Melnick (1968) Serologic diagnosis and fetal involvement in maternal rubella. JAMA, *203:*111–115.

Rorke, L.B. (1973) Nervous system lesions in the congenital rubella syndrome. Arch. Otolaryngol., *98:*249–251.

Rosenberg, H.S., E.H. Oppenheimer, and J.R. Esterly (1981) Congenital rubella syndrome: The late effects and their relation to early lesions. In: Perspectives in Pediatric Pathology. H.S. Rosenberg and J.Bernstein, eds. Vol. 6, pp. 183–202.

Rubenstein, P., M.E. Walker, B. Fedun, M.E. Witt, L.Z. Cooper, and F. Ginsberg-Fellner (1982) The HLA system in congenital rubella patients with and without diabetes. Diabetes, *31:*1088–1091.

Rudolph, A.J., M.D. Yow, C.A. Phillips, M.M. Desmond, R.J. Blattner, and J.L. Melnick (1965a) Transplacental rubella infection in newly born infants. JAMA, *191:*843–845.

Rudolph, A.J., E.B. Singleton, H.S. Rosenberg, D.B. Singer, and C.A. Phillips (1965b) Osseous manifestations of the congenital rubella syndrome. Am. J. Dis. Child., *110:*428–433.

Serdula, M.K., J.A. Frank, Jr., A.C. Curtis, III (1979) Effect of the U.S. rubella immunization program on the rate of the congenital rubella syndrome. Proceedings of the Interscience Conference on Antimicrobial Agents and Chemotherapy, pp. 1203–1205.

Sever, J.L., and G.R. Monif (1965) Limited persistence of virus in congenital rubella. Am. J. Dis. Child., *110:*452–454.

Sever, J.L., K.B.Nelson, and M.R. Gilkeson (1965) Rubella epidemic, 1964: Effect on 6,000 pregnancies. Am.J. Dis. Child., *110:*395–407.

Sever,J.L., J.B. Hardy, K.B. Nelson, and M.R. Gilkeson (1969) Rubella in the Collaborative Perinatal Research Study. II. Clinical and laboratory findings in children through three years of age. Am. J. Dis. Child.,*118:*123–132.

Shaver, K.A. (1983) Congenital rubella syndrome and diabetes: A study of genetic and epidemiologic risk factors. Doctoral dissertation, Genetics Department, Medical College of Virginia.

Shaver, K.A., J.A. Boughman, N. Kenyon, T. Mohanakumar, and W. E. Nance (1984) HLA antigen Associations in the congenital rubella syndrome. Disease Markers, *2:*381–391.

Shewman, D.A., J.D. Cherry, and Sarah E. Kirby (1982) Shedding of rubella virus in a 4 1/2-year-old boy with congenital rubella. Pediatr. Infect. Dis., 1:342–343.

Singer, D.B., M.A. South, J.R. Montgomery, and W.E. Rawls (1969) Congenital rubella syndrome. Lymphoid tissue and immunologic status. Am. J. Dis. Child., *118:*54–61.

South, M.A., and C.A. Alford (1980) The immunology of chronic intrauterine infections. In: Immunologic Disorders in Infants and Children, second edition. E.R. Stiehm and V.A. Fulginiti, eds., W.B. Saunders Co., Philadelphia, pp. 702–714.

Townsend, J.J., J.R. Baringer, J.A. Wolinsky, N. Malamud, J.P. Medick, H.S. Panitch, R.A.T. Scott, L.S. Oshiro, and N.E. Cremer (1975) Progressive rubella panencephalitis. N. Engl. J. Med., *292:*990–993.

Townsend, J.J., W.G. Stroop, J.R. Baringer, J.S. Wolinsky, J.H. McKerrow, and B.O. Berg (1976) Neuropathology of progressive rubella panencephalitis after childhood rubella. Neurology, *32:*185–190.

Ueda, K., Y. Nishida, K. Oshima, and T.H. Shepard (1979) Congenital rubella syndrome: Correlation of gestational age at time of maternal rubella with type of defect. J. Pediatr., *94:*763–765.

Weil, M.L., H.H. Itabashi, N.E. Cremer, L.S. Oshiro, E.H. Lennette, and L. Carnay (1975) Chronic progressive panencephalitis due to rubella virus simulating subacute sclerosing panencephalitis. N. Engl. J.Med., *292:*994–998.

Weller, T.H., and F.A. Neva (1962) Propagation in tissue culture of cytopathic agents from patients with rubella-like illness. Proc. Soc. Exp. Biol. Med., *111:*215–225.

Wolinsky, J.S. (1978) Progressive rubella panencephalitis. In: Handbook of Clinical Neurology. P.J. Vinken and G.W. Bruyn, eds. North-Holland, Amsterdam, Vol. 34, pp. 331–341.

Ziring, P.R., B.A. Fedun, and L.A. Cooper (1975) Thyrotoxicosis in congenital rubella. J. Pediatr., *88:*1002.

Ziring, P.R., G. Gallo, M. Finegold, E. Buimovici-Klein, and P. Ogra (1977) Chronic lymphocytic thyroiditis. Identification of rubella virus antigen in the thyroid of a child with congenital rubella. J. Pediatr., *90:*419–420.

TERATOGEN UPDATE: ENVIRONMENTALLY INDUCED BIRTH DEFECT RISKS, PAGES 93–95 (1986)

Congenital Cytomegalovirus Infection

D.W. REYNOLDS, S. STAGNO, AND C.A. ALFORD
Department of Pediatrics, University of Alabama at Birmingham, Birmingham, Alabama 35294

CLINICAL MANIFESTATIONS

This chronic intrauterine infection occurs in one to two percent of live births in most populations and is recognized as the most common cause of congenital viral infections in man. Only about one to five percent of the infants with congenital cytomegalovirus (CMV) infection have typical cytomegalic inclusion disease; another five percent have atypical illness, and 90 percent have no clinical manifestations at birth. For the unfortunate few symptomatic infants, classic findings comprise hepatitis with direct reacting hyperbilirubinemia, splenomegaly, thrombocytopenia with or without petechiae, either gestational prematurity of intrauterine growth retardation, and encephalitis. Additional manifestations of relatively high frequency include microcephaly, anemia, and intracranial calcifications. Less frequently, chorioretinitis, optic atrophy, hydrocephaly, myocarditis, pneumonitis, and disseminated intravascular coagulopathy may occur in the sick neonate (Figs. 1, 2, and 3). These latter three involvements, along with cerebral infection and bleeding tendency, may be life threatening. For the most part, extraneural pathology is self limited. Clinically apparent infection is usually followed, in decreasing order of occurrence, by psychomotor retardation, hearing loss, and visual impairment. Milder forms of these permanent impairments to the brain and perceptual organs (especially the inner ear) occur in a minority of patients subclinically infected at birth (Fig. 4).

The teratogenic capacity of this virus is likely of low order. Physical defects in virtually every organ system have been associated with intrauterine acquisition of this agent; however, with most structural anomalies only a few case reports exist. Exceptions include inguinal hernias in males, first arch abnormalities, hypoplasia or agenesis of central nervous system structures, and a defect of amelogenesis (enamel) that affects mainly primary dentition (Fig. 5). Assessing the true embryopathic potential of CMV is hampered by the subclinical nature of the maternal infection, thereby making it very difficult to define the time of transmission to the fetus, and by the high frequency of this fetal infection.

EPIDEMIOLOGY

Both primary and recurrent maternal infections during pregnancy can be transmitted to the fetus. In highly immune populations, there is good evidence that the latter (classically thought not to occur at all) is more common than the former. However, congenital CMV infection resulting from primary maternal infection is more likely to be serious than that resulting from recurrent infection. The relative contributions of these two forms of maternal infections to the total incidence of congenital acquisition in various groups and in acute neonatal morbidity and long term sequelae demands better definition in view of current efforts toward vaccine development. If recurrent involvement proves to be a cause of fetal infection but is less likely to cause disease, then it may be possible to develop a vaccine to immunize susceptible women. The modes of transmission to susceptible adults likely include direct contact spread (respiratory and venereal), blood transfusion, and organ transplants. At present too little is understood about these events to effect preventive guidelines.

PATHOGENESIS

The factors responsible for the occurrence of disease in some infants are unclear but include, on a speculative basis, early gestational transmission, primary maternal infection, increased virulence of the infecting strain, and a genetic predisposition of the host. Likewise, the pathologic pathways of tissue injury have yet to be elucidated. Direct and indirect (vasculitis) viral cytolysis and/or immunologic self injury are prominent possibilities. Indeed, the possibility of continued low grade tissue injury is clearly suggested by the following: chronic viral replication as demonstrated by excretion of

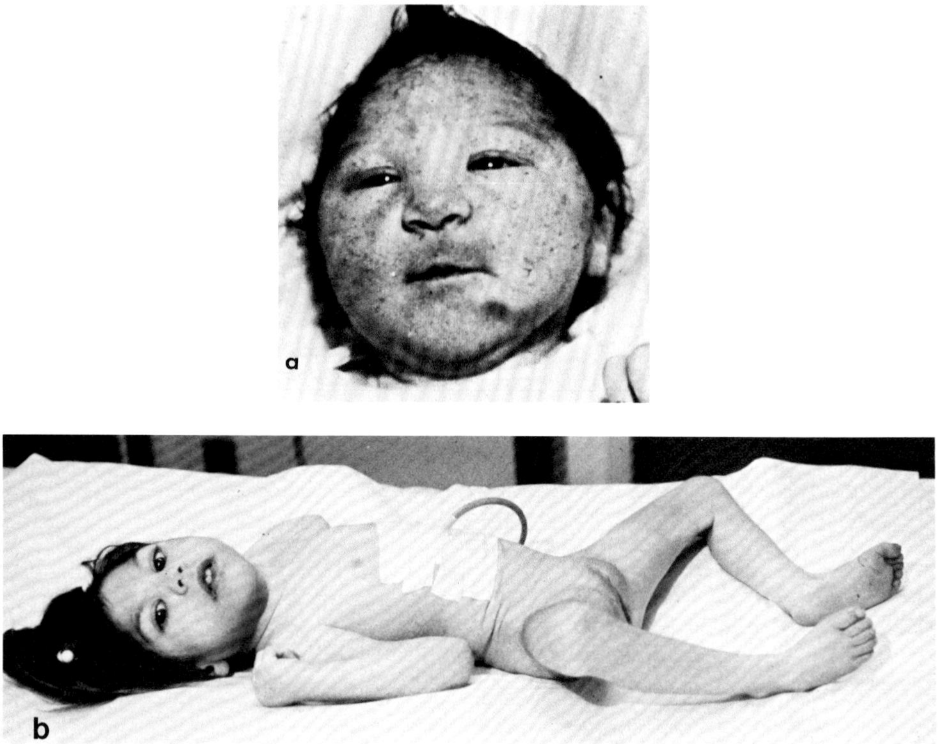

Fig. 1. a) Neonate with congenital cytomegalovirus infection manifesting petechiae and microcephaly. b) Same patient at 8 years of age showing spastic quadriplegia, microcephaly, mental retardation, and chorioretinitis. (Patient is fed through a gastrostomy tube.)

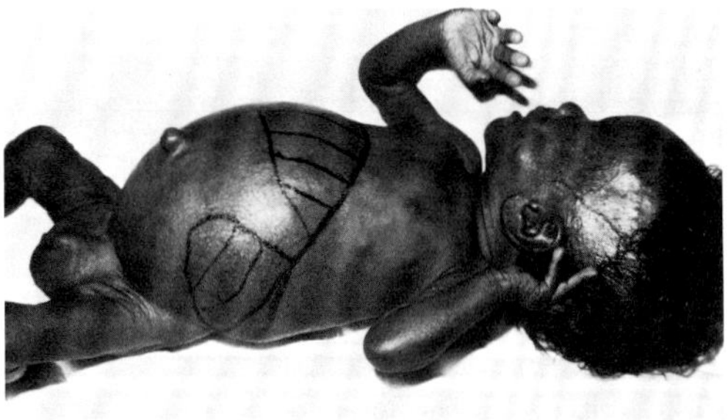

Fig. 2. Four month old with symptomatic congenital infection manifesting severe failure to thrive, hepatitis with hepatosplenomegaly, bilateral inguinal hernias, and micropenis.

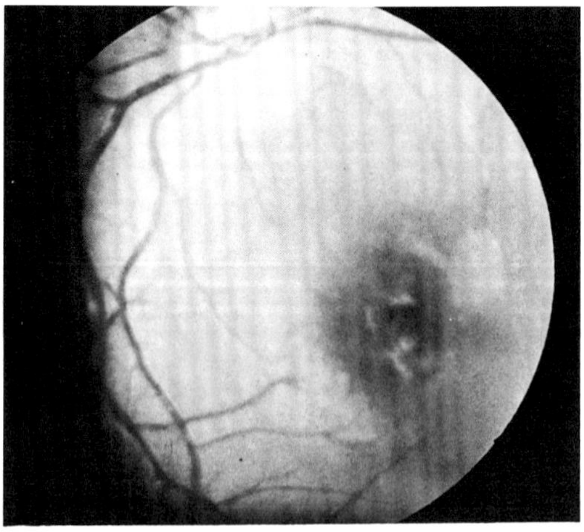

Fig. 3. CMV chorioretinitis. This patient had clinically severe congenital infection.

infectious virus (urine and saliva) lasting for years; intense humoral immune response; diminished or absent in vitro lymphocyte transformation responses to CMV antigens; and immune complex formation. Singly or in combination these pathologic pathways may explain the development of late onset sequelae (hearing loss, mental retardation, chorioretinitis) even among infants who are asymptomatic at the outset.

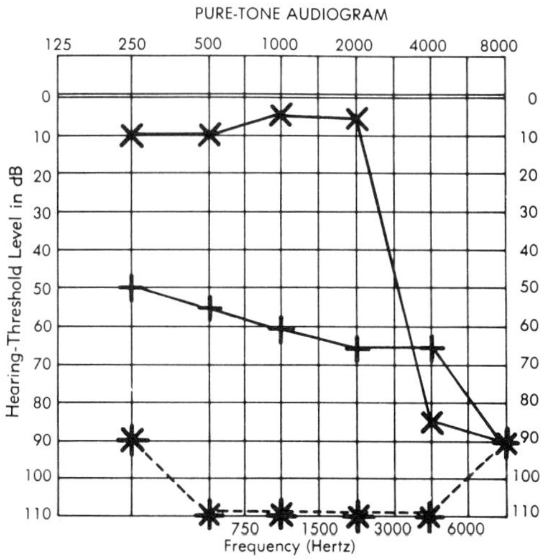

Fig. 4. Hearing deficits in two children with congenital cytomegalovirus infection. Three-year-old white female with neonatal disease and total deafness, (———). Ten-year-old white male with inapparent congenital infection displaying a moderate unilateral functional hearing loss and bilateral high frequency decrements, (– – –). (X) left ear; (+) right ear.

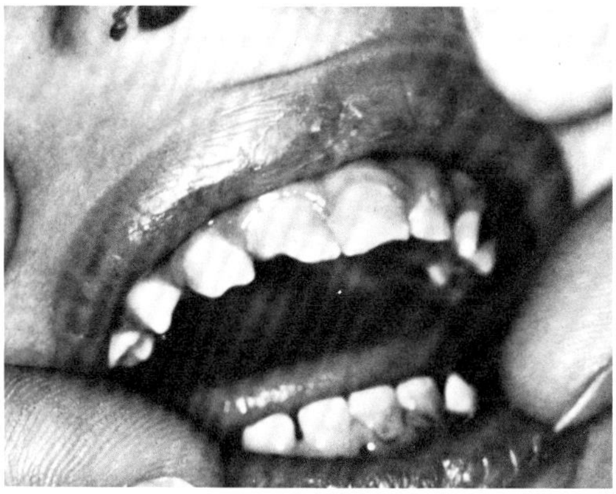

Fig. 5. CMV affected teeth. This patient had clinically severe congenital CMV infection. Note fractured borders and opaque and hypocalcified enamel.

DIAGNOSIS

The isolation of virus from urine during the first week of life remains the most sensitive and specific method of diagnosis. In lieu of definitive virologic confirmation, the demonstration of persistent circulating antibody during the first 6 to 9 months of life is of limited diagnostic significance. Differentiation of fetal from natal acquisition can be difficult with this approach. This can be achieved with assurance only by examination of the cord and monthly serum specimens through six months of age. Stable titers confirm fetal involvement; patterns of waning with subsequent increased production of antibody can be seen with both types of infection. Immunoglobulin M levels or the presence of rheumatoid factors in cord blood can be used as screening methods for inapparent fetal infection. The detection of CMV specific IgM antibody in cord blood has not yet achieved wide acceptibility as most tests still give too many false positive and false negative results.

TREATMENT AND PROGNOSIS

At present, there is no safe and effective chemotherapeutic agent available for the treatment of this infection. Adenine arabinoside, acyclovir, and interferon have proved ineffective. All patients with congenital CMV infection deserve serial assessments of auditory, mental/behavioral, and visual acuity in childhood so that supportive therapy can be instituted at the earliest possible interval once morbidity is recognized.

ACKNOWLEDGMENTS

This work is supported by grants from the General Clinical Research Center #5 MO1 RR32, National Institute of Child Health and Human Development #HD10699, and the March of Dimes Birth Defects Foundation.

LITERATURE CITED

Hanshaw, J.B. (1983) Cytomegalovirus. In: Infectious Diseases of the Fetus and Newborn Infant, 2nd Edition. J.S. Remington and J.O. Klein eds. Philadelphia: W.B. Saunders Company, pp 104–144.

Reynolds, D.W., S. Stagno, K.G. Stubbs, A.J. Dahle, M.M. Livingston, S.S. Saxon, and C.A. Alford (1974) Inapparent congenital cytomegalovirus infection with elevated cord IgM levels. N. Engl. J. Med., *290*:295–296.

Pass, R.F., S. Stagno, G.J. Myers, and C.A. Alford (1980) Outcome of symptomatic congenital CMV infection. Results of long-term longitudinal follow-up. Pediatrics, *66*:758–762.

Stagno, S., R.F. Pass, M.E. Dworsky, and C.A. Alford (1983) Congenital and perinatal cytomegaloviral infections. Semin. Perinatol., *7*:31–42.

TERATOGEN UPDATE: ENVIRONMENTALLY INDUCED BIRTH DEFECT RISKS, PAGES 97–100 (1986)

Congenital Toxoplasmosis

JOHN W. LARSEN, JR.
Department of Obstetrics and Gynecology, The George Washington University School of Medicine and Health Sciences, Washington, D.C. 20037

Toxoplasma gondii is a protozoan parasite named by Nicolle and Manceaux ('09) after a North African rodent, the gondi, in which the organism had been observed in the spleen and liver. The symptom complex of hydrocephaly, microphthalmia, and chorioretinitis due to congenital toxoplasmosis was first recognized by an ophthalmologist, Janku ('23), in Czechoslovakia.

MANIFESTATIONS

The manifestations of fully developed congenital toxoplasmosis are those of multiple organ damage and dysfunction. Overall fetal growth is usually retarded and tissue examination has shown that the *T. gondii* protozoans may be present in virtually every organ. No single clinical finding is pathognomic of the disease. Hydrocephalus, microphthalmus, and chorioretinitis were prominent in the original case described by Janku in 1923 (Fig. 1). Neurological abnormalities present at birth may include microcephalus or hydrocephalus (Fig. 2) and periventricular calcifications. Retinal lesions of variable intensity may be the first clinical sign suggesting the underlying disease (Fig. 3). Newborn infants with active disease may have fever, convulsions, maculopapular skin rash, lymphadenopathy, hepatosplenomegaly, icterus, and thrombocytopenia.

The frequency with which congenitally infected infants are symptomatic at birth is unknown but probably less than 20% have overt evidence of disease. (Remington and Desmonts, '83). When congenital toxoplasmosis is sufficiently advanced to be clinically recognizable at birth, severe damage or a fatal outcome may be expected 40% of the time. The frequency with which infected infants who are asymptomatic at birth subsequently develop significant disease is not known.

The severity of toxoplasmosis in newborn children appears to be related to the trimester of pregnancy during which the acute maternal infection occurred. If the toxoplasmosis is acquired by a pregnant woman during the first trimester, the infection is transmitted to the fetus about 15 to 20% of the time. However, the majority of those fetuses that become infected during the first trimester are likely to have severe manifestations of the disease. The rate of congenital acquisition increases to 25 to 30% during the second trimester and reaches approximately 60% during the third trimester. Approximately 90% of the fetuses that become infected during the third trimester are asymptomatic at birth.

TRANSMISSION

In the great majority of cases congenital toxoplasmosis occurs only when a previously uninfected pregnant woman becomes infected, and hence may transmit the protozoans across the placenta to the fetus (Desmonts and Couvreur, '74). The two ways in which a previously uninfected pregnant woman may acquire toxoplasmosis during pregnancy are by eating raw meat containing toxoplasma cysts, or by ingestion of oocysts excreted in the feces of infected cats.

Chronic maternal toxoplasmosis with myometrial cysts is unlikely to lead to infection of the human placenta (Remington and Desmonts, '83). However, delay of transmission of the parasites from placenta to fetus may occur occasionally, perhaps as late as parturition.

EPIDEMIOLOGY

The incidence of human exposure to *T. gondii* varies widely in different geographical areas; the incidence of women with antibodies to *T. Gondii* is greater than 80% in Paris; the United States average seems to be less than 40%. In the Collaborative Perinatal Project in the United States the incidence of maternal seroconversions during pregnancy was 6.4 per 1,000 pregnancies (Sever, '66). The same study found the incidence of classical clinically severe congenital toxoplasmosis to be one in 4,000 pregnancies. The

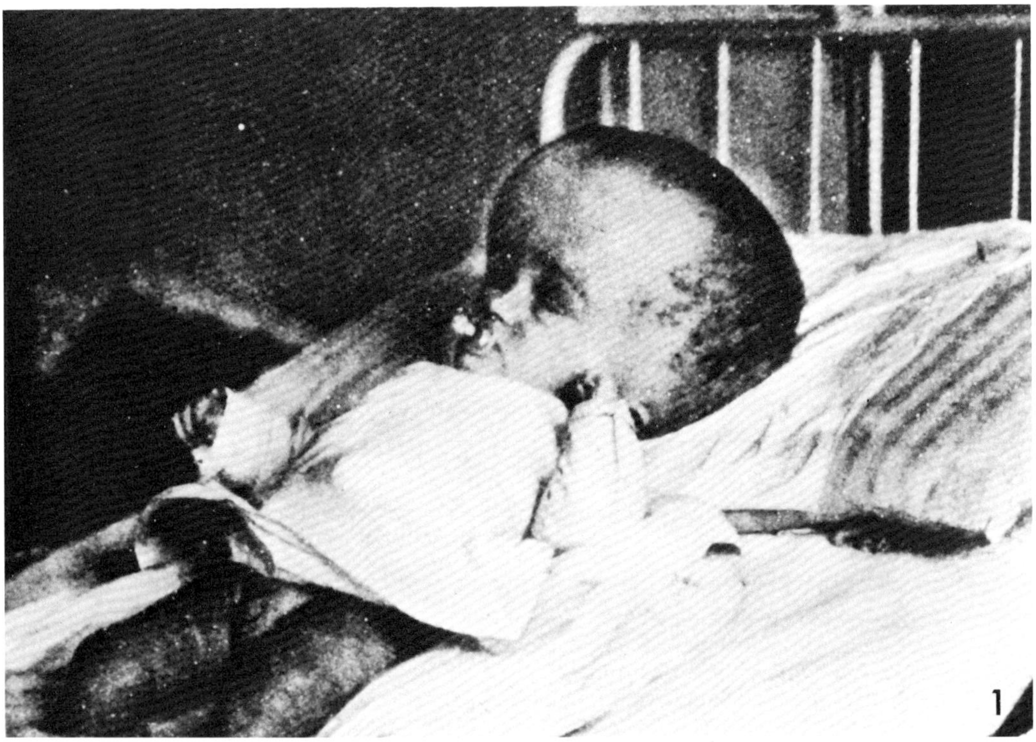

Fig. 1. Hydrocephalic infant with toxoplasmosis. (From Janku, Czech Med. *62:*1021–1143, By permission.)

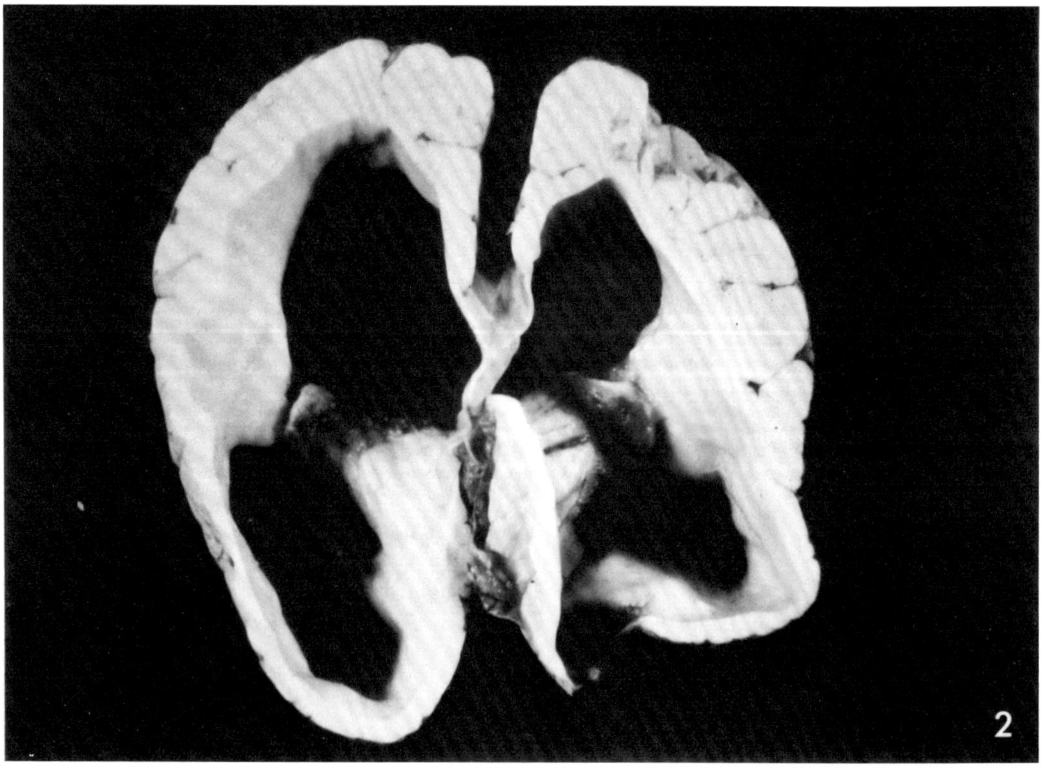

Fig. 2. Transverse section of brain with hydrocephalus due to toxoplasmosis. (By courtesy of B.H. Kean, The New York Hospital-Cornell Medical Center.)

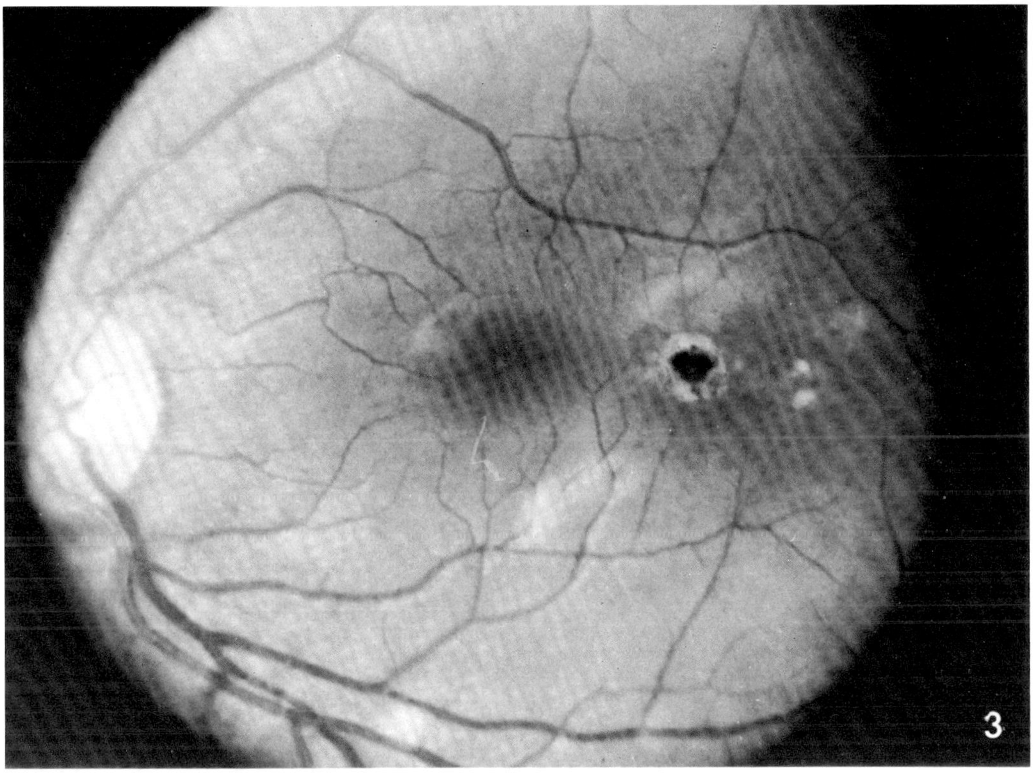

Fig. 3. Retinochoroiditis due to toxoplasmosis. (By courtesy of B.H. Kean, The New York Hospital-Cornell Medical Center.)

probability of maternal acute toxoplasmosis during pregnancy will vary among geographic areas, increasing where exposure is likely and decreasing where the proportion of women with pre-existing antibodies is high.

LABORATORY DIAGNOSIS

Identification of the infecting organisms by animal inoculation techniques is sufficiently costly and cumbersome to preclude its general use for clinical purposes. Furthermore, tissue biopsy or minced placenta rather than simple blood sampling is needed for toxoplasma isolation. Two tests of antibody response, the Sabin Feldman dye test and the fluorescent antibody test, are widely used, although hemagglutination, complement fixation, and skin tests may also be performed. The fluorescent antibody test, which largely measures IgG antibodies, has been modified to measure the IgM antibodies that might be found in sera from acutely infected women or in the cord sera of infected fetuses (Remington et al., '68a, '68b). More recently Naot and associates ('81) have developed a double sandwich IgM-ELISA test for detection of IgM antibodies for toxoplasma. This test appears to have fewer false-positive and false-negative results than the IgM indirect fluorescent antibody test and therefore should become widely used.

Under ideal circumstances it is possible to detect both maternal and fetal asymptomatic infections and to discriminate passive transfer of maternal antibodies to the fetus from true fetal infection. In more practical circumstances the serological titers of toxoplasma antibodies in an asymptomatic infant may be followed; the expectation is that the uninfected child's titer will decrease by 50% each month after birth.

If toxoplasmosis has been suspected prior to delivery, it is useful to examine the placenta histologically for toxoplasma cysts. The placenta should be fixed in formalin and not refrigerated or frozen to avoid lysis of the organisms and false-negative histology. A positive examination of the placenta after term delivery will support the diagnosis of acute maternal infection during pregnancy and has predictive value for ascertaining neonatal toxoplasmosis.

TREATMENT

Management of the pregnant woman or newborn child with suspected or proven toxoplasmosis in the United States is complicated by the absence of a safe, simple treatment for the infection. Although *T. gondii* infection in adults is self-limited without therapy in most cases, when chemotherapy is used the most effective regime available has been a combination of pyrimethamine and sulfonamides (Sever et al., '79, Remington and Desmonts, '83). Both have toxicity that could outweigh their benefits when used during pregnancy. In particular, pyrimethamine, a folic acid antagonist, may be teratogenic during the first trimester; although it should be noted that the drug has been used extensively in malarial areas of the world without having been demonstrated to cause human malformations (Fuchs et al., '74). Sulfonamides used and not cleared before delivery may compete sufficiently for fetal bilirubin binding sites to lead to kernicterus.

Desmonts and Couvreur ('74) reported on treatment of toxoplasmosis during pregnancy with spiramycin. Although the drug does not easily cross the placenta, and therefore should not be expected to cure an affected fetus, Desmonts and Couvreur believed that treatment decreased the number of affected offspring by action of the antibiotic on the placenta.

Fuchs et al. ('74) recommended that pregnancy termination should be considered when acute maternal toxoplasmosis has been diagnosed in early pregnancy. Whether to treat asymptomatic pregnant women who have shown seroconversion during pregnancy remains a matter for individual clinical judgement. At decision-making extremes, the newborn with fulminating disease would be treated, whereas the pregnant symptom-free woman with a chronically positive antibody test would be observed without receiving chemotherapy. It is currently recommended that symptomatic infants with persistent or rising antibody titers receive chemotherapy.

Detection of toxoplasmosis in pregnant women or newborns presumes either a very high index of suspicion for toxoplasmosis or a systematic serological screening program. An ideal serological screening plan would include testing before or early in pregnancy and follow-up testing for seroconversion or rising antibody titers. A discussion of the cost-benefit analysis of such a program can be found in Remington and Desmonts ('83).

PREVENTION

In the United States, it is likely that nearly all congenital toxoplasmosis could be eliminated if susceptible women avoided ingestion of meat that had not been thoroughly cooked or previously frozen, and avoided contact with infected cats (Frenkel and Dubey, '72). Raw meat can contain cysts that become infective when the parasites are liberated during digestion. The cat appears to be the definitive host for *T. gondii*. Infectious oocysts are found in cat feces. Toxoplasmosis in cats may be significantly reduced by their being fed only dry, canned, or cooked food, and by preventing them from ingesting wild rodents that may carry the organism. Further protection for pregnant women who are antibody negative may be obtained by their avoiding exposure to soil or litter containing the feces of infected cats.

LITERATURE CITED

Desmonts, G. and J. Couvreur (1974) Congenital toxoplasmosis: A prospective study of 378 pregnancies. N. Engl. J. Med., *290:*1110–1116.

Frenkel, J.K., and J.P. Dubey (1972) Toxoplasmosis and its prevention in cats and man. J. Infect. Dis., *126:*442–673.

Fuchs, F., A.C. Kimball, and B.H. Kean (1974) The management of toxoplasmosis in pregnancy. Clin. Perinatol., *1:*407–422.

Janku, J. (1923) Pathogenesa a pathologická anatomie tak nazvaného vrozeného kolobomu zluté skvrny v oku normálne velikém a mikrophthalmickém s nálezm parazitu v sítnici. Czech. Med., *62:*1021–1143.

Naot, Y., G. Desmonts, and J.S. Remington (1981) IgM enzyme-linked immunosorbent assay test for the diagnosis of congenital Toxoplasma infection. J. Pediatr., *98:*32–36.

Nicolle, C., and L. Manceaux (1909) Sur un protozoaire nouveau de Gondi, Toxoplasma. Arch. Inst. Pasteur, (Tunis), *2:*97–103.

Remington, J.S., and G. Desmonts (1983) Toxoplasmosis. In: Infectious Diseases of the Fetus and Newborn Infant. J.S. Remington and J.O. Klein, eds. W.B. Saunders Company, Philadelphia, pp 143–263.

Remington, J.S., M.J. Miller, and I. Brownlee (1968a) IgM antibodies in acute toxoplasmosis. I. Diagnostic significance in congenital cases and a method for their rapid demonstration. Pediatrics, *41:*1082–1091.

Remington, J.S., M.J. Miller, and I. Brownlee (1968b) IgM antibodies in acute toxoplasmosis. II. Prevalence and significance in acquired cases. J. Lab. Clin. Med., *71:*855–866.

Sever, J.L. (1966) The prevention of mental retardation through control of infectious diseases. PHS Publ. No. 1692, Washington, D.C., pp 37–68.

Sever, J.L., J.W. Larsen, and J.H. Grossman (1979) Toxoplasmosis. In: Handbook of Perinatal Infections. Little Brown and Company, Boston, pp 157–163.

TERATOGEN UPDATE: ENVIRONMENTALLY INDUCED BIRTH DEFECT RISKS, PAGES 101–105 (1986)

Congenital Varicella

DAVID A. FUCCILLO
Microbiological Associates, Bethesda, Maryland 20816

Varicella (chickenpox) and herpes zoster (shingles) are caused by the same virus. Primary infection with varicella-zoster virus (VZV) results in the characteristic chickenpox infection. The virus then apparently enters a latent phase within the nuclei of neurons and basal root ganglia. Garland was the first to propose that reactivation of the virus results in the clinical manifestations characteristic of zoster (Garland, '43). The virus was isolated in tissue culture in 1953 at which time the common etiology for both diseases was confirmed (Weller, '53). A live attenuated vaccine for varicella developed by Japanese investigators has been shown to stimulate antibodies in seronegative children (Takahashi et al., '74).

EPIDEMIOLOGY

VZV infection usually occurs in the winter or spring with epidemics occurring every 2–5 years. Children to 8 years of age are the group primarily affected but any susceptible individual may become infected. This disease is highly contagious with an 80–90% clinical attack rate. Immunity to varicella is lifelong; however, humoral antibody in the containment of primary infection is not clear since it has been recognized that reinfection does occur at a variable rate. Also, antibodies do not protect against the reactivation and clinical expression of zoster. In the United States the immunity to VZV is about 100% by age 60 (Gershon et al., '81). It is estimated that at least 2.8 million cases occur annually (Preblud, '81). Approximately 32% of varicella cases occur between 1 and 4 years of age; 50% occur between 5 and 9 years of age. This is not true in less developed nations where 46% can occur in individuals 15 years or older (Jezek et al., '81). Geographical location can greatly influence the susceptibility to infection. A recent study of women at childbearing age in New York revealed that 4.5% were not immune whereas 16% from tropical areas, immigrants to New York, were susceptible (Gershon et al. '76).

Information on the frequency of zoster infection is not readily available; however, a recent study indicated that the incidence was approximately 130 cases per 100,000 of population and that the total number of zoster cases appearing annually in the United States was at least 300,000 (Ragozzino et al., '82; Preblud and D'Angelo, '79).

CLINICAL ASPECTS

The incubation of varicella is usually 14 to 17 days. It is thought that two episodes of viremia take place during this period of time. From day 0 to 6 of the incubation period, infection can take place at the conjuctivae and/or mucosa of the upper respiratory tract and is probably the portal of entry for the virus. Viral replication occurs in the regional lymph nodes, tonsils, or salivary glands; then a primary viremia takes place. From day 6 to 14, viral replication occurs in the liver, spleen, or other organs and then a secondary viremia occurs. This leads to widespread cutaneous infection; characteristic exanthem occurs when virus in high titer is released from the internal sites of multiplication (Grose, '81). A prodrome period of headache, fever, and malaise may occur at 1 to 3 days prior to the eruption of the red macular rash, which progresses to papules, vesicles, and pustules. The eruption crusts over and involves the trunk more heavily than the extremities. Additional lesions continue to appear in the same general area for 2 to 6 days.

Complications of varicella include an interstitial pneumonitis, especially in adults. Central nervous system involvement is another complication, which most commonly includes acute cerebellar ataxia, encephalitis, septic meningitis, and myelitis. Other complications include Reye's syndrome, nephrosis, nephritis, arthritis, and myocarditis. Increased risks of complications appear in immunosuppressed individuals.

The first sign of zoster infection is neuralgia, which can continue for a few days to weeks, followed by the characteristic rash of small, fluid-filled blisters typically confined to 1 or more adjacent dermatomes. The blisters or lesions are usually limited to a band spanning one side of the trunk or clustered to one side of the face. Zoster usually involves the thoracic dermatomes followed in frequency by lumbar, cervical, and trigeminal nerve distributions. Severity of infection increases with age. Older patients have persistent neuralgia that can be severe and last from several months to a year.

FETAL AND NEONATAL VARICELLA-ZOSTER INFECTION

VZV infection during pregnancy can result in serious maternal illness and may cause serious damage to the fetus or to the newborn. Congenital defects have been reported after severe maternal varicella or herpes zoster but are so uncommon that analyses to determine rates are plagued with problems. As previously mentioned, 4.5 to 16% of women of childbearing age are susceptible to varicella infection and some of those infected during pregnancy have produced children with congenital defects. In one study, a tabulation of the prevalence of defects in 11 cases from the literature was performed (Williamson, '75). Cataracts, microphthalmus, Horner syndrome, anisocoria, optic atrophy, nystagmus, and chorioretinitis were reported in nine infants; brain damage was seen in seven; and skin scars and hypoplasia of limbs and trunk appeared in six. It was suggested that the hypoplasia of the specific parts could have been due to the degeneration of the nerve supply to that particular area (Fig. 1). It has been very difficult to determine the incidence of such abnormalities in an infected pregnant women population as compared to a control population. There has been only one prospective study to estimate the incidence of such abnormalities. An 8-year study has been reported encompassing approximately 190,000 pregnancies annually in New York City (Siegal, '73). Only four malformations among babies born to 135 mothers who had chickenpox during pregnancy were identified. These compared with five malformations during this period in the 146 matched controls. Only 27 of the pregnancies complicated by chickenpox occurred during the first trimester and, of these, two were associated with congenital anomalies (7.4%) compared with three anomalies among 87 pregnancies in the control population (3.4%). One child whose mother had varicella at 8 weeks of gestation had a unilateral cataract. The second infant whose mother had varicella during the ninth week of gestation had microcephaly.

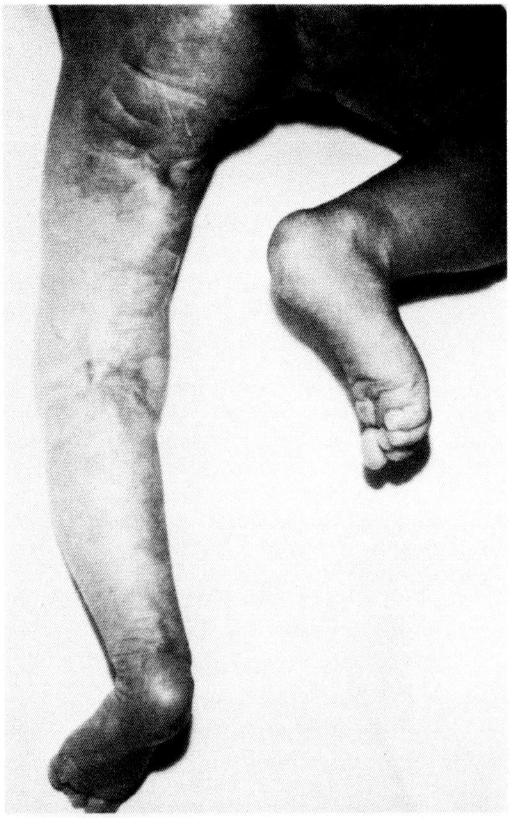

Fig. 1. The photograph shows the lower extremities of a 3-day-old girl delivered two weeks postmature by cesarean section. The mother had varicella in the sixteenth week of pregnancy. The findings at birth were: a red, indurated, scarred lesion in the gluteal region and along the dorsal part of the left leg down to the heel approximating the region of the sciatic nerve. The surface was partly moist and there was an open wound in the gluteal fold. The scar caused slight contractures of the knee and hip. The left leg was smaller than the right one and the fifth toe was rudimentary. The small leg had a blue tinge and felt cold. The deep tendon reflexes could not be elicited and there seemed to be a severe sensory loss in the leg. (By courtesy of Dr. Marta Donner, Helsinki University Central Hospital, Helsinki, Finland.)

Other summaries have called attention to reports of related congenital disease typically consisting of some combination of limb deformity, cicatricial skin lesions, cortical atrophy, and ocular abnormalities (Srabstein et al., '74; Brunell, '83). Most of the cases occurred following maternal VZV infections during the first trimester of pregnancy, typically at 8 to 15 weeks gestation.

Infection relatively late in pregnancy is often manifested at birth or in the newborn period by the presence of the characteristic chickenpox skin lesion plus severe pneumonia with other complications. Zoster lesions with their characteristic segmental distribution have also been observed. Often zoster in children under 2 years of age will elicit a history of intrauterine exposure to VZV. The presence of zoster at this early age should stimulate a search for the residual of congenital damage, especially chorioretinitis. Maternal infection 5 to 10 days before delivery may produce disease in the infant and symptoms usually develop within 4 days of delivery (Meyers, '74). These infants usually escape severe effects of infection, presumably due to maternal antibody conferring some protection. However, maternal infection to 4 days before delivery may result in infection of the infant; approximately 30% of infected children die of disseminated disease or have severe neurological damage. Several reports of zoster during pregnancy have been described (Duehr, '55; Webster, '77; Brazin et al., '79). Statistics are not adequate to calculate attack rates but gestational zoster is less common than varicella.

LABORATORY DIAGNOSIS

Isolation of the virus is usually very difficult. Attempts at isolation should be made from the vesicular fluid of skin lesions within 4 days of their appearance. The passage or storage of virus should be made with whole infected cells of WI-38 cultures or other human cell lines. Some investigators, however, have reported that virus can be isolated using cultures of guinea pig cells (Harbour and Caunt, '75; Edmond et al., '81).

Antibody to varicella, in the past, has been usually measured by the complement fixation (CF) antibody technique. This antibody can be demonstrated in primary infections by the beginning of the second week after onset of the rash. CF antibodies, however, are not long term or lifelong antibodies and will drop to undetectable levels in many individuals after a few months convalescence. Therefore, this antibody test should not be used for determining previous exposure or susceptibility to varicella. The serological tests that can be used to determine immunity with reasonable accuracy include the fluorescent antibody membrane antigen test (FAMA) and the new enzyme linked immunosorbent assay (ELISA) (Williams et al., '74; Forghani et al., '78; Gershon et al., '81). Antibodies usually appear 2 to 5 days after onset of rash and reach maximum titers during the second and third weeks. These include IgG, IgM, and IgA antibodies. Thereafter IgG will decline but persist at low levels for life, whereas IgA and IgM will disappear and are usually not detectable 12 months after the illness (Cradock-Watson et al., '79).

CONTROL AND PREVENTION

It is unknown whether passive immunization of pregnant women with varicella-zoster immune globulin (VZIG) can prevent fetal infection. However, previous studies have shown that passive immunization of pregnant women against rubella still resulted in infants being born with congenital rubella (Cooper, '68). Primary indication for VZIG use in pregnant women should be to prevent complications of varicella in a susceptible adult host rather than preventing intrauterine infection. VZIG has been shown to prevent chickenpox when given to susceptible children within 96 hours of exposure and is recommended for use in new-born infants whose mothers have had the onset of varicella within 5 days prior to or 2 days following delivery (Center for Disease Control, '84). VZIG can be obtained from the regional offices of the American Red Cross. Detailed recommendations for VZIG have recently been published by the American Academy of Pediatrics (AAP, '83).

Interferon and transfer factor has been shown to prevent chickenpox when given to children with leukemia in advance of exposure (Merigan et al., '78; Steele et al., '80). There has been no reported experience in prevention of varicella with these materials in pregnant women. Neither material has been licensed for use. Anti-viral agents have been used for treatment but not prevention of varicella-zoster infection (Whitley et al., '76; '82). Beneficial effects have been noted with the use of these agents in immunocompromised hosts but no information is available of experience in pregnant women and newborns.

It has been reported that a live varicella-zoster vaccine developed in Japan, called the OKA strain, when given within 3 days following exposure, has prevented infection in susceptible children following household and hospital exposure (Asano et al., '82). The vaccine is not licensed in the United States at the present time and can only be used for investigational studies. It has not been used in the newborn nor administered to pregnant women. Reactions with the vaccine were usually mild or absent. Some of the vaccinated subjects develop low grade fevers 10 to 14 days after inoculation and occasionally some have mild vesicular rashes. Zoster has developed in a few vaccinated children with leukemia; however there is no indication of a vaccine-associated increase in the severity or the frequence of zoster. Studies done in the United States with this vaccine would indicate that results are good (Arbeter et al., '82). A second vaccine, the KMcG strain, cultivated in WI 38 cells, has been developed in the United States (Neff et al., '81). Vaccine studies with material passed less than 40 times produced some generalized rashes and seroconversion. Vaccine made at 60 passages, however, was found to be over attenuated and now studies are in progress to produce an intermediate passage (Arbeter et al., '83). Although results look promising with the vaccines available, it will be many years before investigations are complete enough to determine what the possible consequences could be of producing a latent infection with vaccine virus.

SUMMARY

Maternal varicella during pregnancy may have a variety of outcomes on the fetus and the newborn infant. Management of the options and choices by the physician and patient in this situation is rather difficult since recommendations must be made on the basis of very limited data. Convincing evidence of teratogenic effects from VZV has come from a number of studies documenting infection in the first trimester of pregnancy. What is difficult to assess is the incidence of congenital abnormalities during this early gestational period. Information is very limited but does indicate there is about a 4% chance of congenital abnormalities occurring when varicella infection takes place during the first trimester. Additional important information is that maternal infection 5 to 10 days before delivery may produce disease in the infant that will usually develop within 4 days of delivery. Most of these infants will escape the severe effects of infection, presumably due to protection of the maternal antibody. However, if maternal infection is 0 to 4 days before delivery, infection of the infant may result and approximately 30% of the infected children will die of disseminated disease. The use of high titer VZIG in these newborns shortly after birth may prevent disseminated disease.

LITERATURE CITED

American Academy of Pediatrics (AAP), Committee on Infectious Diseases (1983) Expanded guidelines for use of varicella-zoster immune globulin. Pediatrics, *72:* 886–9.

Arbeter, A.M., S.E. Starr, R.E. Weibel, and S.A. Plotkin (1982) Live attenuated varicella vaccine: Immunization of healthy children with OKA strain. J. Pediatr., *100:*886–93.

Arbeter, A.M., S.E. Starr, R.E. Weibel, B.J. Neff, and S.A. Plotkin (1983) Live attenuated varicella vaccine: The KMcC strain in healthy children. Pediatrics, *71:*307–12.

Asano, Y., S. Hirose, S. Iwayama, T. Miyata, T. Yazaki, and M. Takahashi (1982) Protective effect of immediate inoculation of a live varicella vaccine in household contacts in relation to the viral dose and interval between exposure and vaccination. Biken. J., *25:*43–5.

Brazin, S.A., J.W. Simkovich, and W.T. Johnson (1979) Herpes zoster during pregnancy. Obstet Gynecol., *53:*175–181.

Brunell, P.A. (1983) Fetal and neonatal varicella-zoster infections. Semin. Perinatol., 7 *1:*47–56.

Center for Disease Control (1984) Varicella-zoster immune globulin distribution — United States and other countries, 1981–1983. MMWR, *33:*81–100.

Cooper, L.C. (1968) Rubella: A preventable cause of defects. Alan R. Liss, Inc. for the National Foundation—March of Dimes. New York, BD:OAS *IV:*23–25.

Cradock-Watson, J.E., M.K.S. Ridehalgh, and M.S. Bourne (1979) Specific immunoglobulin responses after varicella and herpes zoster. J. Hyg. (Lond), *82:* 319–36.

Duehr, P.H. (1955) Herpes zoster as a cause of congenital cataract. Am. J. Opthalmol., *39:*157–161.

Edmond, B.J., C. Grose, and P.A. Brunell (1981) Varicella-zoster virus infection of diploid and chemically transformed guinea-pig embryo cells; factors influencing virus replication. J. Gen. Virol., *54:*403–7.

Forghani, B., N.J. Schmidt, and J. Dennis (1978) Antibody assays for varicella-zoster virus: Comparison of enzyme immunoassay with neutralization, immune adherence agglutination, and complement fixation. J. Clin. Microbiol., *8:*545–52.

Garland, J. (1943) Varicella following exposure to herpes zoster. N. Engl. J. Med., *228:*336–7.

Gershon, A.A., R. Raker, S. Steinberg, B. Topf-Olstein, and L.M. Drusin (1976) Antibody to varicella-zoster virus in parturient women and their offspring during the first year of life. Pediatrics, *58:*692–6.

Gershon, A.A., H.M. Frey, S.P. Steinberg, M.D. Seeman, D. Bidwell, and A. Voller (1981) Determination of immunity to varicella using an enzyme-linked-immunosorbent assay. Arch. Virol., *70:*169–172.

Grose, C. (1981) Variation on a theme by Fenner: The pathogenesis of chickenpox. Pediatrics, *68:*735–737.

Harbour, D.A. and A.E. Caunt (1975) Infection of guinea pig embryo cells with varicella zoster virus. Arch. Virol., *49:*39–47.

Jezek, Z., W. Hardjotanojo, A.G. Rangaraj (1981) Facial scarring after varicella: A comparison with variola major and variola minor. Am. J. Epidemiol., *114:*798–803.

Merigan, T.C., K.H. Rand, R.B. Pollard, P.S. Abdallah, G.W. Jordan, and R.P. Fried (1978) Human leukocyte interferon for the treatment of herpes zoster in patients with cancer. N. Engl. J. Med., *298:*981–7.

Meyers, J.D. (1974) Congenital varicella in term infants: Risks reconsidered. J. Infect. Dis., *129:*215–217.

Neff, B.J., R.E. Weiber, V.M. Villarejos et al. (1981) Clinical and laboratory studies of K McC strain live atten-

uated varicella virus. Proc. Soc. Exp. Biol. Med., *166:*339–47.
Preblud, S.R. and L.J. D'Angelo (1979) Chickenpox in the United States, 1972–1977. J. Infect. Dis., *140:*257–60.
Preblud, S.R. (1981) Age-specific risks of varicella complications. Pediatrics, *68:*14–17.
Ragozzino, M.W., L.J. Melton III, L.T. Kurland, C.P. Chu, and H.O. Perry (1982) Risk of cancer after herpes zoster: A population-based study. N. Engl. J. Med., *307:* 393–7.
Siegel, M. (1973) Congenital malformations following chickenpox, measles, mumps and hepatitis. JAMA, *226:*1521–1524.
Srabstein, S.C., R.P. Morris, R.P. Lark, et al. (1974) Is there a congenital varicella syndrome? J. Pediatr., *84:*239–243.
Steele, R.W., M.G. Myers, and M.M. Vincent (1980) Transfer factor for the prevention of varicella-zoster infection in childhood leukemia. N. Engl. J. Med., *303:*355–9.
Takahashi, M., T. Otsuka, Y. Okuno, Y. Asano, T. Yazaki, and S. Isomura (1974) Live vaccine used to prevent the spread of varicella in children in hospital. Lancet, *2:*1288–90.
Webster, M.H. (1977) Congenital abnormalities and maternal herpes zoster. Br. Med. J., *2:*1193.
Weller, T.H. (1953) Serial propagation in vitro of agents producing inclusion bodies derived from varicella and herpes zoster. Proc. Soc. Exp. Biol. Med., *83:*340–6.
Whitley, R.J., L.T. Ch'ien, R. Dolin, G.J. Galasso, and C.A. Alford Jr., eds. (1976) Adenine arabinoside therapy of herpes zoster in the immunosuppressed: NIAID Collaborative Antiviral Study. N. Engl. J. Med., *294:*1193–9.
Whitley, R., M. Hilty, R. Haynes, et al. (1982) Vidarabine therapy of varicella in immunosuppressed patients. J. Pediatr., *101:*125–31.
Williams, V., A. Gershon, and P.A. Brunell (1974) Serologic response to varicella-zoster membrane antigens measured by indirect immunofluorescence. Infect. Dis., *130:*669–672.
Williamson, A.P. (1975) The varicella zoster virus in the etiology of severe congenital defects. Clin. Pediatr., *14:*553–559.

TERATOGEN UPDATE: ENVIRONMENTALLY INDUCED BIRTH DEFECT RISKS, PAGES 107–111 (1986)

Venezuelan Equine Encephalitis: Its Relation to Severe Cerebral Malformations

FRANZ WENGER
Emeritus, Department of Pathology, University Hospital and Medical School, University of Zulia State, Maracaibo, Venezuela

Epidemics of equine encephalitis among animals in Venezuela have been related to seasons of heavy rain, because of the proliferation of insect vectors, especially *Aedes taeniorynchus*; the epidemics caused the death of horses and donkeys. The first description was given by Beck and Wyckhoff ('38). The Venezuelan type of equine encephalitis virus was isolated by Kubes and Rios ('39). The disease is not limited to Venezuela—there are reports of isolated cases and epidemics from Colombia, Trinidad, Brasil, Ecuador, and Texas. Human cases have been laboratory infections, of such a mild course that Tigerett et al. ('62), who observed arrest of uterine cancer in women affected by Venezuelan type of encephalitis, proposed vaccination with the virus as treatment of advanced cancer, especially lymphomas. Sporadic cases in humans, by natural infection, were only suspected of being encephalitis (Negrette, '60). In 1962, after a season of unusually heavy rains, which flooded the country, there was a severe epidemic of encephalitis in the North-Western part of Venezuela (Zulia State, Peninsula of Goajira), which clearly affected humans as well as animals; there were quick passages of the virus from sick animals, mostly equine, through insect vectors to man, from man through insects to man, and probably even from human to human directly.

During this epidemic, the population, living in small rural communities, was affected by an acute, usually benign infectious disease (Castillo, '64). The correct diagnosis was made by culture of the virus and by neutralizing antibody tests (Fossaert, '63; Sellers et al., '65). From October to December there were 6,762 officially registered cases, 389 of which were classified clinically as severe, showing significant neurological symptoms; 43 patients died, mostly children (Avilan Rovira '64, '71). The pathological findings in 16 autopsy cases were reported (Wenger '63).

From the very beginning of the epidemic, frequent abortions were observed in women who lived in the affected district and who were pregnant from 1 to 3 months. Later I had the opportunity to examine seven deceased newborns, whose mothers had suffered a severe attack of encephalitis between the thirteenth and thirty-sixth week of pregnancy (Wenger, '67). In these cases, the fetuses had kept on living and developing to full term, despite the fact that the virus had produced severe damage to the brain. Table 1 shows a summary of the lesions related to months of pregnancy, the attack of encephalitis, and clinical findings of mother and child. The fetal abnormalities seem to be the result of a short attack of the virus of Venezuelan equine encephalitis with destruction of the cerebral cortex in the fetus. In cases 5, 6, and 7, time had permitted removal of the necrotic tissue and transformation of the necrotic cerebrum into a cystic mass, a condition similar to "hydro-anencephaly." In cases 1–4, of only 2 weeks to 1 month from the maternal disease to the birth of the child, only hemorrhage and necrotic softening of the brain were found. Clinically, no severe damage in the cerebrum was suspected, and the diagnosis was just "dyspnea." It also seems remarkable that in case 5, the child lived, in poor condition, for 2 days, in the absence of practically any cerebrum. In case 6, there were no active movements at al, including no active breathing at any time; the child lived only by artificial breathing through an intratracheal catheter, which was closed after 4 hours in the absence of any improvement. Case 7 was stillborn.

After 1962 only small outbreaks and sporadic cases (especially in 1964) were seen perhaps because of immunity against infection, or because never since have there been such heavy rains as in 1962. In any case, we had no more autopsy cases like those reported, although we continued to received the large autopsy material at the Maracaibo University Hospital, Division of Pathology, from the maternity wards, where many women from the Northern part of Zulia State, Goajira Peninsula, are attended. As far as I know,

TABLE 1. Clinical findings in seven cases of equine encephalitis

Identification	Case 1 (8610)	Case 2 (8725)	Case 3 (8736)	Case 4 (8792)	Case 5 (10513)	Case 6 (11513)	Case 7 (10754)
Interval between maternal encephalitis and birth	2 weeks	1 month	1 month	1 month	4 months	5 months	5 months
Months of pregnancy at attack of encephalitis	8 1/2 months	8 months	8 months	8 months	5 months	5 months	3 months
Weight at birth	2,800 gr	2,500 gr	2,700 gr	3,050 gr	3,200 gr	3,550 gr	1,400 gr
Clinical aspects of newborn	Dyspnea, convulsions	Dyspnea, omphalitis septicemia	Dyspnea, omphalitis	Severe dyspnea, jaundice	Dyspnea	No active movements; no active respiration; no osteo-tendinous reflexes	Premature, microcephalic microphthalmic; luxation of hip
Age at death	2 days	5 days	7 days	15 min	2 days	4 hours	Stillborn
Cause of death by post-mortem	Broncho-pnemonia	Broncho-pneumonia	Broncho-pneumonia	Atelectasis of lungs	Pulmonary atelectasis broncho-pneumonia	Asphyxia	—
Brain: macroscopic findings	Extensive softening and hemorrhage	Massive necrosis of cerebrum, focal necrosis of cere-bellum.	Massive cerebral necrosis	Necrosis and hemorrhage	Cystic transformation of cerebral hemispheres. Only rudimentary basal ganglia	Only rudimentary foci of cerebrum and basal ganglia; no cerebellum.	Only thin membranes, few small foci of rudimentary nervous tissue; hypoplasia of medulla (2 mm)
Brain: histological findings	Massive necrosis of nervous tissue and necrosis of the wall of blood vessels; thrombosis, infiltration by leuco-cytes.	Necrosis and hemorrhage. perivascular lymphocytic infiltration.	Necrosis, many histiocytes with phagocytosis.	Necrosis and hemorrhage. Granulation tissue progressing from meninges	Connective tissue with phagocytic histocytes. Only small foci of residual nervous tissue	Rudimentary foci of nervous tissue, with neuroglia, but very few ganglion cells. Small foci of calcification.	Neuroglia with few ganglion cells; retina formed only by two layers of epithelium

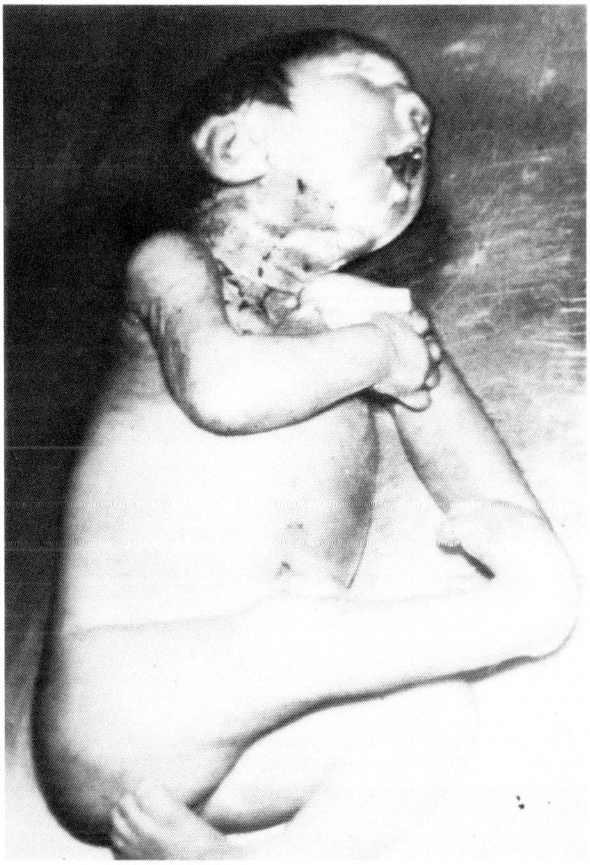

Fig. 1. Stillborn fetus, thirty-third week of pregnancy. 20 weeks after attack of maternal encephalitis: microcephalus, microphthalmia, luxation of hip.

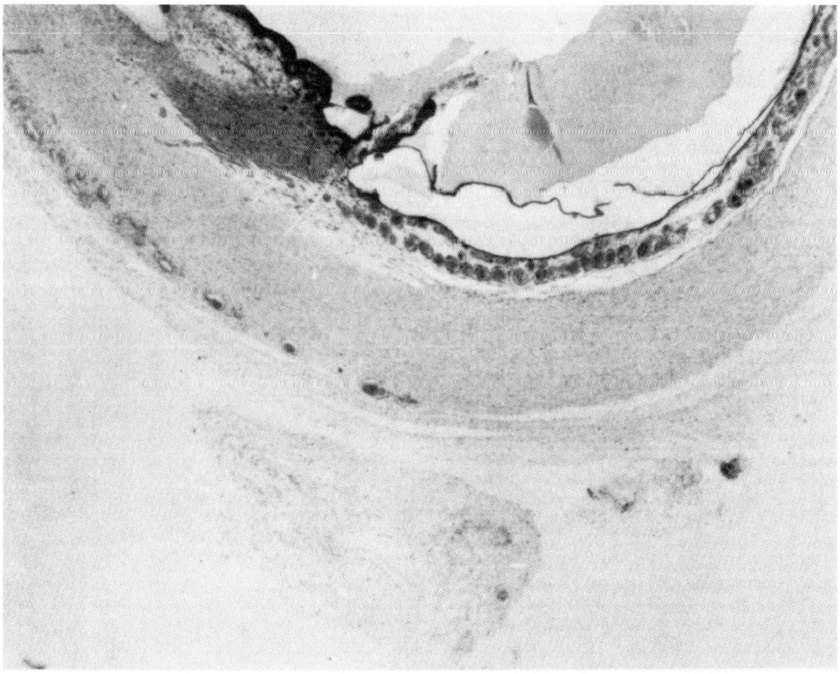

Fig. 2. The same case as Figure 1: Low power view of eye, which is well developed except for the retina, which consists only of two sheets of pigmented, single-layered epithelium.

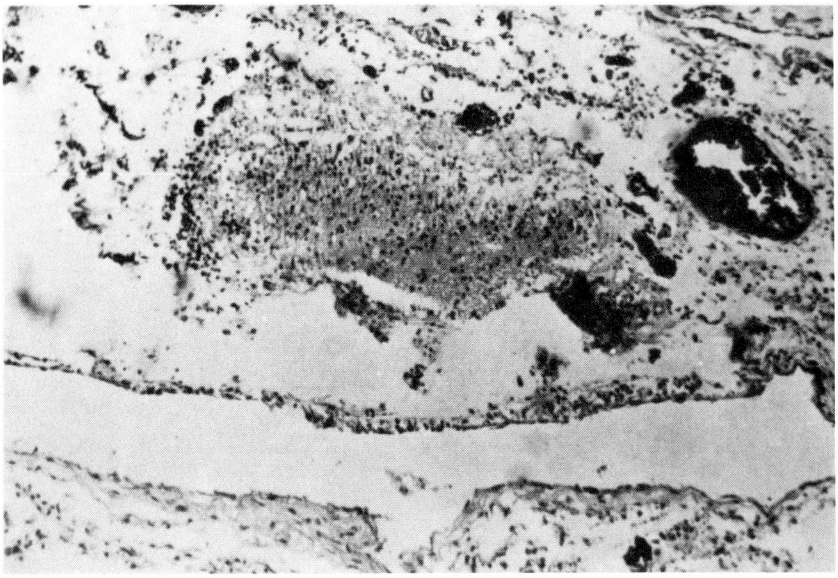

Fig. 3. Infant born at term, encephalitis at 20 weeks of pregnancy with hydroanencephaly. A small remainder of cerebral tissue, which had survived, is seen surrounded by proliferated meningeal tissue.

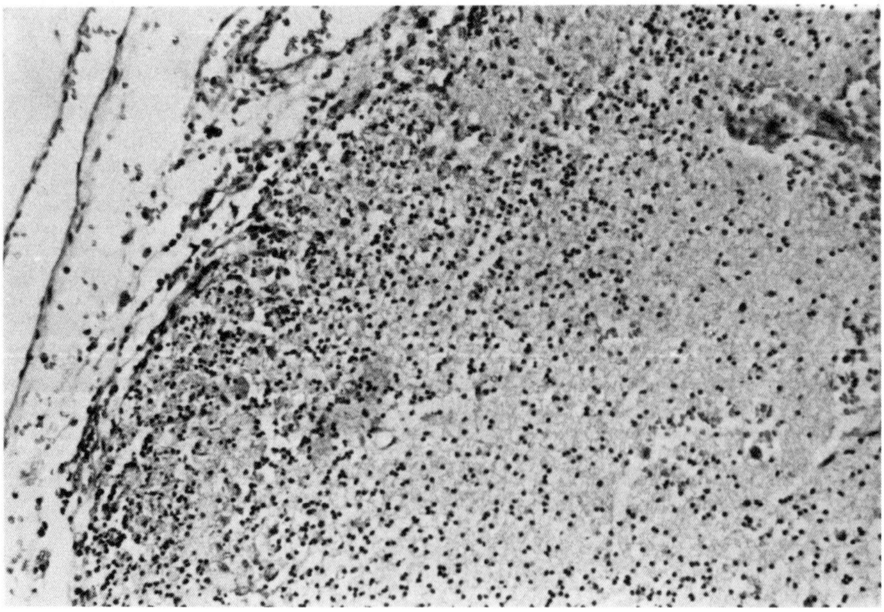

Fig. 4. Infant born on term, encephalitis 1 month earlier: there is necrosis of the cerebral cortex, with beginning resorption.

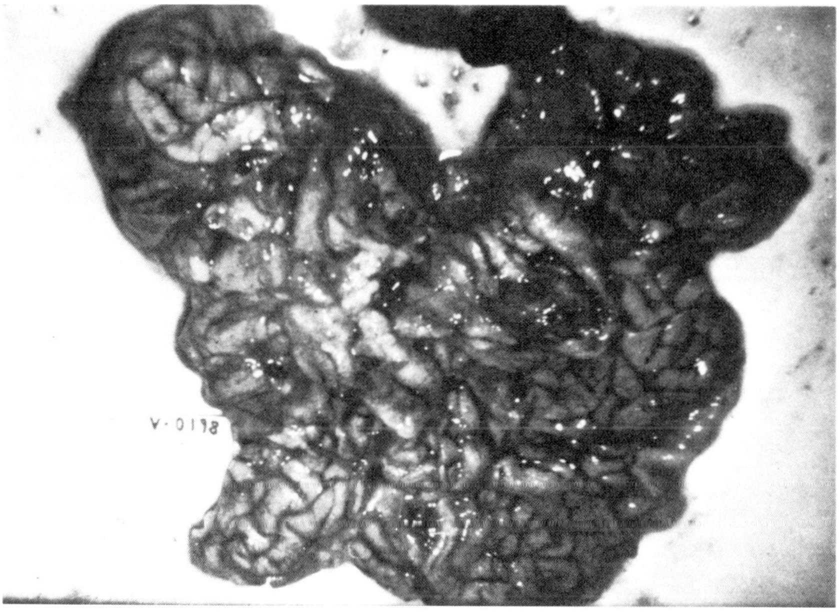

Fig. 5. Infant born nearly on term; encephalitis 2 weeks earlier: gross view of cerebrum, showing diffuse softening and hemorrhage.

there were no reports of hydro-anencephaly-like cases after maternal encephalitis. Yet London et al. ('77) reported cerebral and ocular malformations induced in Rhesus monkey fetuses by injection of Venezuelan encephalitis virus, thus giving experimental support to the pathological and clinical observation of this virus being a potential teratogen. Therefore, pregnant women should be advised to move away from areas of epidemics of encephalitis—especially those due to the Venezuelan type of virus—as a means of prevention of malformations in the offspring.

LITERATURE CITED

Avilan Rovira, J.M. (1965): El brote de Encephalitis Equina Venezolana al Norte del Estado Zulia a fines de 1962. Rev. Venez. de Sanidad y Asistencia Social, Vol 29, *3:*291.

Avilan Rovira, J.M. (1971): Epidemiología, de las Encephalitis en Venezuela, según las estadísticas de mortalidad. Publicaciones del Depto. de Demografia y Epidemiología, Ministerio de Sanidad y Asistencia Social, Caracas.

Beck, C.E. and Wyckhoff (1938): Science, *88:*530.

Castillo, C.E. (1964): Informe sobre una reciente epidemia de encefalitis equina Venezolana, en la Zona Norte del Estado Zulia. Rev. Venez. San. y Asist. Soc., *29:*325.

Fossaert H. (1963): Symposium sobre Virología en la Encephalitis Equina Venezolana. 10a Convención Anual de la Asoc. Venezol. para el avance de la Ciencia, Caracas.

Kubes, V. and F.A. Rios (1939): The causative agent of infectious equine encephalo-myelitis in Venezuela. Science, *90:*20.

London, W.T., N.H. Levitt, S.G. Kent, V.G. Wong, and J.L. Sever (1977): Congenital cerebral and ocular malformations induced in Rhesus Monkeys by Venezuelan equine encephalitis virus. Teratology, *16:* 285.

Negrette, A. (1967): Encefalitis epidemica. Investigaciones Clínicas *1:*11.

Sellers, R.F., G.H. Bergold, O.M. Suarez, and A. Morales (1965): Investigations during Venezuelán equine encephalitis outbreaks in Venezuela. Am. J. Trop. Med. Hyg., *14:*460.

Tigerett, W.D., W.H. Crosby, T.O. Berge, D.L. Howie, S. Kress, H.G. Dangerfield, J.W. Ross, and W. Frank (1962): The virus of Venezuelan equine encephalo-myelitis as an anti-neoplastic agent in man. Cancer *15:*628.

Wenger, F. (1963): Hallazgos de Anatomía Patológica en la reciente epidemia de encefalitis equina Venezolana. Investigaciones Clinicas, *7:*21.

Wenger, F. (1967): Necrosis cerebral masiva del feto en casos de encefalitis equina Venezolana. *21:*13.

TERATOGEN UPDATE: ENVIRONMENTALLY INDUCED BIRTH DEFECT RISKS, PAGES 113–117 (1986)

Congenital Syphilis

JOHN H. GROSSMAN III
Department of Obstetrics and Gynecology, George Washington University Medical Center, Washington, D.C. 20037

The damage due to fetal infection with *Treponema pallidum,* untreated during pregnancy, ranges from fulminent neonatal sepsis and death to asymptomatic infection persisting in childhood and culminating in tertiary syphilis in early adolescence. By convention, clinicians classify congenital syphilis as "early" and "late." This terminology specifically refers to the time in the child's life when the diagnosis of syphilis is made.

MANIFESTATIONS

Early congenital syphilis is an infectious, life threatening disease apparent in children under 2 years of age. The children are often small for gestational age, or premature with hemolytic anemia, hepatosplenomegaly, and occasionally hydrops. The placenta is frequently large (feto-placental ratios less than 5:1) with villitis and perivasculitis. Spirochetes may be demonstrable using special staining techniques. A maculopapular or vesiculobullous rash may be present. Fluid from skin lesions may be found to contain spirochetes when studied using darkfield microscopy. Over 50% of these infants have "snuffles," a thick white or blood-tinged nasal discharge (Fig. 1) teeming with treponemes. Periosteitis and long bone osteochondritis can cause Parrott's pseudoparalysis, due to bone and joint pain. Meningitis and cerebrospinal fluid abnormalities are not uncommon.

Late congenital syphilis appears in children over 2 years of age and is asymptomatic in two-thirds of all cases. Serology is invariably positive. Those with findings have the more classical "stigmata" of congenital syphilis. These include interstitial keratitis, VIII nerve deafness, dental and bony deformities (Hutchinson's teeth, mulberry molars, sabre shins, saddle nose, frontal bossing, palatal perforation, Clutton's joints), cutaneous lesions (rhagades and gummas), and, rarely, neurologic and cardiovascular defects (Figs. 2–4).

EPIDEMIOLOGY

Although congenital syphilis appears less prevalent than a decade ago, several hundred cases continue to occur in the United States annually. It is difficult to know how many of the 5,000 reported cases among women of childbearing age in 1980 (Taber, '82) actually resulted in infections among offspring. Recent series reporting pregnancy outcome following antepartum diagnosis of maternal syphilis (Jones and Harris, '79; Srinivasan et al., '83) suggest that more than three-fourths of infants delivered under these circumstances are asymptomatic at birth. This suggests that serosurveillance during pregnancy coupled with aggressive treatment of suspected cases greatly reduces the likelihood of symptomatic disease at birth. It also suggests the potential for late congenital syphilis (which should be a preventable disease) in cases where inadequately-treated infants fail to receive careful followup. Compliance with followup of infants is frequently poor among at-risk groups; Srinivasan et al. ('83) reported that less than one-half of affected newborns returned for followup after discharge. Fortunately, antepartum detection and aggressive postpartum treatment makes late congenital syphilis uncommon in the majority of cases.

Dissemination of syphilis to the fetus is possible at all stages of maternal infection, including the late latent stage, when asymptomatic patients remain persistently seropositive. Most frequently, however, dissemination is associated with a placentitis arising from hematogenous spread of the spirochetes between the first and second stage of infection in the mother. Untreated syphilis results in congenital infection in 75–95% of all cases (Taber, '82).

Contrary to previous thought, pregnancies are not impervious to treponemal invasion during the first half of gestation. Careful histologic examination has demonstrated spirochetes in products of conception in the first trimester (Harter and Benirschke, '76). Dissolution of the cytotrophoblast was previously postulated as the cause of fetal susceptibility to infection after the eighteenth week; however, electron microscopy has failed to demonstrate any loss of tissue integrity. Recently, immunologic immaturity in fetuses has been proposed to explain

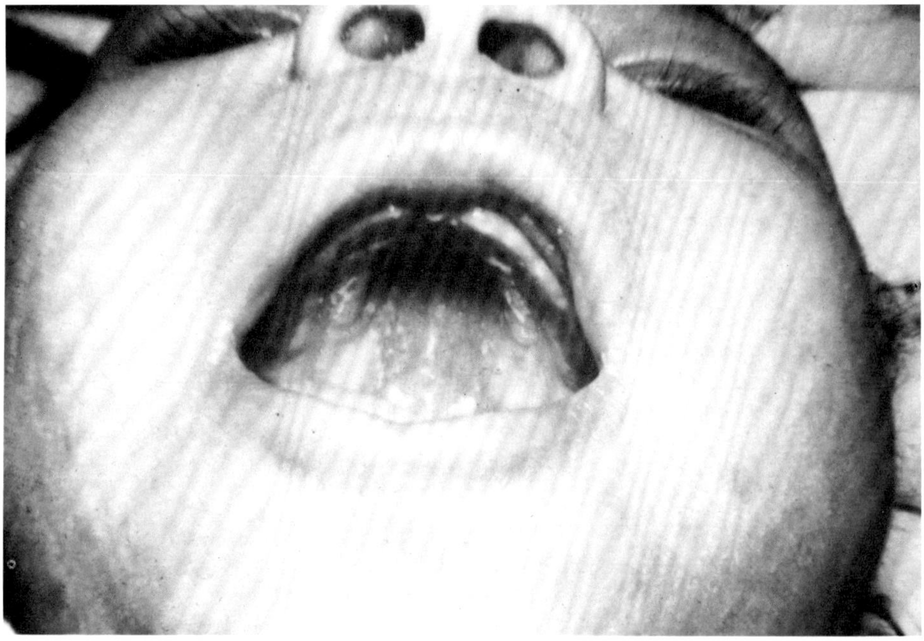

Fig. 1. Nasopharyngeal discharge of early congenital syphilis.

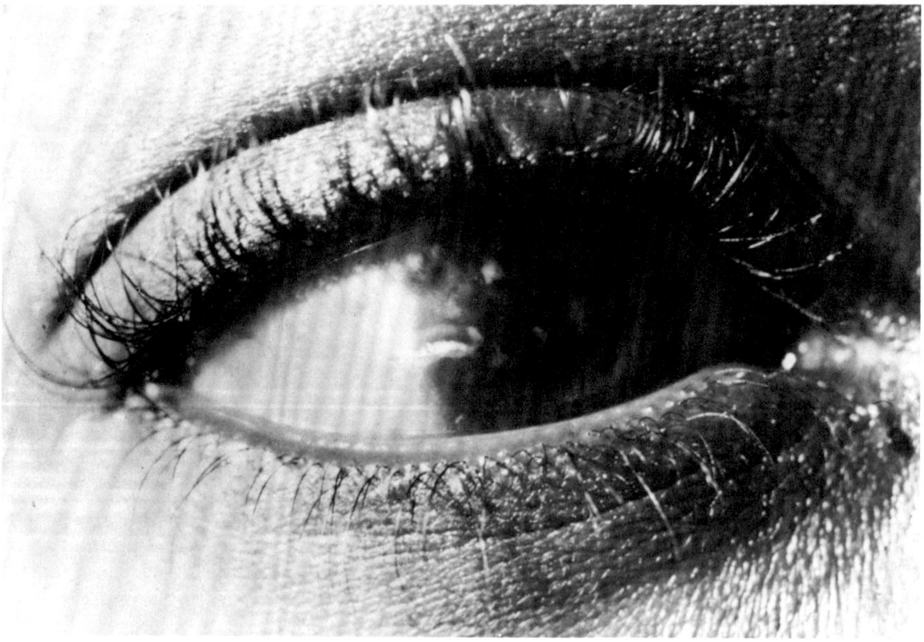

Fig. 2. Interstitial keratitis of late congenital syphilis.

the absence of any apparent fetal inflammatory response to infection during the first twenty gestational weeks (Taber, '82). Signs of congenital syphilis are uncommon before the infant is three weeks old; indeed if they are present at birth, the prognosis is usually unfavorable (Jones and Harris, '79; Srinivasan et al., '83).

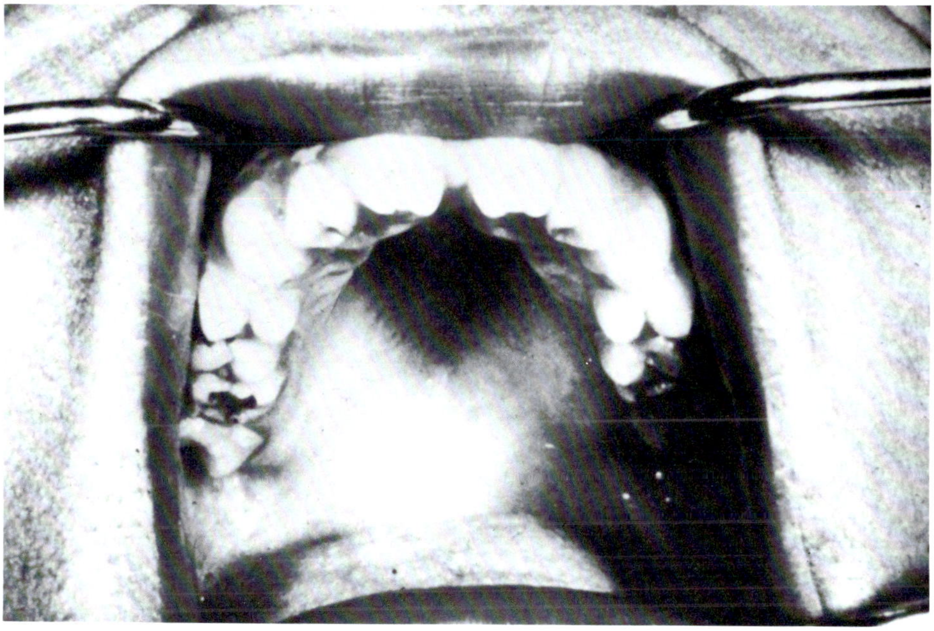

Fig. 3. Notched incisors (Hutchinson's teeth) of late congenital syphilis.

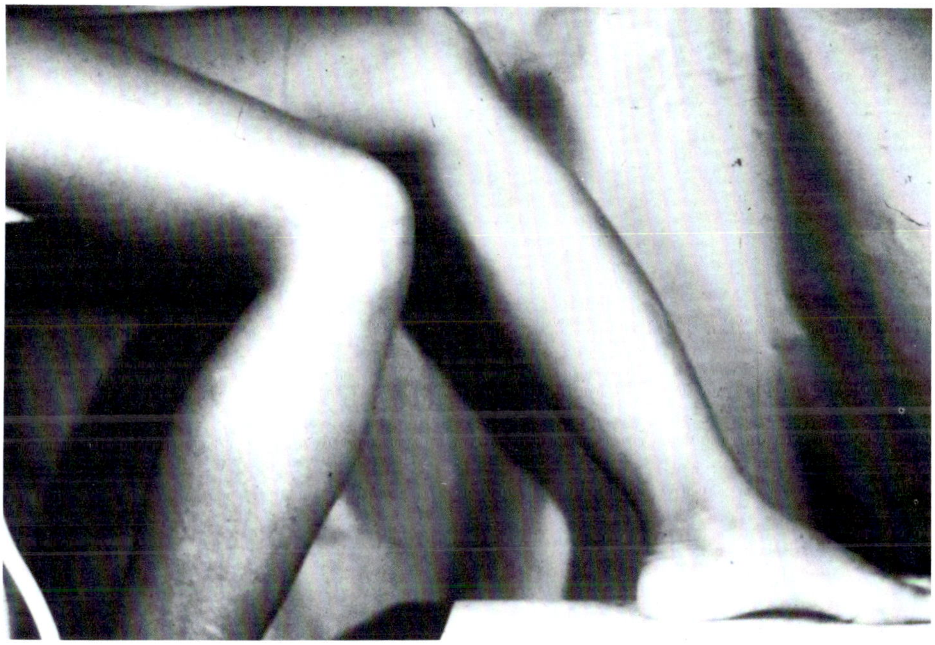

Fig. 4. Sabre shins of late congenital syphilis.

DIAGNOSIS

Congenital syphilis is preventable if maternal infection is detected and adequately treated early in pregnancy. The presence of an indurated painless ulcer should suggest the possibility that a syphilitic chancre is present. Subtle lesions missed during a cursory genital examination or unobserved extragenital lesions, especially oral chancres, may incorrectly exclude the diagnosis. Since serologic reactivity may have not developed among individuals with primary syphilis, a darkfield microscopic examination of secretions from the lesions is mandatory. Women who are not treated should receive followup serologic testing in 4 to 6 weeks to detect seroconversion.

The presence of a diffuse maculopapular rash, especially when accompanied by generalized lymphadenopathy, mucous patches, and condylomata lata, should prompt suspicion of syphilis and initiate appropriate serologic testing. Unfortunately, this is not always the case. Chapel ('81) reported 34 cases of secondary syphilis seen by 36 physicians. One-third of these practitioners failed to consider the diagnosis of syphilis but routine serologic screening ultimately established the diagnosis. Nearly one-seventh failed to establish the correct diagnosis either clinically or by laboratory testing.

District of Columbia Health Regulations require serologic screening for syphilis at all initial registration prenatal visits or within 30 days thereafter. Additionally, the Commission of Public Health strongly recommends that a second serology be performed during the last trimester. Since serologic screening may produce biologic false positive tests during pregnancy, confirmation of seroreactivity should be made using a syphilis-specific test such as the fluorescent treponeme absorption (FTA-ABS) test or the microhemagglutination test for *Treponema pallidum* (MHA-TP). These tests remain positive lifelong after initial infection and are thus not useful in the diagnosis and management of individuals with known previous infections (Wood, '76). In contrast, with prompt treatment, most reaginic tests for syphilis revert to negative. Following treatment during pregnancy, we perform monthly VDRL (Venereal Disease Research Laboratories) titers and retreat if titers subsequently rise again later in gestation. Infants of treated mothers require careful serologic and clinical scrutiny at and following birth.

Diagnosis of symptomatic neonatal infection can be accomplished in several ways. Demonstration of spirochetes in skin lesions or nasal discharge is diagnostic as is a cord VDRL antibody titre 4-fold greater than that of maternal serum. Unfortunately, most cases present without physical signs. These are more difficult diagnostic problems and often the only clue consists of a vague history of maternal venereal disease treated during pregnancy.

Cord blood IgM testing has been proposed as a general screening test for congenital infections and FTA-ABS-IgM (Fluorescent Treponeme Antibody Absorption-Immunoglobulin M) as a specific test for congenital syphilis. The latter assay is not generally available and it has been suggested that false positives may arise from fetal IgM directed against maternal IgG (Reimer et al., '75). In such instances, maternal IgG antibody elaborated in response to infection is acquired passively by the fetus, which then produces an IgM anti-antibody. The absence of a reactive cord blood FTA-ABS-IgM does not exclude congenital syphilis; 10% of infants with congenital infection are seronegative at birth (Kaufmann et al., '75).

Asymptomatic seropositive offspring of mothers who were treated for syphilis during pregnancy present a problem in clinical management. More specific treponemal tests or IgM assays can be employed if available. If the titer is due to passive maternal transfer of IgG without congenital infection, serial VDRLs should show a quantitative decrease with time and revert to negative by 6 months of life (Taber, '82).

Srinivasan et al. ('83) have said that the likelihood of asymptomatic neurosyphilis among newborns is low. McCracken and Kaplan ('74) failed to detect FTA-ABS-IgM in the spinal fluid of 16 asymptomatic infants. On the other hand, Jones and Harris ('79) found seroreactivity in the spinal fluid of 2/18 infants despite documented antepartum treatment of the mother. In view of the notoriously poor followup of potentially infected infants, aggressive diagnostic evaluation and/or therapy seems warranted. Certainly, examination of spinal fluid for pleocytosis, elevated protein, or positive serology is indicated in suspicious cases.

TREATMENT

Early in vitro studies have shown 0.03 mcg/ml of penicillin to be treponemicidal; however, the long replication time of the spirochete necessitates maintaining these levels for periods of 1 to 2 weeks for adequate therapy. Benzathine penicillin is well-suited for maternal therapy and the CDC recommends intramuscular injection of 2.4 million units in a single dose for adult syphilis of less than 1 year's duration. The same dose given weekly for 3 weeks is adequate therapy for syphilis of more than 1 year's duration. In the latter instance, neurosyphilis must be specifically excluded by lumbar puncture.

Positive cerebrospinal fluid findings require parenteral penicillin-G (aqueous or procaine) since benzathine penicillin crosses the blood/brain barrier poorly. Doses administered for neurosyphilis should range from 12 to 24 million units per day given for at least 10 days. Some authorities have theorized that single dose benzathine penicillin therapy of women with primary syphilis may be inadequate for treating intrauterine neurosyphilis in their babies. As discussed earlier, careful evaluation of even apparently normal newborns of such women seems prudent.

Penicillin-allergic pregnant women with syphilis should not receive tetracycline therapy due to potential adverse effects upon fetal dentition and bone. Oral erythromycin stearate, ethylsuccinate, or base in doses of two grams per day for 15 to 20 days should be effective for the mother. Congenital syphilis has been reported in infants after such therapy, however, perhaps due to inconsistent transplacental distribution of erythromycin.

We follow women treated for syphilis during pregnancy with monthly VDRLs until delivery and their children are examined and followed carefully after birth. All infants with suspected congenital syphilis are evaluated for evidence of neurosyphilis by lumbar puncture. Neonatal syphilis with neurologic involvement requires parenteral aqueous or procaine penicillin G—50,000 units per kilogram every day for a minimum of 10 days. Infants with normal cerebrospinal fluid should receive a single dose of intramuscular benzathine penicillin G, 50,000 units per kilogram.

PREVENTION

One half of the cases of congenital syphilis reported each year have received no serologic screening during pregnancy. A proportion of such cases have received no prenatal care. Others are missed because screening was not performed during both the first and third trimesters of pregnancy, the later being especially appropriate in "high risk" patient populations. All patients with positive serologies in pregnancy require followup consisting of a history for recent or past syphilis exposure, a thorough re-examination for mucocutaneous lesions, a treponemal test for syphilis, and evaluation for neurosyphilis with appropriate chemotherapy as indicated. Serologic testing must be repeated monthly for the remainder of pregnancy. It is important to trace contacts and consider the possibility of re-infection, as well. Infants of mothers who have been diagnosed and treated require careful scrutiny at birth and they should be treated if there is any question concerning the adequacy of previous therapy in utero. Finally, even in the absence of positive maternal serology, congenital syphilis should be part of the differential diagnosis of any seriously infected child and appropriate steps should be instituted to establish or exclude the diagnosis.

Untreated intrauterine syphilis can cause abortion, stillbirth or neonatal infection with or without symptoms and signs. Thus the infection poses a threat to human pregnancy at all stages of gestation. Although it is generally presumed that early diagnosis and treatment of syphilis complicating the first 20 weeks of pregnancy is rarely associated with long-term perinatal damage, late treatment (for example, at birth or later) will prevent further damage but will not reverse damage already done. In general, early diagnosis and treatment of perinatal syphilis provides the best outlook. Serosurveillance, followup, and aggressive use of antibiotic therapy are crucial to assure a successful pregnancy outcome.

LITERATURE CITED

Chapel, T.A. (1981) Physician recognition of the signs and symptoms of secondary syphilis, JAMA, *246:*250–251.

Harter, C.A. and K. Benirschke (1976) Fetal syphilis in the first trimester. Am. J. Obstet. Gynecol., *124:*705–711.

Jones, J.E. and R.E. Harris (1979) Diagnostic evaluation of syphilis during pregnancy. Obstet. Gynecol., *54:*611–614.

Kaufman, R.E., D.C. Olansky, and P.J. Weisner (1975) The FTA-ABS (IgM) test for neonatal syphilis. A critical review. J. Am. Vener. Dis. Assoc., *1:*79–84.

McCracken, J.H. and J.M. Kaplan (1974) Penicillin treatment for congenital syphilis, JAMA, *228:*855–860.

Reimer, C.B., C.M. Black, D.J. Phillips, L.C. Logan, E.F. Hunter, B.J. Pender, and B.E. McGrew (1975) The specificity of fetal IgM: Antibody or anti-antibody? Ann. NY Acad. Sci., *254:*77–93.

Srinivasan, G., R.S. Ramamurthy, A. Bharthi, S. Voora, and R.S. Pildes (1983) Congenital syphilis: A diagnostic and therapeutic dilemma. Pediatr. Infect. Dis., *2:*436–441.

Taber, L.H. (1982) Evaluation and management of syphilis in pregnant women and newborn infants. Pediatr. Infect. Dis., *1:*224–227.

Wood, R.M. (1976) Tests for Syphilis. In: Manual of Clinical Immunology. N.R. Rose and H. Friedman, eds. American Society for Microbiology, Washington, D.C.

TERATOGEN UPDATE: ENVIRONMENTALLY INDUCED BIRTH DEFECT RISKS, PAGES 119–121 (1986)

Methylmercury Poisoning

BERNARD WEISS AND RICHARD A. DOHERTY
Division of Toxicology and Environmental Health Sciences Center, Department of Radiation Biology, and Department of Pediatrics, University of Rochester School of Medicine, Rochester, New York 14642

MANIFESTATIONS

Methylmercury is the most toxic compound of mercury. Its toxic properties are most clearly evidenced by neurological and behavioral disturbances. Sensory malfunctions include paresthesias, astereognosis, and apparent constriction of the visual fields. Motor manifestations range from impairment of fine coordination to gross ataxia, depending upon the degree of exposure. A variety of nonspecific symptoms have also been described. Fetal and neonatal intoxication can impair behavioral development and produce severe brain damage. Congenital malformations are rare. The consequences most difficult to ascertain, however, are postnatal functional (behavioral) deficits that may require advanced behavioral methods to characterize and that may not be detectable for many years owing to compensatory mechanisms within the central nervous system (Weiss, '83).

EPIDEMIOLOGY

Toxic exposure of populations has occurred mainly in two ways. Methylmercury is a cheap and effective fungicide frequently used in the past to treat seed wheat and other seed grains. Several poisoning episodes have resulted from consumption of homemade bread prepared from methylmercury-treated seed wheat. The most severe and best studied was a major disaster in Iraq in the winter of 1971–72 (Bakir et al., '73; Amin-Zaki et al., '81).

Other populations have been exposed by consuming fish containing high concentrations of methylmercury. In the Japanese cities of Minamata and Niigata, industrial discharge of mercury into local waterways resulted in high fish concentrations and poisoning of local fish-eating families (Tsubaki and Irukayama, '77).

Certain fish from inland lakes in the United States, Canada, and Sweden, contaminated by mercury effluent from chloralkali plants and paper mills, also have demonstrated high methylmercury concentrations. Microorganisms in bottom sediment convert the inorganic mercury to the highly toxic methyl form. Recent studies of the impact of acid precipitation indicates that its ability to leach metals from soil, combined with its lowering of pH, sharply elevates the concentration of methylmercury in fish from affected lakes, as in the Adirondacks.

Other fish-eating populations take in substantial quantities from the consumption of predatory oceanic species, such as swordfish and shark. The source of methylmercury in pelagic fish is unclear, but it appears to arise from geologic sources and cumulates through the food chain. Except for the Japanese outbreaks, however, clinical poisoning from fish ingestion has not arisen as a serious public health threat. Much more worrisome is the prospect of subtle functional impairment in some members of populations that consume contaminated fish. The fetal brain is the source of this concern.

Methylmercury is known to pass freely from mother to fetus and both human and animal observations suggest that the developing fetal brain is the most sensitive organ. Infants may also be exposed to significant amounts of mercury through suckling if the mother has consumed methylmercury. Adding to the hazard, infants excrete mercury less rapidly than adults. Dose-response calculations based on the data from Iraq (Clarkson et al., '81) suggest that the fetus is at least 4–10 times as sensitive as the adult to methylmercury toxicity, displaying evidence of both motor and intellectual retardation. Methylmercury profoundly interferes with brain development in all species investigated experimentally (Spyker, '75).

DIAGNOSIS

The only way definitively to confirm a diagnosis of methylmercury poisoning, if neurologic criteria are consistent, is to establish exposure, particularly by chemical assay. Atomic absorption methods are probably the most useful for routine determinations of blood and hair mercury levels. Hair is espe-

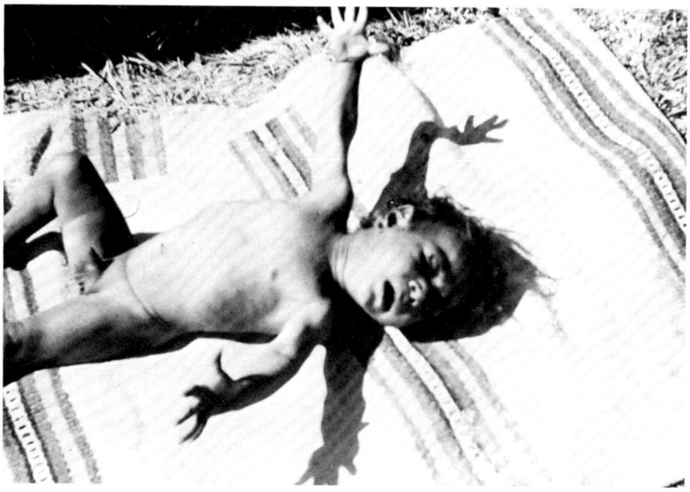

Fig. 1. Congenital methylmercury poisoning—cerebral syndrome dominated by hypertonicity, mental retardation and blindness at 20 months of age. (Amin-Zaki et al., '74. By permission.)

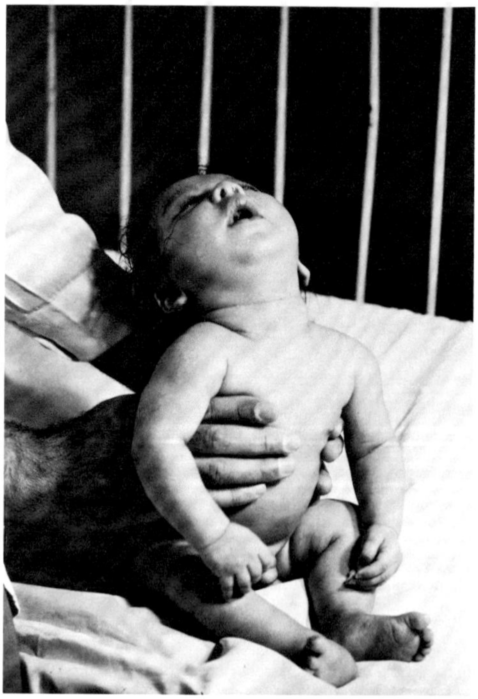

Fig. 2. Congenital methylmercury poisoning—cerebral palsy syndrome with severe motor and mental handicap, blindness, and deafness. (Amin-Zaki et al., '74. By permission.)

cially useful for recapitulating exposure history since it grows approximately 1 cm/month, and the amount incorporated into growing hair is directly proportional to concurrent mercury concentration in blood (Clarkson et al., '81)

TREATMENT

No totally satisfactory method of treatment has yet been established, and treatment remains a difficult problem. Several new techniques appear promising, however, but only for acute treatment. The chelating agent DMPS (2,3-dimercaptopropane sulfonate) was used with some success in Iraq and has shown its effectiveness in animal studies. Since the main public health threat stems from fetal exposure, however, prevention is the main therapeutic strategy. Given the long half-life of methylmercury (50–140 days), women anticipating pregnancy should avoid fish from contaminated areas and also marine fish, such as swordfish, with high flesh concentrations of methylmercury.

PREVENTION

Methylmercury poisoning can be prevented only by insuring that the contaminant does not enter food supplies. This requires that it no longer be used as a fungicide and that industrial discharge of mercury into the environment be halted. Since inorganic mercury and certain of its compounds can be converted by microorganisms in bottom sed-

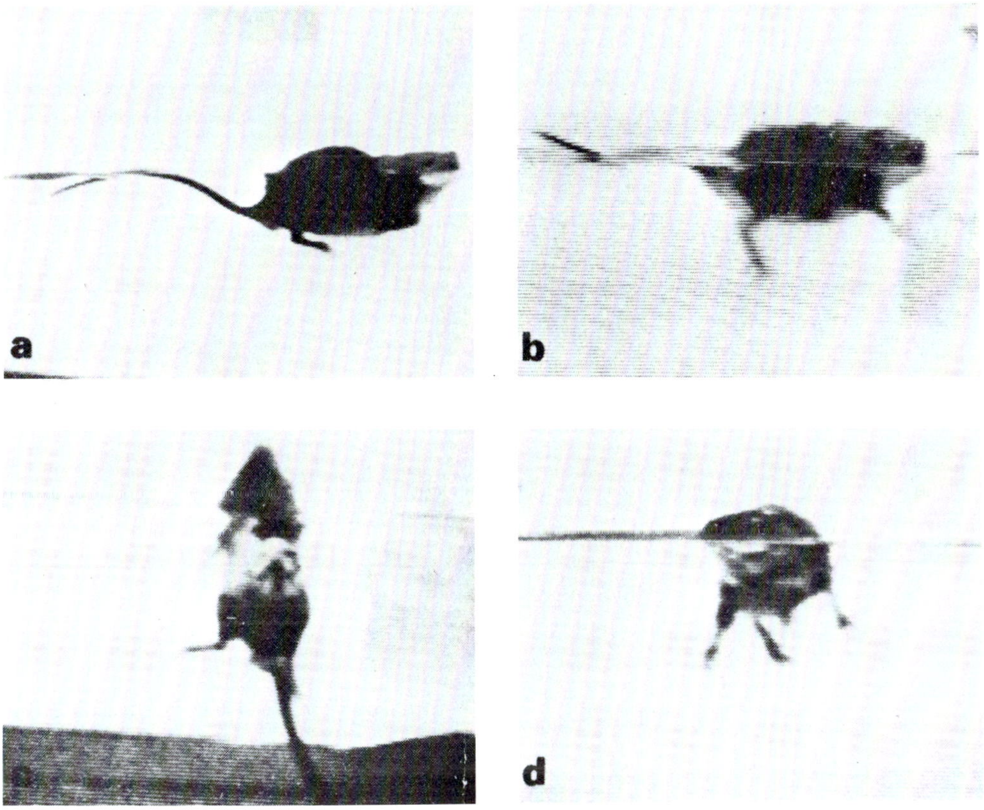

Fig.3. Comparison of swimming postures in control and methylmercury dicyandiamine-treated mice (prenatal administration). Controls a) swim with front legs tucked, hind legs alternately kicking to turn or propel, and tail under water for balance and propulsion. Figures, b), c), and d) show characteristic swimming postures of methylmercury-treated mice. The "freezing" posture with all legs extended is shown in b), floating suspended in a vertical position with only the head above water in c), and swimming with legs askew and inability to maintain normal orientation in water in d). (From Weiss and Spyker, Pediatrics, *53*:851–853, 1974. By permission.)

iment to the most toxic methyl form, which ascends the food chain to organisms consumed by humans, current and future waste mercury deposits may represent a long-term threat to health. In addition, the long-range hazards posed by the consequences of acid rain must be dealt with on almost a global scale if prevention is to be considered seriously.

ACKNOWLEDGMENTS

This paper was supported in part by NIH grants ESO1247 and ESO1248 to the University of Rochester Environmental Health Sciences Center as well as a contract with The U.S. Energy Research and Development Administration at the University of Rochester Biomedical and Environmental Research Project under which it has been assigned Report No. DOE/EVO/3490-2396

LITERATURE CITED

Amin-Zaki, L., M.A. Majeed, M.R. Greenwood, S.B. Elhassani, T.W. Clarkson, and R.A. Doherty (1981) Methylmercury poisoning in the Iraqi suckling infant: A longitudinal study over five years. J. Appl. Toxicol., *1*:210–214.

Bakir, F., S.F. Damluji, L. Amin-Zaki, M. Murtadha, A. Khalidi, N.J. Al-Rawi, S. Tikriti, H.I. Dahir, T.W. Clarkson, J.C. Smith, and R.A. Doherty (1973) Methylmercury poisoning in Iraq. Science *181*:230–241.

Clarkson, T.W., C. Cox, D.O. Marsh, G.J. Myers, S.K. Al-Tikriti, L. Amin-Zaki, and A.R. Dabbagh (1981) Dose-response relationships for adult and prenatal exposure to methylmercury. In: Measurement of Risks. G.G. Berg and H.D. Maillie, eds. Plenum, New York, pp.111–130.

Spyker, M.J. (1975) Behavioral teratology and toxicology. In: Behavioral Toxicology. B. Weiss and V.G. Laties, eds. Plenum, New York, pp.311–344.

Tsubaki, F. and K. Irukayama, eds. (1977) Minamata Disease. Elsevier, New York.

Weiss, B. (1983) Behavioral toxicology of heavy metals. In: Neurobiology of the Trace Elements. I. Dreosti and R. Smith, eds. Humana Press, pp.1–50.

Congenital Minamata Disease: Intrauterine Methylmercury Poisoning

MASAZUMI HARADA
Department of Epidemiology, Institute for Medical Genetics, Kumamoto University Medical School, Kumamoto 862 Japan

In 1955, many cases of severe neurological disease were found in the Minamata area of Kyushu, Japan. In 1959 it was demonstrated that the symptoms were due to poisoning by methylmercury, an effluent from an acetaldehyde plant of the Chisso Corporation. The toxin was transmitted through ingestion of seafood taken in Minamata Bay, hence the term "Minamata disease" (Study Group of Minamata Disease, Kumamoto University, 1968).

Meanwhile, in 1958, Professor Kitamura had discovered that in the district there were many infants, born after 1955, who showed symptoms resembling those of cerebral palsy. He stated: "It is possible that the substance causing the poisoning was transferred to the infants through the placenta or mother's milk, producing symptoms similar to those of Minamata disease" (Kitamura et al., '59; Kitamura et al., '60).

Thereafter, careful epidemiological and clinical studies were conducted (Harada, '64; Harada, '68), and pathological research as well (Matsumoto et al, '65; Takeuchi, '77), so that by 1962 the disease was identified as methylmercury poisoning via placenta. Subsequently, experimental findings confirming the fact have been made public successively (Morikawa, '61; Moriyama, '67; Fujita, '69). A long time was needed for reaching that conclusion because it was contrary to prevailing beliefs. It was thought that, as in the case of the blood-brain barrier, poison could not easily pass through the placenta, and that the fetus was thus protected. However, some poisons actually not only pass through the placenta but can also afflict the fetus without causing serious damage to the mother.

Congenital Minamata disease was first elucidated clinically in Minamata, but there have been some similar reports. Cases of cerebral palsy with mental deficiency are described in a report concerning poisoning caused by eating seed grain treated with alkyl mercury, announced in Sweden by Engleson and Herner in 1952. They suspected in this case that alkyl mercury had passed through the placenta. Perhaps this was the first description of what is now known as congenital Minamata disease. Reported thereafter were many cases in Minamata; one in Niigata, Japan (Harada, '76); one in New Mexico (Synder, '71); and six cases in Iraq (Amin-Zaki et al., '74). Judging from these facts, congenital Minamata disease is not the problem of Minamata alone.

MANIFESTATIONS

During pregnancy or at birth, no abnormality has been observed in mothers of affected children. No conspicuous abnormality has been seen in newborns' weight at birth or number of months in utero. Breast-fed infants were most numerous, and some had mixed feeding. It was at the beginning of the sixth month after birth that abnormalities were recognized. Symptoms were instability of neck, convulsion, and failure of the eyes to follow. Patients developed severe neurological symptoms as well as mental symptoms. Observed at a high rate were common symptoms such as intelligence disturbance (100%), primitive reflex (100%), cerebellar symptoms (100%), disturbance of body growth and nutrition (100%), dysarthria (100%), deformity of limbs (100%), hyperkinesia (chorea, athetosis) (95%), hypersalivation (95%), paroxysmal symptom (82%), strabismus (77%), and pyramidal symptom (75%). Clinically, they showed similar clinical pictures with each other (Figs. 1–4).

Such diffuse cerebral damage can be recognized not only in congenital Minamata disease but also in cerebral palsy caused by other factors. However, some symptoms are characteristic of the former.

Compared with cases of cerebral palsy as a group caused by other factors, congenital Minamata disease cases exhibit a more marked degree of intelligence disturbance; cerebellar symptoms and strabismus are more common. Symptoms on the right and

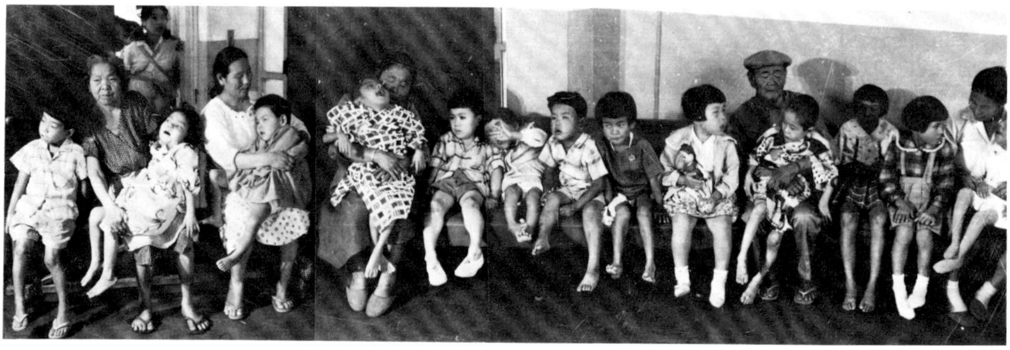

Fig. 1. Congenital Minamata disease patients in Minamata area. The patients showed very similar clinical picture to each other. (Photographed by M. Harada in 1962).

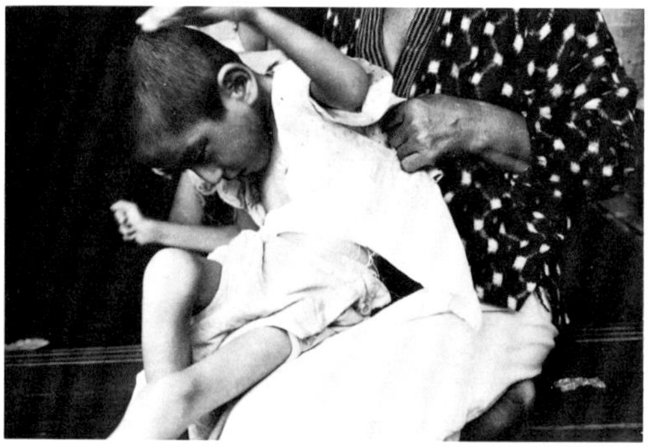

Fig. 2. Neck is unsteady, inability to sit up. Male aged six years, born in 1956, died in 1969 without any improvement of symptoms.

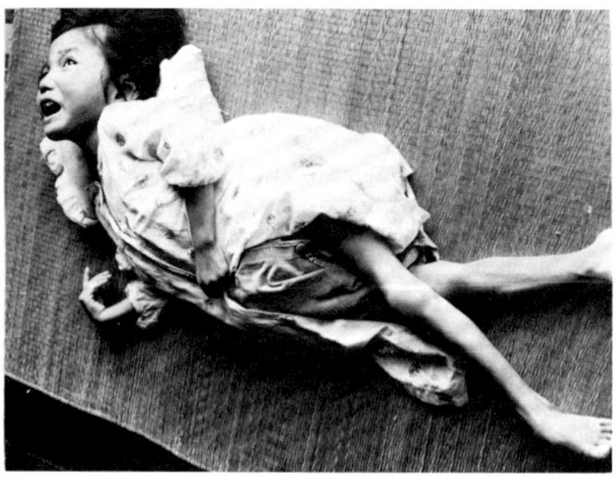

Fig. 3. Deformities of limbs, nutritional deficiency, a condition resembling akinetic mutism. Female aged six years, born in 1956, died in 1962.

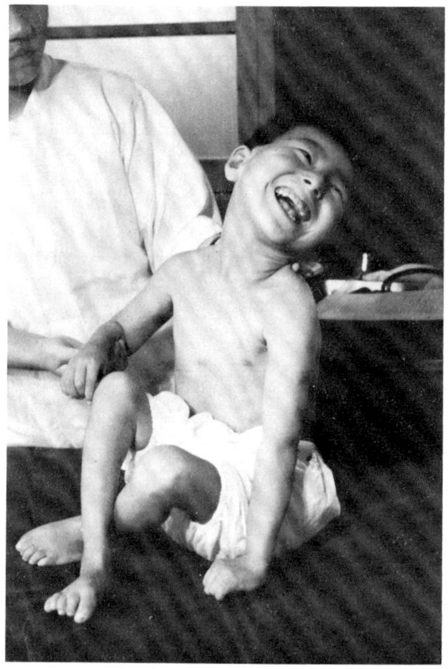

Fig. 4. Forced laughter, a condition resembling akinetic mutism. Female aged six years, born in 1956, died in 1977.

left side are undifferentiated, and no factors that might have caused abnormality were noticed during perinatal period.

Also, degenerative signs and malformations are rare, but microcephaly is observed in 60% of congenital Minamata disease cases. Abnormality of chromosomes has not yet been recognized.

During 15 years of follow up research, improvement of motor function has been more noticeable in mild cases than in those of medium degree. Especially, paroxysmal symptoms, hypersalivation, primitive reflex and cerebellar symptoms have been relatively susceptible to improvement, and in some cases only clumsiness of movement remains apparent. But even in light cases, intelligence disturbance was left unimproved.

PATHOLOGY AND EXPERIMENT

General atrophy and hypoplasia of the brain cortex and abnormality of the cytoarchitecture, remaining matrix cells, hypoplasia of the corpus callosum, intramedullary preservation of the nerve cells, and dysmyelination of the pyramidal tract have been observed. In the cerebellum, hypoplasia of the granular cell layer and other layers as well as degeneration of granular cells (characteristic of Minamata disease) were observed (Takeuchi, '77).

Researchers succeeded in causing brain disturbances in fetuses of pregnant cats or mice by giving methylmercury experimentally (Morikawa, '61; Moriyama, '67). Further, transplacental passage of organic mercury was confirmed by means of radioautography (Fujita, '69). The possibility of brain damage through mother's milk was also confirmed (Deshimaru, '69).

EPIDEMIOLOGY

In the diagnosis of congential Minamata disease, epidemiological factors are very important. In the three most heavily contaminated areas, Yudo, Modo, and Tsukinoura, which are fishermen's villages of Minamata City, 220 infants were born during 1955 through 1958. Among them, 13 were suffering from severe congenital Minamata disease, and the morbidity rate was high at 6.9%. Incidence of infantile and adult cases coincided, both in region and time. Later research revealed that the disease existed in a broader region, and 40 cases have been officially registered until 1976. In many families, Minamata disease affected two or more members. However, the symptoms of mothers were relatively light. Of 28 affected mothers, all showed peripheral sensory disturbance, but such symptoms as mild incoordination (79%), constriction of the visualfield (57%), dysarthria (43%) and tremor (39%) were not observed in all of the cases (Harada, '76). In Minamata cases, mercury values in the hair of the parents of affected infants was not known at time of birth, but two to five years afterward patients and their parents showed high level of mercury in the hair (Minamata Disease Study Group of M.D., '68). In the Niigata case, one mother showed 293 ppm of mercury in the hair during pregnancy. Also, a mother of a New Mexico case had a mercury value of 2.91 ppm in her blood, and her affected infant had 2.77 ppm in its urine. Therefore, for the diagnosis of congenital Minamata disease it is valuable that mercury contents in the hair, blood or urine were high in the postnatal period.

In cases at Minamata, methylmercury values in the umbilical cords of patients were more than 1.0 ppm in many cases (Harada, '76, '77).

Sometimes, the mercury value does not necessarily coincide with the usual clinical symptoms, but a correlation with the degree of environmental pollution is observed. Mental retardation (excluding cases of congenital Minamata disease) of children born between 1955 and 1958 in the heavily polluted Minamata area was 29.1%, and was 17.5% in pupils of lower secondary school in the Minamata area. Both figures were significantly higher than those of control areas. Furthermore, clumsiness in movements of fingers and other motor functions were seen in these mental retardation cases, and in these infants mild or incomplete cases of congenital Minamata disease are suspected (Harada, '76).

RECENT FINDINGS

It is not definitely known what amount of the methylmercury-contaminated foods eaten by mothers causes congenital Minamata disease. In Minamata, patients were discovered 2 to 5 years after falling ill (Harada, '64; Study Group of Minamata disease, '68). The congenital Minamata disease that occurred in New Mexico in 1969 was due to the mother's intake of pork containing 27.5 ppm of methylmercury during a 3-month period starting in the sixth month of pregnancy (Pierce et al., '70; Synder, '71; Harada, '76). In Iraq in 1972, newborns showed three times as high a methylmercury concentration in the blood as their mothers, who for 2 months had eaten the bread that had a mean mercury content of 9.1 ppm. Serious brain damage was observed in the newborns whose methylmercury concentration exceeded 2,500 ng/ml. The methylmercury concentration in the mother's milk was 3 to 6% of that in their blood. The methylmercury concentration in the blood of the infants who were taking mothers' milk was, however, slightly lower than or equal to the mothers. It exceeded 1,000 ng/ml for some of the infants (Bakir et al., '73).

Both maternal blood and mother's milk are sources of methylmercury in what is clinically named congenital Minamata disease. Once taken up, methylmercury remains in the brain for a long period. In the autopsied cases in Minamata, 0.4 and 0.7 ppm of methylmercury were detected from the cerebrum of the congenital Minamata disease patients who died 2 years and 6 months and 6 years and 3 months, respectively, after birth (Takeuchi, '77). Symptoms may also progress for a long period.

Whether or not the mercury safety standards for adults suffice for the fetus is unknown. The World Health Organization has urged stricter regulation on behalf of pregnant females.

In Niigata the females with hair mercury contents of more than 50 ppm were advised to terminate their pregnancies. This was so effective a measure that only one case of congenital Minamata disease took place there. However, it still remains possible that mild (mental retardation) cases occurred and were unrecognized.

Methylmercury is generally believed to damage fetuses, not embryos. Recent animal experiments, however, have demonstrated embryo damage due to methylmercury (Khera, '73; Fuyuta et al., '78). Does this occur in humans? It is possible that human embryo damage would cause spontaneous abortions. The author and others investigated, by interview, mothers who lived in one of the most heavily polluted districts during the period (1956–1961) when the greatest pollution was occurring. We determined that out of 272 pregnancies, there were 32 abortions, nine stillbirths, four deaths within 1 week after birth, four congenital Minamata disease patients, and four infant Minamata disease patients. In this population stillbirths and abortions occurred at the somewhat high rate of 15.0%.

There was also the possibility that congenital abnormalities were being overlooked or congenital Minamata disease was unrecognized because of unusual symptoms. It became clear, however, through the investigation that the district was also subject to high rates of congenital abnormalities. They included high palates, auditory canal defects, syndactylia, congenital retinochoroidal colobomata, congenital heart abnormalities (septal defects), congenital pupil malformations, microcornea, microcephalia, hydrocephalia, archynoid cysts, and so forth (Fujino et al., '80). Thus as described before, methylmercury is not only fetotoxic but it also may be embroyotoxic.

LITERATURE CITED

Amin-Zaki, L., S. Elhassani, M.A Majeed, T.W. Clarkson, R.A. Doherty and M. Greenwood (1974) Intra-uterine methylmercury poisoning in Iraq. Pediatrics, *54:*587–595.

Bakir, F., S.F. Damiluji, L. Amin-Zaki, M. Murtadha, A. Kahlidi, N.Y. Al-Rawi, S. Tikriti, H.I. Dhahiv, T.W. Clarkson, J.C. Smith, and R.A. Doherty (1973) Methylmercury poisoning in Iraq. An inter-university report. Science, *181:*230–241.

Deshimaru, M. (1969) Electron microscopic studies on experimental organic mercury poisoning in nursling rat brain. Psychiat. et Neurol. Jap., *71:*506–513 (Japanese edition).

Engleson, G., and T. Herner (1952) Alkyl mercury poisoning. Acta Paediat. *41:*289–294.

Fujino, T., Y. Itai, and M. Harada (1980) Congenital malformations and organic mercury poisoning. Constitutional Med. (Japanese edition), *44:*103–115.

Fujita, E. (1969) Experimental studies of organic mercury poisoning, on the behaviors of Minamata disease causal agent in the maternal bodies and its transference to their infants via either placenta or breast milk. J. Kumamoto Med. Soc., *43:*37–62 (Japanese edition).

Fuyuta, M., T. Fujimoto, and S. Hirata (1978) Embryotoxic effects of methylmercuric chloride administered to mice and rats during organogenesis. Teratology, *18:*353–366.

Harada, M. (1964) Neuropsychiatric disturbances due to organic mercury poisoning during the prenatal period. Psychiat. et Neurol. Jap., *66:*426–468 (Japanese ed., English summary).

——(1976) Intrauterine poisoning, clinical and epidemiological studies and significance of the problem. Bulletin. Institute of Constitutional Medicine, Kumamoto University, Suppl. *25:*1–60.

——(1977) Study on methylmercury concentration in the umbilical cords of the inhabitants born in the Minamata area. Brain and Develop.,, *9:*79–84 (Japanese edition).

Harada, Y. (1968) Congenital Minamata disease. In: Minamata Disease. Study Group of Minamata Disease, Kumamoto University, Japan, pp. 93–117.

Khera, K.S. (1973) Teratogenic effects of methylmercury in the cat. Note on the use of this species as a model for teratogenicity studies. Teratology, *8:*293–304.

Kitamura, S., Y. Hirano, Y. Noguchi, T. Kojima, T Kakita and H. Kuwaki (1959) The epidemiological survey on Minamata disease (No. 2). J. Kumamoto Med. Soc., *33* (Suppl. 3):569–571 (Japanese edition).

Kitamura, S., T. Kakita, J. Kojoo, and T. Kojima (1960) A supplement to the results of the epidemiological survey on Minamata disease (No. 3). J. Kumamoto Med. Soc., *34* (Supple. 3):476–480 (Japanese edition).

Matsumoto, H., G. Koya, and T. Takeuchi (1965) Fetal Minamata disease. A neuropathological study of two cases of intrauterine intoxication by a methylmercury compound. J. Neuropathol. Exp. Neurol., *24:*563–574.

Matsumoto, H., and T. Takeuchi (1965) Fetal Minamata disease, a neurological study of two cases of intrauterine intoxication by a methyl-mercury compound. J. Neuropath. and Experiment. Neurol., *24:*563–574.

Minamata Disease (1968) Study Group of Minamata Disease. Kumamoto University, Kumamoto City, Japan.

Morikawa, N. (1961) Pathological studies on organic mercury poisoning. I. Experimental organic mercury poisoning in cats and its relation to the causative agent of Minamata disease. II. Experimental production of congenital cerebellar atrophy by bimethylmercuric sulfide in cats. Kumamoto Med. J., *14:*71–93.

Moriyama, H. (1967) A study on the congenital Minamata disease. J. Kumamoto Med. Soc., *41:*506–532 (Japanese edition).

Synder, R.D. (1971) Congenital mercury poisoning. New Eng. J. Med., *284:*1014–1016.

Takeuchi, T. (1977) Pathology of fetal Minamata disease. Paediatrican, *6:*69–87.

TERATOGEN UPDATE: ENVIRONMENTALLY INDUCED BIRTH DEFECT RISKS, PAGES 127–130 (1986)

PCBs and Cola Colored Babies: Japan, 1968, and Taiwan, 1979

WALTER J. ROGAN
Epidemiology Branch, National Institute of Environmental Health Sciences, Research Triangle Park, North Carolina 27709

In 1968, the use of rice bran cooking oil contaminated with polychlorinated biphenyls (PCBs) and other chemicals caused an outbreak of severe acne among residents of Kyushu, Japan (Kuratsune et al., '72). The health ministry eventually included over 1,000 persons as cases; reports are available on 13 children born to affected women (Taki et al., '69). Two children were stillborn, one of whom was deeply, diffusely pigmented (cola colored). The other children tended to have low birthweight, elevated bilirubin, conjunctivitis with enlargement of the sebaceous glands of the eyelid, pigmentation of the gums, nails, and groin, and hypoplastic deformed nails. Two children had scalp calcifications and natal teeth (Funatsu et al., '71). Some developed chloracne, which is follicular plugging with comedone and cyst formation. Previously, chloracne was thought to result only from dermal contact with PCBs and other halogenated polycyclics, like the naphthalenes (Crow, '70); it was familiar to occupational physicians as "cable handler's itch," from the pruritic bands produced by PCB-insulated electric wire.

In 1979, a very similar outbreak occurred on Taiwan (Lan et al., '81), which was rapidly shown to involve PCB-laden cooking oil processed in machinery of Japanese manufacture similar to that leading to the 1968 poisonings. This time, more than 2,000 cases have been recorded, many of them young women, since the exposed included boarders at a school attached to the food processing plant. Thus far, eight babies have been described who were born to cases (Wong and Hwang, '81; Law et al, '81); these children show signs very similar to the Japanese Yusho (oil disease) babies (Table 1). Four children had a peculiar black pigmentation of the nose that had not been seen in 1968.

PCBs are clear oily substances that resist thermal, metabolic, or environmental degradation. They were sold as mixtures of the variously chlorinated congeners of the biphenyl rings. Since the 1930s, 886 million pounds have been produced (Brinkman and deKok, '80), used, and disposed of in relatively uncontrolled ways. In 1966, Jensen (Anon., '66) found PCBs in hair from his wife and child and the tissues of a dead eagle. This implied that PCBs were a widespread environmental contaminant. Yusho had followed epizootics—chick edema disease and X disease in cattle—that showed the toxicity of halogenated hydrocarbons like PCBs, and US manufacturing ceased in the 1970s. Current use and disposal are strictly regulated by the Toxic Substances Control Act of 1976; the only remaining use is as the insulating dielectric material in heavy, closed electrical equipment.

Neither in Japan nor in Taiwan has there been a clear relationship between symptoms of those affected or fetopathy and dose. The amount of oil consumed had to be reconstructed, of course, but blood levels of the chemicals drawn relatively soon after exposure have been difficult to interpret clinically (Umeda et al., '78). This is due in part to the technical difficulty of chemical analysis for substances present in the part per billion range and also to the variable relationships among exposure, "body burden," and blood or fat level. In addition, in both cases the PCBs had seen service as heat transfer agents and had undergone some thermal degradation (Chen et al., '81; Nagayama et al., '77). The resulting mixtures are contaminated with the highly toxic dibenzofurans, as well as tri- and quatraphenyls, which have the same potential toxicity (in the laboratory at least), but are active at much lower doses. Thus measurable PCBs may be only a surrogate for what is actually the toxic agent.

Animal studies have more or less confirmed the fetotoxicity of the chemicals, at least in susceptible species (McConnell, '80). The Rhesus is one such, and females fed 2.5 parts per million of commercial grade PCBs in the diet have difficulty conceiving and give birth to small offspring. The infants develop chloracne (Allen and Barsotti, '76), do not learn mazes well (Bowman et al., '78), and suffer increased mortality (Allen and Barsotti, '76). Most studies show that exposure

TABLE 1. Neonatal signs in Japanese and Taiwanese** outbreaks*

Case	LB/SB[1]	Country	Sex	BW[2]	Stained skin	Stained gingiva	Stained nail	Conjunctival hypersecretion	Acne	Jaundice
1	LB	Japan	M	N	?[3]	–	–	–		+
2	LB	Japan	F	N	+	–	–	+		+
3	LB	Japan	M	N	?	–	–	+		++
4	LB	Japan	M	SFD	+	+	–	+		?
5	LB	Japan	F	N	+	+	+	+		+
6	LB	Japan	M	N	+	–	+	+		+
7	LB	Japan	M	SFD	+	–	–	+		?
8	LB	Japan	M		+	–	–	+		+
9	LB	Japan	M	SFD	+	+	+	+		?
10	LB	Japan	F	N	?	–	–	–		+
11	LB	Japan	M	N	+	+	+	+		+
12	SB	Japan	?	?	+	?	?			
13	SB	Japan	F	SFD	+	?	?			
14	LB	Taiwan	M	3600g	+	–	+	++	–	
15	LB	Taiwan	M	2500g	–	–	–	–	–	+
16	LB	Taiwan	F	2400g	+++	–	+	+++	++	
17	LB	Taiwan	M	3600g	++	+	++	+	–	
18	LB	Taiwan	F	1800g	++	+	++	+	–	
19	LB	Taiwan	F	1800g	++	+	++	+	–	
20	LB	Taiwan	F	2820g	+		+	+		
21	LB	Taiwan	F	1800g	+		+	+		

*Kuratsune et al., '72.
**Cases 14–19 from Wong and Hwang, '81. Cases 20–21 from Law et al., '81.
[1]LB/SB, livebirth, stillbirth.
[2]BW, birthweight—N, normal; SFD, small for dates.
[3]?, noted as ? in reference.

to PCBs in utero causes slow growth, altered immune function, and slowed development, although the usual tests for teratogenesis are negative. The immune dysfunction is a T cell lesion, with histologic depletion and/or hypoplasia of the thymus (McConnell, '80).

Some follow-up information is available on the Japanese children. The growth disturbance tended to disappear a few years after exposure ceased (Yoshimura and Ikeda, '78), but some pigmentation remained. Harada ('76) examined some of the children at ages 7 to 9 who were in utero or sucklings during the episode; he found them to be apathetic and listless, with "soft" neurological signs. Formal IQ or developmental tests have not been reported, and, of course, no followup is yet available from Taiwan.

In the US, accidents and residues on foods have led to ubiquitous population exposure to PCBs. Sensitive chemical analysis shows PCBs in the majority of adipose tissue (Kutz and Strassman, '76) or (because of their fat content) breast milk samples (Rogan et al., '80) from unselected populations. The PCBs are highly lipophilic, and small doses accumulate in body fat over a lifetime. The only circumstance in which substantial amounts of PCBs are excreted is lactation, thus exposing the suckling, who is known to accumulate PCBs (Abe et al., '75; Kuwabara et al., '78; Masuda et al., '78). For the weaned, the sole remaining dietary source of importance is probably sport fish from contaminated waters; commercial foods are regulated by the Food and Drug Administration (FDA, '78).

Human beings are likely to remain contaminated by PCBs for decades; the tissue half lives of the heavier congeners is very long. Accidental exposure from poorly controlled disposal of used PCBs will likely continue also. Thus far, acute human illness is thought to be limited to chloracne, with or without non-specific laboratory disturbances, such as elevated triglycerides or liver enzymes. Some adults in Taiwan have shown diffuse hyperpigmentation without chloracne (Cheng et al., '81), and the high sensitivity attributed to that condition as a "marker" of exposure is thus brought into question. No reports of PCB fetopathy or illness attributable to PCBs in breast milk exist outside these two outbreaks, although several groups are looking.

Questions of management arise when a pregnant woman is exposed, or thinks she may have been exposed, to PCBs. A blood sample sent to a commercial facility will likely show measurable levels whether there has been special exposure or not. There are no "normal" or "threshold" values worked out for such cases, and there is no quality assurance program among laboratories to promote comparability. Blood (or fat or milk) testing thus seems of minimal value for the individual. In most cases, women who had affected children had chloracne themselves, and exposure to amounts insufficient to produce some effect in the mother probably lessens the chance of fetopathy considerably. In the newborn, low birthweight and hyperbilirubinemia are non-specific, but pigmented hypoplastic nails, pigmented gums, or natal teeth should prompt suspicion.

The toxicity of PCBs is an active research area for both toxicologists and public health workers. The very low levels of PCBs to which everyone is exposed probably have little or nothing to do with noticeable birth defects, but it can be argued that such exposures decrease the margin of safety for reproduction in general. Besides, accidents involving relatively high exposures will likely recur, as the massive amounts of PCB containing equipment now in use wear out and must be discarded. On a more basic level, PCBs are one of the relatively few known human teratogens that are also (laboratory) carcinogens (IARC, '78), and thus mechanisms of disease processes may be found that are of wider import (Miller, '77).

FOLLOWUP—1984

There were three international meetings on the toxicity of PCB and similar compounds in 1983; at two of them, new findings about the fetopathy were presented. Proceedings of all three have appeared as volumes 59 and 60 of "Environmental Health Perspectives."

At the Japanese meeting, Hsu et al. ('85) reported that there are now 39 cases of congenital Yucheng (of whom 8 died), as the illness has come to be called in Taiwan. At a later meeting in North Carolina, Miller ('85) reviewed the teratologic findings. He emphasized some differences between the Japanese and Taiwanese children, the peculiar black noses have continued to appear in Taiwan, but were not seen in Japan, and some of the affected Taiwanese children had normal birthweights, whereas all of the Japanese babies were small. McNulty ('85) reported on dental abnormalities in a primate animal model that may explain the natal teeth; the monkeys have cysts beneath the gingival surface. There is still no understanding of the mechanisms involved in the fetopathy, nor of the precise roles of the contaminant chemicals, although there is agreement that the highly toxic dibenzofuran contaminants are responsible for some of the toxicity seen. A clinical field survey of the transplacentally exposed Taiwanese children was done in 1985, but results are not yet available.

Little can be added that is useful for counseling patients. No critical period has been identified; indeed, since PCBs are excreted so slowly, affected babies have been seen years after exposure ceased. While there are still no reports of fetopathy outside of the two epidemics, there are now two reports of subtle neurological dysfunction associated with transplacental exposure to PCBs in the U.S. (Jacobson et al., '84; Rogan et al., '86). It remains unlikely that exposure to PCBs in the doses usually encountered in this country would cause major defects in the offspring.

LITERATURE CITED

Abe, S., Y. Inoue, and M. Takamatsu (1975) Polychlorinated biphenyl residues in plasma of Yusho children born to mothers who had consumed oil contaminated by PCB. Fukuoka Acta. Med., *66:*605–9 (in Japanese).

Allen, J.R., and D.A. Barsotti (1976) The effects of transplacental and mammary movement of PCBs on infant Rhesus monkeys. Toxicology, *6:*331–40.

Anonymous (1966) Report of a new chemical hazard. New Scientist, *32:*612.

Bowman, R.E., M. Heironimous, and J.R. Allen (1978) Correlation of PCB body burden with behavioral toxicology in monkeys. Pharmacol. Biochem. Behav., *9:*49–56.

Brinkman, U.A. Th., and A. deKok (1980) Production, properties, and usage. In: Halogenated Biphenyls, Terphenyls, Naphthalenes, Dibenzodionins and Related Products. R. Kimbrough, ed. Elsevier/North Holland, New York, pp. 1–40.

Chen, P.H., K.T. Chang, and Y.D. Lu (1981) Polychlorinated biphenyls and polychlorinated dibenzofurans in the toxic rice bran oil that caused PCB poisoning in Taichung. Bull. Environ. Contam. Toxicol., *26:*489–95.

Cheng, P-C, C-J Chen, C-K Wong, and P-H-S Chen (1981) Dermatologic survey of 122 PCB poisoning patients in comparison with blood PCB levels. Clin. Med. (Taipei), *7:*15–22 (in Chinese).

Crow, K.D. (1970) Chloracne. Transact. St. John's Hosp. Dermatol. Soc., *56:*79–99.

Food and Drug Administration (1978) Action levels for poisonous or deleterious substances in human food and animal feed. FDA, Industry Guidance Branch, Washington.

Funatsu, I., F. Yamashita, T. Yoshinake, T. Funatsu, Y. Ito, S. Tsugawa, M. Hayashi, T. Kato, M. Yakashiji, G. Okamato, A. Arima, N. Adachi, K. Takahashi, M. Miyahara, Y. Tashiro, M. Shimomura, S. Yamasaki, T. Arima, T. Kuno, H. Ide, and I. Ide (1971) A chlorobiphenyl induced fetopathy. Fukuoka Acta. Med., *62:*139–49 (in Japanese).

Hsu S.T., Ma C.I., Hsu S.K-H, Wa S.S., Hsu N.M., Yeh C.C., and Wu S.B. (1985) Discovery and epidemiology of PCB poisoning in Taiwan: A four year follow up. Environ. Health Perspec., *59:*5–10.

Harada, M. (1976) Intrauterine poisoning. Bull. Institute Constitutional Medicine Kumamoto University, *25(supplement):*1–60.

International Agency for Research on Cancer (1978) Polychlorinated biphenyls and polybrominated biphenyls. IARC monographs on the evaluation of carcinogenic risk of chemicals to humans, *18:*43–85.

Jacobson, J.L., S.W. Jacobson, P.M. Schwartz, G.G. Fein, and J.K. Dowler (1984) Prenatal exposure to an environmental toxin: A test of the multiple effects model. Developmental Psychol., *20:*523–532.

Kuratsune, M., T. Yoshimura, J. Matsuzaka, and A. Yamaguchi (1972) Epidemiologic study on Yusho, a poisoning caused by ingestion of rice oil contaminated with a commercial brand of polychlorinated biphenyls. Environ. Health Perspec. Exp. *Vol 1:*119–28.

Kutz, F.W., and S.C. Strassman (1976) Residues of polychlorinated biphenyls in the general population of the U.S. National Conference on Polychlorinated Biphenyls. EPA-560/6-75-004:139–43.

Kuwabara, K., T. Yakushiji, I. Watanabe, S. Yoshida, K. Koyama, N. Kunita, and I. Hara (1978) Relationship between breast feeding and PCB residues in blood of the children whose mothers were occupationally exposed to PCBs. Int. Arch. Occup. Environ. Health, *41:*189–97.

Lan, C-F, H-S Chen, L-L Shieh, and Y-H Chen (1981) An epidemiologic study on polychlorinated biphenyls poisoning in Taichung area. Clin. Med. (Taipei), *7:*96–100 (in Chinese).

Law, K-L, B-T Hwang, and I-S Shaio (1981) PCB poisoning in newborn twins. Clin. Med. (Taipei), *7:*88–91 (in Chinese).

Masuda, Y., R. Kagawa, H. Kuroki, M. Kuratsune, T. Yoshimura, I. Taki, M. Kusuda, F. Yamashita, and M. Hayashi (1978) Transfer of polychlorinated biphenyls from mothers to fetuses and infants. Fd. Cosmet. Toxicol., *16:*543–6.

McConnell, E.E. (1980) Acute and chronic toxicity, carcinogenesis, reproduction, teratogenesis and mutagenesis in animals. In: Halogenated Biphenyls, Terphenyls, Naphthalenes, Dibenzodioxins and Related Products. R. Kimbrough, ed. Elsevier/North Holland, New York, pp. 109–50.

McNulty, W.P. (1985) Toxicity and fetotoxicity of TCDD, TCDF, and PCB isomers in rhesus macaques *(Macaca mulatta).* Environ. Health Perspec., *60:*77–88.

Miller, R.W. (1977) Relationship between human teratogens and carcinogens. J Nat. Cancer. Inst., *58:*471–4.

Miller, R.W. (1985) Congenital PCB poisoning: A reevaluation. Environ. Health Perspec., *60:*211–214.

Nagayama, J., Y. Masuda, and M. Kuratsune (1977) Determination of polychlorinated dibenzofurans in tissues of patients with Yusho. Fd. Cosmet. Toxicol., *15:*195–8.

Rogan, W.J., A. Bagniewska, and T. Damstra (1980) Pollutants in breast milk. N. Engl. J. Med., *302:*1450–3.

Rogan, W.J., B.C. Gladen, J.D. McKinney, N. Carreras, P. Hardy, J. Thullen, J. Tinglestad, and M. Tully (1986) Neonatal effects of transplacental exposure to PCBs and DDE. J. Pediatr., *109:*(in press).

Taki, I., S. Hisanaga, and Y. Amagase (1969) Report on Yusho (chlorobiphenyls poisoning) pregnant women and their fetuses. Fukuoka Acta. Med., *60:*471–4 (in Japanese).

Umeda, G., H. Nakajima, and K. Yatsuki (1978) Some problems on health effects of polychlorinated biphenyls. Ecotoxicol. Environ. Safety, *1:*437–46.

Wong, K-C, and M-Y Hwang (1981) Children born to PCB poisoning mothers. Clin. Med. (Taipei), *7:*83–7 (in Chinese).

Yoshimura, T., and M. Ikeda (1978) Growth of school children with polychlorinated biphenyl poisoning or Yusho. Environ. Res., *17:*416–25.

Smoking and Pregnancy

MARTHA M. WERLER, BARBARA R. POBER, AND LEWIS B. HOLMES
Embryology-Teratology Unit, Children's Service, Massachusetts General Hospital (M.M.W., B.R.P., L.B.H.) and the Department of Pediatrics, Harvard Medical School (B.R.P., L.B.H.), Boston, Massachusetts 02114

Cigarette smoking during pregnancy is still common despite warnings that it is harmful to the fetus. Although estimates of cigarette smoke exposure indicate a decrease over the past decade in both the proportion of pregnant women who smoke and the number of cigarettes smoked (1), cigarette smoking continues to be the most common known harmful exposure during pregnancy. An estimated 30.9% of women are smoking cigarettes before pregnancy and 25.5% are estimated to continue to smoke during pregnancy (2).

Since Simpson first reported an association between maternal smoking and decreased birthweight (3) many effects on the offspring of smokers have been investigated.

INTRAUTERINE GROWTH RETARDATION

Intrauterine growth retardation is the most consistently observed effect of maternal smoking. Decreased birthweight has been observed in virtually all studies of smoking mothers. This relationship remains after accounting for maternal age (4,5,10,11, 13), parity (5,7,10,11), maternal weight gain (5,6), prepregnant weight and/or height (4,5,10,11,13), gestational age (4–7,10), socioeconomic status (4–7, 10,11,13), and race (8,9). Meyer et al. controlled for the effects of all of these potential confounders simultaneously using a multiple regression model and found that a dose response relationship between cigarette smoking and reduced birth weight persisted (5). Smoking ten to 20 cigarettes per day throughout pregnancy reduces birthweight approximately 200 gm; this amount varies (92–316 gm) from study to study depending on the population and which, if any, cofactors were also considered (7,10–13). Women who stop smoking during the first half of their pregnancy deliver infants with birthweights averaging close to those of nonsmokers (10,13).

The medical significance of low birthweight is not totally understood. It is known that perinatal mortality increases exponentially with decreasing birthweight for both smokers and nonsmokers (8). Morbidity among infants of smokers due to low birthweight alone is not clearly documented. It would require analysis of birthweight, gestational age, and morbidity, controlling for known antepartum causes of morbidity, e.g., abruptio placentae or maternal infection and for postnatal smoke exposure.

Several mechanisms of action by which smoking exerts its growth retardant effect on the fetus have been hypothesized, including the following:

Nicotine as a vasoconstrictor

Nicotine has been shown to be a vasoconstrictor in adult smokers (14). Accordingly, it has been postulated that nicotine-mediated uteroplacental vessel constriction causes growth retardation through decreased perfusion of fetal tissues.

Placental blood flow has been estimated by measuring the rate of dehydro-epiandrosterone sulfate (DHA-S) conversion to estriol by the placenta (15). Blood levels of estriol were determined in smokers and nonsmokers before and after DHA-S loading. Following a 3-hour period of smoking abstinence, smokers had lower percentage increases in serum estriol in comparison to nonsmokers. Four days later, smokers were reloaded with DHA-S immediately after smoking two cigarettes. Among these women, serum estriol increases were even less after smoking two cigarettes than the levels observed after smoking abstinence. These results suggest that smokers have chronically decreased placental flow as well as an acute decrease of even greater magnitude.

Uteroplacental flow has also been measured with radionuclides. After injection with Indium-113m-transferrin, the placental blood inflow rate of 20 smokers was compared to 20 nonsmokers of similar age and stage of pregnancy (16). Smokers abstained from smoking the morning of the study and then smoked two cigarettes prior to placental inflow measurements. Placental inflow of radioactive blood was observed to be significantly slower ($P < .005$) among smokers than nonsmokers. Also, the number of cigarettes smoked daily by smokers correlated with the degree of slowed blood flow ($P < .023$). A similar study which used ^{133}Xenon compared the intervillous blood flow of former smokers before and after smoking one cigarette (17). Blood flow decreased ($P < .05$) after the cigarette was smoked.

The effect of nicotine on uterine blood flow has been evaluated in pregnant rhesus monkeys (18). The rate of blood flow was measured continuously by a cuff-type electromagnetic flowmeter applied to a uterine artery. A significant decrease in uterine blood flow was observed during 20 minutes of nicotine infusion and continued for 10 minutes following infusion, after which the flow rate rose to the baseline preinfusion rate.

Prostacyclins (PGI-2) which are known for their antithrombotic and vasodilator properties have been studied in endothelial cells from umbilical arteries of smokers and nonsmokers (19). Endothelial cells from the infants of smokers produced less PGI-2 than those cells from infants of nonsmokers. This group also cultured umbilical artery endothelial cells of smokers and nonsmokers immediately following delivery (20). In vitro growth was successful in fewer smokers than nonsmokers ($P < .01$). Among the successful cell cultures (six smokers > 15 cig./day and 17 nonsmokers), PGI-2 levels were less for smokers than nonsmokers ($P < .01$). These results suggest that the effect of smoking on PGI-2 production remains after removal of the cigarette smoke exposure.

Decreased placental perfusion as observed by these varying methods of study may prevent optimal fetal growth.

A direct effect of nicotine on fetal tissue

There is evidence that nicotine readily crosses the human placenta (21). A study of rhesus monkeys found that it persists in higher concentration and has a longer half-life in the fetus than in the mother (22). Also, nicotine was found to accumulate in specific fetal organs when these pregnant rhesus monkeys were injected with nicotine, although the total accumulated amount was a small fraction of the nicotine which crossed the placenta. Perhaps nicotine exerts a growth-inhibiting effect on fetal tissue.

Carboxyhemoglobin and fetal hypoxia

The carbon monoxide (CO) content of cigarette smoke also crosses the placenta and produces an increase in fetal carboxyhemoglobin (HbCO) levels (6,23,24). Among 105 infants of women who had smoked during labor, cord blood HbCO concentrations were 2.55 times higher than simultaneous maternal blood concentrations. The time of last cigarette before delivery ranged from less than 1 hour to 10 hours among these women. The fetal HbCO to maternal HbCO ratio increased as the time between last cigarette and delivery increased. This increasing ratio reflects the longer half-life of HbCO in fetal blood in comparison to maternal blood.

Adults will compensate for chronic carbon monoxide exposure by becoming polycythemic and by increasing oxygen saturation. Bureau et al. studied a group of smoking and nonsmoking women and their newborns for compensatory alterations in oxygen carrying capacity following CO exposure (25). HbCO was higher in both smoking mothers and their newborns ($P < .0005$). Although smoking mothers had increased hematocrit levels their hemoglobin, P_{50}, and 2,3-diphosphoglycerate (2,3-DPG) were similar to nonsmokers, suggesting that pregnant women have less CO compensation than do nonpregnant adults. Cord blood analysis of infants of smokers did demonstrate increased hemoglobin, hematocrit, and fetal hemoglobin (HbF), decreased P_{50}, and unaltered 2,3DPG level when compared to offspring of nonsmokers. It appears that some amount of compensation occurs in fetuses who are chronically exposed to CO, although it is small in comparison to nonpregnant adults. Exposed nonpregnant adults experience a seven to 12 times greater decrease in P_{50} and three to six times greater increase in hematocrit than fetuses. The lesser ability of the fetus to adapt to chronic CO exposure may result in decreased birthweight.

Thiocyanate toxicity in the fetus

Increased blood thiocyanate levels have been measured in cord blood of infants of smokers as well as in the serum of pregnant smokers (26). McGarry and Andrews hypothesized that the supply of vitamin B_{12} in smokers is depleted since it is used in the detoxification of cyanide to thiocyanate (4). Additionally, sulfur-containing amino acids are also required for detoxification of cyanide (27). A depleted supply of these vitamins and/or amino acids may inhibit protein synthesis and in turn retard growth of the fetus.

Nutritional deficit among smokers

It has been postulated that the reduced birthweight of infants of smokers may be secondary to nutrient starvation assuming smokers eat less. Studies have addressed this issue by controlling for maternal weight gain and/or prepregnant weight in smoking-birthweight analyses (4,6,28–33). No difference in maternal weight gain was found between smokers and nonsmokers in the majority of studies (4,6,28–30,33). Some investigators have concluded that the nutrition effect has a greater role than smoking in predicting birthweight (31,32) although they have been criticized for inadequate adjustment for maternal weight gain. Since the fetus accounts for 40% of maternal weight gain, women carrying low-birthweight fetuses will have less weight gain. Ounsted and Scott (33) evaluated this problem by using net weight gain calculated as final weight less prepregnant, placental, and birthweights rather than "total weight gain." Net weight gain did not differ for smoking and nonsmoking women who delivered small-for-gestational-age babies. Among the women who delivered large babies, smokers had greater net gain than did nonsmokers. A food and calorie intake study has also found that smoking mothers do not consume less food or calories than nonsmokers (34). Conversely, diet supplementation for pregnant women increased birthweights among smokers but not among nonsmokers (35).

Anthropometric indices of subcutaneous fat deposition and lean body mass in the newborn infant have been studied in relation to maternal smoking (28). Measurements of skinfold thickness of biceps, triceps, abdomen, and subscapular area were used as indices of subcutaneous fat deposition, and midarm cross-sectional fat and nonfat areas were calculated from measurements of midarm circumference and midarm skinfold thickness using the formula of Gurney and Jelliffe. A multivariate analysis which controlled for gestational age, gender, parity, maternal height, weight gain in pregnancy, and weight at term found smoking was not associated ($P > .05$) with a reduction in head circumference, ponderal index, fat area of the arm or subcutaneous fat. Smoking was found to be associated ($P < .01$) with a reduction in birthweight, length, arm circumference, and nonfat area of the arm. A dose-response relationship for number of cigarettes smoked per day was observed with birthweight and nonfat area of arm. It is postulated that smoking has a targeted effect on lean, but not fat, tissue growth. In support of this hypothesis, it has been observed that well-nourished infants are fatter when born at high altitudes than low altitudes (36) and that hypoxia results in increased lipid/protein ratios in in vitro studies (37,38). These findings add credence to the theory that reduced birthweight among smokers is not mediated by undernourishment since undernourishment of the fetus equally effects both fat and lean tissue.

EARLY FETAL DEATH

An association between smoking among pregnant women and the occurrence of spontaneous abortions has been established in several studies (39–43). The association persists after adjusting for confounding factors, such as maternal age (39,40), parity (41), history of previous abortions (39,42), alcohol use (43), and exposure to waste anesthetic gases (39). A dose-response relationship has also been reported (39,43). Smoking during pregnancy is associated with chromosomally normal abortuses (42,44). This may be indicative of an increased rate of abortions among otherwise viable products of conception due to smoking. However, Kline et al. (40) found an interaction between smoking and maternal age in relation to chromosomally abnormal fetuses. Smoking women under the age of 30 are less likely to have a chromosomally abnormal abortus than nonsmokers whereas smokers over 30 are more likely to have a chromosomally abnormal abortus than nonsmokers. It is unclear whether this interaction indicates that smoking affects meiosis or the survivability of an embryo/fetus *in utero* or both.

Three hypotheses have been proposed to explain the excess of spontaneous abortions among smokers: smoking acts as a lethal teratogen, smoking acts as an abortifacient, or smoking acts as a fetotoxin. It is not possible to test these hypotheses without making assumptions about the fetal age at death, the duration of survival *in utero* with ultimately lethal malformations, changes in fetal vulnerability through gestation (45), and about cigarette smoke as an accumulating chronic exposure.

PERINATAL MORTALITY

There is a controversy regarding the relationship between smoking and perinatal mortality (PNM), the latter usually being defined as a reproductive loss after the 20th week of gestation and before the seventh day of life. Three studies show an adverse effect of smoking on PNM after adjusting for many of the maternal and demographic cofactors (5,46,51,52), although there are many studies which have not controlled for these factors that found both positive (4,11,47) and negative (8,48–50) associations between smoking and increased PNM. Factors other than smoking are known to be important predictors of PNM such as social class, previous history of PNM, maternal age, and parity (52). These factors must be considered in analyses of smoking and PNM or the associations may be spurious. For example, maternal smoking seems to affect the fetus of a mother in a high socioeconomic status (SES) group less than the fetus of a mother in a low SES group (51); studies that have a greater proportion of high SES women will demonstrate fewer adverse effects of smoking on PNM. Women who are at high risk for PNM (low social class, advanced maternal age, and history of a previous loss) have an even greater risk for PNM if they smoke. It has also been observed that low-birthweight infants born to smokers have a lower PNM rate than those born to nonsmokers (4,8). This is due to a higher mean birthweight for low-birthweight babies (<2,500 gm) born to smokers than observed for nonsmokers. Some studies had found no associations between smoking and PNM, possibly due to lower risk samples (8,48–50). Also, smoking has been observed to be protective for toxemia (48). If perinatal deaths due to toxemia are included in a study, a possible smoking effect could be diluted. Among a large sample of women from all social classes, women who decrease or stop smoking during pregnancy have been found to have infants with lower rates of PNM than women who do not reduce their cigarette consumption (10).

Abruptio placentae (52,53), placenta previa (52), prematurity alone (4), and pneumonia (4) have been found to be the cause of PNM in a greater proportion of the offspring of smokers than nonsmokers.

PLACENTAL FUNCTION AND MORPHOLOGY

Smoking in association with placenta previa and abruptio placentae has been well documented, independent of many maternal cofactors (5,54). In one large study (54) women who stopped smoking during pregnancy had a decreased risk for abruptio placentae and placenta previa, although it was not clear when these women changed their smoking habits. It has been hypothesized that a cumulative effect of smoking is fibrosis of the uterine artery walls as in the arteries of other organs. Decreased blood flow through those arteries could explain the excess of abruptions and infarcts in placentas. In support of this, the number of years a woman smokes is associated with the occurrence of large placental infarcts and abruptio placentae (54).

Placental weight does not differ between smokers and nonsmokers; therefore the placental/birthweight ratio is greater for smokers in comparison to nonsmokers (30,55,56).

Many structural changes have been observed in the placentas of smokers, including large and small infarcts, fibrinoid changes in arteries, avascular stem villi, fibrotic peripheral villi and necrosis at the margin of the placenta (54), and thickened basement membranes of trophoblasts, and smaller vessels in terminal villi (56,57). Van der Velde et al. (57) suggest that the cadmium component of cigarette smoke causes decreased density of terminal villi vessels based on the finding of cadmium accumulation in human placentae and comparable effects in the systems of cadmium-exposed rats. They also point out that hypoxia causes an increase in the exchange area of the terminal villi. However, they observed the opposite in the 20 placentas reviewed, suggesting hypoxia is not the cause of reduced birthweight.

Placental function was studied serially in 124 women between 28 and 40 weeks gestation (15). Blood levels of human placental lactogen (hPL), lactic dehydrogenase (LDH), and copper were used as indicators of placental metabolic activity. Only hPL levels differed significantly between heavy smokers (>20 cig./day) and nonsmokers.

CONGENITAL MALFORMATIONS

There are conflicting results with regard to whether there is an association between maternal smoking and the occurrence of congenital malformations. Methodologic and analytic differences make it difficult to compare studies. Specific differences and limitations include the following:

1) lack of uniform definition of a congenital malformation — terms have included "severe congenital anomaly" (8), "non-skin abnormalities" (39), and "severe, moderate and trivial malformations" (58);

2) failure to identify or enumerate specific etiologic causes—some studies list chromosomal abnormalities (58,59), whereas others do not mention them (4,39,47);

3) failure to confirm diagnoses and/or sole use of medical record based diagnoses (4,39,41,47,58–60);

4) indirect or absent documentation of the smoking exposure (47,59);

5) variability in the method and timing of collecting exposure information—antepartum (58), postpartum (4,10,60), or no direct data collection (47,59);

6) absent or incomplete control of potential confounders and risk factors (4,47,58,61).

Furthermore, the three large studies reporting a positive association between maternal smoking and the occurrence of all major malformations had ascertained (or analyzed) only live births (39,58,60); the studies finding no such association appear to have ascertained both live births and stillbirths (4,47,61,62). The spectrum of malformations has varied with the birth status of the study population; this ascertainment difference may also contribute to the discrepant results.

No clear relationship has been established between maternal smoking and specific types of malformations. Six studies have examined the association between neural tube defects and maternal smoking (4,59,61,63–65); three additional studies have examined the relationship between smoking and "central nervous system defects" (41,58,60). Results from four studies support an association especially between heavy smoking and neural tube defects (60,61,63,64), whereas five refute it (4,41,58,59,63). Of note, virtually all the studies neglect to control for important confounders (e.g., socioeconomic status). In the two studies that do stratify for SES, only a weak association remains (61,65). Hearey et al. suggest a possible link between paternal (but not maternal) smoking and the occurrence of neural tube defects (63). The smoking status of both parents was not taken into account in this analysis. This is necessary to identify whether each parent's smoking status has an independent or an interactive effect on the fetus.

The possibility of an association between the occurrence of orofacial clefts and smoking has also been evaluated. Four studies report varying degrees of a positive association (4,59,60,66) and two find no association (41,61). Results from the single largest "positive" study become nonsignificant when the relationship is analyzed according to the specific type of cleft (66).

Suggestions that smoking is associated with congenital heart disease (67), limb reduction defects (68), and the prevention of musculoskeletal abnormalities (41,58) remain essentially isolated reports that have not been substantiated by other studies (4,60,61,69).

Animal experiments of cigarette exposure and malformations have produced conflicting results. Nicotine injected into chick embryos in doses equivalent to the amount absorbed in humans from smoking one cigarette has induced vertebral anomalies (70,71). However, pregnant rats exposed to smoke equivalent to 30 cigarettes twice a day did not have an increased frequency of skeletal anomalies as observed after fixing and staining the fetuses (72). Studies of cattle and pigs who ingested tobacco plants while grazing show epidemic proportions of newborns with musculoskeletal anomalies (73,74), although the specific exposures to the fetus are likely to be different than those in cigarette smoke.

These contradictory results make it difficult to conclude that smoking is an important teratogen or that it is entirely free of teratogenic effects. Part of the current uncertainty is attributable to the many exposure, disease, and analytical interstudy differences. Additional well-designed research may resolve these issues.

PATERNALLY MEDIATED EFFECTS

Little attention has been given to the effects of paternal cigarette smoking on the fetus. A prospective study relating parental factors to reproductive outcomes found that infants born to fathers who smoke more than ten cigarettes per day and nonsmoking mothers have an increased risk for perinatal mortality and serious malformations (75). Many important factors were not included in this analysis.

It has been suggested that smoking among males is associated with abnormal spermatogenesis. Many studies of sperm quality and smoking select their populations from infertility clinics, which unfortunately creates a potential selection bias. Reductions in sperm motility (76,77), sperm counts (76,77), and increased frequencies of morphologically abnormal sperm (77) have been reported among smokers. The findings are not consistent across studies and many potential confounders (e.g., alcohol, occupational exposures, heat exposure) were not considered (76–78). Serial sperm analyses among smokers and nonsmokers are needed to further evaluate these reported effects and to establish whether a dose-response relationship exists.

MORBIDITY AND BEHAVIORAL EFFECTS

Passive exposure to maternal cigarette smoke has been documented for the fetus through studies of nicotine and cotinine in human amniotic fluid (21) and studies of nicotine accumulation in fetal tissues of smoke-exposed animals (22). Substantial amounts of nicotine have been measured in breast milk of nursing mothers (79) and increased levels of cotinine have been measured in the urine of children exposed to smoke at home (80). A study of hospital discharge diagnoses found childhood illnesses—primarily respiratory disorders—are linked to maternal smoking (81–84). Behavioral problems and decreased physical growth among children of smokers have been observed in large follow-up studies of offspring of smokers and nonsmokers (85,86). Many important cofactors were controlled, although IQ of parents and general care of children at home have not always been considered. These behavioral and physical problems may be due to smoke exposure during childhood and not exposure *in utero*. It is unclear whether the presence or absence of smoking during pregnancy alters the risk for these problems. An analysis of women who smoked during pregnancy but stopped after delivery would be necessary to resolve this.

An analysis of 605 women enrolled in the Collaborative Study of the Antenatal Administration of Dexamethasone to Lower the Incidence of Respiratory Distress Syndrome (RDS) found an association between maternal smoking and absence of RDS (87). The association remained after adjusting for steroid or placebo treatment, premature rupture of membranes, preeclampsia, gestational age, race, method of delivery, sex, and tocolytic therapy.

In utero exposure to the products of cigarette smoke may exert chronic stress on the fetus that stimulates early lung maturation (87,88).

CONCLUSIONS

Cigarette smoking during pregnancy is clearly harmful to the fetus. Infants of smoking mothers have on the average a 200-gm reduction in birthweight. Women who stop smoking during the first half of pregnancy have infants with birthweights closer to those of nonsmokers. Recent studies have focused on the mechanism of action of cigarette smoke. Decreased placental blood flow is well documented by several methods of study. This nicotine-mediated effect may result in hypoxia which, in turn, causes intrauterine growth retardation. Other components of cigarette smoke have also been implicated as causing growth retardation (carbon monoxide and thiocyanate) although these have not been as thoroughly studied. It is possible that intrauterine growth retardation results from toxic effects of more than one component of cigarette smoke. The evidence is in favor of a direct smoking effect rather than nutrient starvation among smokers.

Epidemiologic data indicates that smoking during pregnancy increases the risk for spontaneous abortion. As yet it is unclear how smoking affects the viability of the fetus and/or the maternal/placental ability to support the fetus.

Women who are already in high-risk groups for perinatal mortality are at an even greater risk if they smoke during pregnancy. Smoking does not substantially increase the risk for perinatal mortality among women who are at low risk to begin with. Abruptio placentae and placenta previa have been linked to smoking during pregnancy. Excess perinatal death has partly been attributed to these two placental abnormalities. There is physical and biochemical evidence showing that structural changes and decreased functions occur more frequently in the placentas of smokers.

There is no conclusive evidence that maternal smoking causes congenital malformations. Both human and animal studies have produced conflicting results. Inconsistencies in results of human studies can be attributed to differences in study design.

Follow-up studies have found increased risks for both physical and behavioral problems among children whose mothers smoked during pregnancy. It is unknown if this is due to postnatal exposure only or if antenatal exposure has an independent effect.

Women seeking prenatal care should be advised that their smoking may reduce birthweight, as well as increase their risk for miscarriage and placental disorders. Women of low socioeconomic status, advanced maternal age, or with a history of a previous loss who smoke should be made aware of their increased risk for perinatal mortality. Caretakers should encourage women to stop smoking since the risk of decreased birthweight is reduced after cessation. Postnatally, parents should be made aware that studies indicate that infants exposed to smoke at home are at risk for illness and behavior problems in childhood.

ACKNOWLEDGMENTS

This work was supported in part by funds provided by Merrell-Dow Pharmaceuticals, Inc., Cincinnati, Ohio.

LITERATURE CITED

1. Streissguth, A.P., B.L. Darby, H. Barr, J. Smith, and D. Martin (1983) Comparison of drinking and smoking patterns during pregnancy over a six year interval. Am. J. Obstet. Gynecol., *145:*716–723.
2. Prager, K., H. Malin, D. Speigler, P. Van Natta, and P. Placek (1984) Smoking and drinking behavior before and during pregnancy of married mothers of liveborn infants and stillborn infants. Public Health Rep., *99 (2):*117–127.
3. Simpson, W.J. (1957) A preliminary report of cigarette smoking and the incidence of prematurity. Am. J. Obstet. Gynecol., *73:*808–815.
4. Andrews, J. and J. McGarry (1972) A community study of smoking in pregnancy. J. Obstet. Gynaecol. Br. Commwlth., *79:*1057–1073.
5. Meyer, M., B. Jonas, and J. Tonascia (1976) Perinatal events associated with maternal smoking. Am. J. Epidemiol., *103:*464–476.
6. Meyer, M. (1978) How does maternal smoking affect birth weight and maternal weight gain? Am. J. Obstet. Gynecol., *131:*888–893.
7. Frazer, T., G. Davis, H. Goldstein, and I. Goldberg (1961) Cigarette smoking and prematurity: a prospective study. Am. J. Obstet. Gynecol., *81:*988–996.
8. Yerushalmy, J. (1971) The relationship of parent's cigarette smoking to outcome of pregnancy—implication as to the problem inferring causation from observed associations. Am. J. Epidemiol., *93:*443.
9. Lubs, M. (1973) Racial differences in maternal smoking effects on the newborn infant. Am. J. Obstet. Gynecol., *115:*66–76.
10. Butler, N., H. Goldstein and E. Ross (1972) Cigarette smoking in pregnancy: Its influence on birth weight and perinatal mortality. Br. Med. J. [Clin. Res.], *2:*127–130.
11. Russell, C., R. Taylor, and E. Law (1968) Smoking in pregnancy, maternal blood pressure, pregnancy outcome, baby weight and growth, and other related factors. Br. J. Prev. Soc. Med., *22:*119–126.
12. Bailey, R. (1970) The effect of maternal smoking on the infant birth weight. N.Z. Med. J., *71:*293–294.
13. Rush, D., and P. Cassano (1983) Relationship of cigarette smoking and social class to birth weight and perinatal mortality among all births in Britain 5–11 April 1970. J. Epidemiol. Community Health, *37:*249–255.
14. Trease, G.E., and W.C. Evans (1983) The pharmacological action of plant drugs. In: Pharmacognosy. 12th edition. Baillière Tindall, London, p. 150.
15. Mochizuki, M, T. Maruo, K. Masuko, and T. Ohtsu (1984) Effects of smoking on the fetoplacental-maternal system during pregnancy. Am. J. Obstet. Gynecol., *149:*413–420.
16. Philipp, K., N. Pateisky, and M. Endler (1984) Effects of smoking on uteroplacental blood flow. Gynecol. Obstet. Invest., *17:*179–182.
17. Lehtovirta, P., and M. Forss (1978) The acute effect of smoking on intervillous blood flow of the placenta. Br. J. Obstet. Gynaecol., *85:*729–731.
18. Suzuki, K., L. Minei, and E. Johnson (1980) Effect of nicotine upon uterine blood flow in the pregnant rhesus monkey. Am. J. Obstet. Gynecol., *136:*1009–1013.
19. Dadak, G., C. Leithner, H. Sinzinger, and K. Silberbauer (1981) Diminished prostacyclin formation in umbilical arteries of babies born to women who smoke. Lancet, *1:*94.
20. Busqcca, M., G. Balconi, A. Pietra, M. Vergarq-Dauden, G. de Gaetano, and E. Dejana (1984) Maternal smoking and Prostacyclin production by cultured endothelial cells from umbilical arteries. Am. J. Obstet. Gynecol., *148:*1127–1130.
21. Van Vanukis, H., J. Langone and A. Milunsky (1977) Nicotine and cotinine in the amniotic fluid of smokers in the second trimester of pregnancy. Am. J. Obstet. Gynecol., *120:*64–66.
22. Suzuki, K., T. Horiguchi, AC. Comas-Urrutia, E. Mueller-Heubach, H.O. Morishima, and K. Adamsons (1974) Placental transfer and distribution of nicotine in the pregnant rhesus monkey. Am. J. Obstet. Gynecol., *119:*253–262.
23. Bureau, M.A., J. Monette, D. Shapcott, C. Pare, J.L. Mathieu, J. Lippé, D. Blovin, Y. Berthiaume, and R. Begin (1982) Carboxyhemoglobin concentration in fetal cord blood and in blood of mothers who smoked during labor. Pediatrics, *69:*371–373.
24. Bartlett, D. (1968) Pathophysiology of exposure to low concentrations of carbon monoxide. Arch. Environ. Health, *16:*719–727.
25. Bureau, M.A., D. Shapcott, Y. Berthiaume, J. Monette, D. Blouis, P. Blanchard, and R. Begin (1983) Maternal cigarette smoking and fetal oxygen transport: A study of P50, 2, 3, diphosphoglycerate, total hemoglobin, hematocrit, and type F hemoglobin in fetal blood. Pediatrics, *72:*22–26.
26. Bottoms, S.F., D.D. Kuhnert, P.M. Kuhnert, and A.L. Reese (1982) Maternal passive smoking and fetal serum thiocyanate levels. Am. J. Obstet. Gynecol., *144:*787–791.
27. Sophian, J. (1968) Preeclamptic toxaemia in smokers. Lancet, *1:*1249–1250.
28. Harrison, G.G., K.S. Branson, and Y.E. Vaucher (1983) Association of maternal smoking with body composition of the newborn. Am. J. Clin. Nutr., *38:*757–762.
29. Spira, A., and B. Servent (1976) Smoking and the fetus. Lancet *1:*1416–1417.
30. Mulcahy, R. J. Murphy, and P. Martin (1970) Placental changes and maternal weight in smoking and

non-smoking mothers. Am. J. Obstet. Gynecol., *106:*103.
31. Davies, D., O. Gray, P. Ellwood, and M. Abernathy (1976) Cigarette smoking in pregnancy: Association with maternal weight gain and fetal growth. Lancet, *1:*385–387.
32. Rush, D. (1974) Birth weight, smoking and pregnancy weight gain. J. Obstet. Gynaecol. Br. Comm. *81:*746–752.
33. Ounsted, M., and A. Scott (1982) Smoking during pregnancy—its association with other maternal factors and birthweight. Acta Obstet. Gynecol Scand., *61:*367–371.
34. Picone, T.A., L.H. Allen, M.M. Schramm, and P.N. Olsen (1982) Pregnancy outcome in North American women. I. Effects of diet, cigarette smoking and psychological stress on maternal weight gain. Am. J. Clin. Nutr. *32:*1205–1213.
35. Rush, D., Z. Stein, and M. Susser (1980) Diet in Pregnancy; A Randomized Controlled Clinical Trial of Nutritional Supplements. Alan R. Liss, Inc., New York.
36. Haas, J.D., G. Moreno-Black, E.A. Frongillo, A.J. Pabon, L.G. Pareja, U.J. Ybarnegary, and G.L. Hurtado (1983) Altitude and infant growth in Bolivia: A longitudinal study. Am. J. Phys. Anthropol., *59:*251–262.
37. Kittlick, P.D. (1977) Hypoxia in fibroblast cultures. Exp. Pathol., *13:*217–225.
38. Gordon, G.B., N.A. Barcza, and M.E. Bush (1977) Lipid accumulation in hypoxic tissue culture cells. Am. J. Pathol., *88:*663–674.
39. Himmelberger, D., B. Brown, and E. Cohen (1978) Cigarette smoke during pregnancy and the occurrence of spontaneous abortion and congenital abnormality. Am. J. Epidemiol. *108:*470–479.
40. Kline, J., B. Levin, P. Shrout, Z. Stein, M. Susser, and D. Warburton (1983) Maternal smoking and trisomy among spontaneously aborted conceptions. Am J Hum. Genet. *35:*421–431.
41. Hemininki, K., P. Mutanen, and I. Soloniemi (1983) Smoking and the occurrence of congenital malformations and spontaneous abortions: Multivariate analysis. Am. J. Obstet. Gynecol., *145:*61–66.
42. Kline, J., Z. Stein, M. Susser, and D. Warburton (1977) Smoking: A risk factor for spontaneous abortion. N. Engl. J. Med., *297:*793–796.
43. Harlap, S., and P. Shiono (1980) Alcohol, smoking and incidence of spontaneous abortion in first and second trimester. Lancet, *2:*173–176.
44. Alberman, E., M. Creasy, M. Elliott, and C. Spicer (1976) Maternal factors associated with fetal chromosomal anomalies in spontaneous abortions. Br. J. Obstet. Gynecol., *83:*621–627.
45. Holmes, L.B., S.E. Vincent, C. Cook, and K.R. Cote (1981) Surveillance of newborn infants for malformations due to spontaneous germinal mutations. In: Population and Biological Aspects of Human Mutation. E.B. Hook and I.H. Porter, eds. Academic Press, New York, pp 351–359.
46. Butler, N., and E. Alberman (1969) Perinatal Problems. Livingstone, Edinburgh.
47. Mulcahy, R. (1968) Effect of age, parity and cigarette smoking on outcome of pregnancy. Am. J. Obstet. Gynecol., *101:*844–849.
48. Rantakallio, P. (1978) Relationship of maternal smoking to morbidity and mortality of the child up to the age of five. Acat Paediatr. Scand., *67:*621–631.
49. Underwood, P., K. Kesler, J.M. O'Lane, and D. Callagan (1967) Parental smoking emperically related to pregnancy outcome. Obstet. Gynecol. *29:*1–8.
50. Niswander, K.R., and M. Godon (1972) The Women—Their Pregnancies. US Department of Health, Education and Welfare, Washington D.C.
51. Comstock, G., F. Shah, M. Meyer, and H. Abbey (1971) Low birth weight and neonatal mortality rate related to maternal smoking—socioeconomic status. Am. J. Obstet. Gynecol., *111:*53–59.
52. Meyer, M.B., J.A. Tonascia, (1977) Maternal smoking, pregnancy complications, and perinatal mortality. Am. J. Obstet. Gynecol., *128:*494.
53. Goujard, J., E. Rumeau and D. Schwartz (1975) Smoking during pregnancy, stillbirth and abruptio placentae. Biomedicine *23:*20–22.
54. Naeye, R., W. Harkness and J. Utts (1979) The duration of maternal cigarette smoking, fetal and placental disorders. Early Hum. Dev., *3:*229–237.
55. Spira, A., N. Spira, J. Goujard, and D. Schwartz (1975) Smoking during pregnancy and placental weight. A multivariate analysis on 3759 cases. J. Perinat. Med., *3:*237–241.
56. Van der Veen, F., and H. Fox (1982) The effects of cigarette smoking on human placenta: A light and electron microscopy study. Placenta, *3:*243–256.
57. Van Der Velde, W.J., J.H.J. Copius Peereboom-Stegeman, P.E. Treffers, and J. James (1983) Structural changes in the placenta of smoking mothers: A quantitative study. Placenta, *4:*231–240.
58. Christensen, R. (1980) The relationship between maternal smoking and the incidence of congenital anomalies. Am. J. Epidemiol, *112:*684–695.
59. Ericson, A., B. Kallen, and P. Westerholm (1979) Cigarette smoking as an etiologic factor in cleft lip and palate. Am. J. Obstet. Gynecol. *135:*348–351.
60. Kelsey, J., T. Dayer, T. Holford, and M. Bracken (1978) Maternal smoking and congenital malformations: An Epidemiologic Study. J Epidemiol. Community Health, *32:*102–107.
61. Evans, D., R. Newcombe, and H. Campbell (1979) Maternal smoking habits and congenital malformations. Br. Med. J. [Clin. Res.], 2:171–173.
62. Chung, C.S., and N. Myrianthopoulos (1975) Factors affecting risks of congenital malformations. I. Epidemiologic analysis. Birth Defects, *XI:*1–21.
63. Hearey, L.D., J.A. Harris, M.S. Usatin D.M. Epstein, H.K. Ury and R.R. Neutra (1984) Investigation of a cluster of anencephaly and spina bifida. Am. J. Epidemiol. *120:*559–564.
64. Naeye, R.L. (1978) Relationship of cigarette smoking to congenital anomalies and perinatal death. Am. J. Pathol. *90:*289–293.
65. Golding J., and N.R. Butler, (1983) Maternal smoking and anencephaly. Br. Med. J. [Clin. Res.], *287:*533–534.
66. Saxen, I. (1974) Cleft lip and palate in Finland: Parental histories, course of pregnancy and selected environmental factors. Int. J. Epidemiol., *3:*263–270.
67. Fedrick, J., E.D. Alberman, and H. Goldstein (1971) Possible teratogenic effect of cigarette smoking. Nature, *231:*529–530.
68. Aro, T. (1983) Maternal diseases, alcohol consumption and smoking during pregnancy associated with reduction limb defects. Early Hum. Dev., *9:*49–57.
69. Yerushalmy, J. (1973) Congenital heart disease and maternal smoking habits. Nature, *242:*262–264.
70. Upshall, D.G. (1972) Correlation of chick embryo teratogenicity with the nicotine activity of a series of tetrahydropyrimidines. Teratology, *5:*287–294.
71. Landauer, W. (1960) Nicotine-induced malformations of chick embryos and their bearing on the phenocopy problem. J. Exp. Zool., *143:*107–122.
72. Reckzeh, G., W. Dontenwill, and F. Leuschner (1975)

Testing of cigarette smoke for teratogenicity in rats. Toxicology, *4:*289–295.
73. Crowe, W., and H.T. Pike (1973) Congenital arthrogryposis associated with ingestion of tobacco stalks by pregnant sows. J. Am. Vet. Med. Assoc., *162:*453–455.
74. Keeler, R.F., J.L. Shupe, M.W. Crowe, A. Olson, and L.D. Balls (1981) Nicotiania glauco-induced congenital deformities in calves: Clinical and pathologic aspects. Am. J. Vet. Res., *42:*1231–1234.
75. Knorr, K. (1979) Influence of tobacco and alcohol on pregnancy and child development. Bull. Schweiz. Akad. Med. Wiss., *35:*137–146.
76. Campbell, J.M., and K.L. Harrison (1979) Smoking and infertility. Med. J. Aust., *1:*342–343.
77. Shearway, M., and K.Z. Mahmoud (1982) Smoking and fertility. Fertil. Steril., *38:*255–257.
78. Rodriguez-Rigau, L.J., K.D. Smith, E. Steinberger (1982) Cigarette smoking and semen quality. Fertil. Steril., *38:*115–116.
79. Luck W., H. Nau (1984) Nicotine and cotinine concentrations in serum and milk of nursing smokers. Br. J. Clin. Pharmacol. *18:*9–15.
80. Greenberg, R., N. Haley, R. Etzel, and F. Loda (1984) Measuring exposure of infants to tobacco smoke. N. Engl. J. Med., *310:*1075–1078.
81. Colley, J.R., W. Holland, and R. Corkhill (1974) Influence of passive smoking and parental phlegm on pneumonia and bronchitis in early children. Lancet, *2:*1031–1034.
82. Yarnell, J., and A. St. Leger (1979) Respiratory illness, maternal smoking habit and lung function in children. Br. J. Dis. Chest., *73:*230–236.
83. Rantakallio, P. (1978) Relationship of maternal smoking to morbidity and mortality of the child up to the age of five. Acta. Paediatr. Scand., *67:*621–631.
84. Harlap, S., and A. Davies (1974) Infant admissions to hospital and maternal smoking. Lancet *1:*529–532.
85. Butler, N.R., and H. Goldstein (1973) Smoking in pregnancy and subsequent child development. Br. Med. J. [Clin. Res.], *4:*573–575.
86. Dunn, H.G., A.K. McBurney, S. Ingram, and C.M. Hunter (1976) Maternal cigarette smoking during pregnancy and the child's subsequent development. Can. J. Public Health, *67:*499–605.
87. Curet, L.B., A.V. Rao, R.D. Zachman, J. Morrison, G. Burkett, and W.K. Polle (1983) Maternal smoking and respiratory distress syndrome. Am. J. Obstet. Gynecol., *147:*446–450.
88. Cluck, L., and M.V. Kulovich (1973) Lecithin/sphingomyelin ratios in amniotic fluid in normal and abnormal pregnancy. Am. J. Obstet. Gynecol., *115:*539–546.

TERATOGEN UPDATE: ENVIRONMENTALLY INDUCED BIRTH DEFECT RISKS, PAGES 141–143 (1986)

Small Head Size After Atomic Irradiation

ROBERT W. MILLER AND JOHN J. MULVIHILL
Clinical Epidemiology Branch, National Cancer Institute, NIH, Bethesda, Maryland 20892

In 1920 reports began to appear about children born with small head circumference and who developed mental retardation, after therapeutic exposure of women to X-rays during pregnancy. These cases and others—a total of 16 in the world literature—were reviewed by Goldstein and Murphy in 1929. By then it was known that these effects occurred only when radiation was given early in pregnancy. The information available had been obtained by retrospective study, as is usual in first identifying new human teratogens.

A prospective study became possible when the atomic bombs were exploded over Hiroshima and Nagasaki in 1945. In 1952 Plummer described microcephaly and mental retardation in 7 of 11 Hiroshima chldren exposed within 1200 m of the hypocenter. Further studies revealed 4 more cases, excluding 2 with Down syndrome, and the effect was related to the distance from the hypocenter (i.e., dose) and to gestational age (Miller, '56). At intermediate dose-levels the effects were intermediate between normal and the pronounced effects seen in the heavily exposed, with no increase in the frequency of gross mental retardation. The last-mentioned evaluation was made when the children were 9 years old.

The scientific design of the study was then improved, with observations limited to children who came for examination between 10 and 19 years of age. Some affected children seen earlier did not appear at the clinics during this interval, and were excluded from the analysis. Careful estimates of dose had been made (Milton and Shohoji, '68), and the new data showed small head size and mental retardation when exposure was at under 18 weeks of gestational age, the frequency of these effects being related to the dose (Miller and Blot, '72; Blot and Miller, '73). In Hiroshima an increase in the frequency of small head circumference was detectable even when the dose in air to the pregnant woman ws 10-19 rad. Her body screened out some of the radiation, so an even smaller dose reached the fetus. The dose-response relation was dramatically shown in a chart published by Blot in 1975 (Fig. 1).

A new three-dimensional graphic portrayal of the Hiroshima data (Fig. 2) shows the frequency of small head circumference with respect to dose and gestational age. It should be noted that each point is based on only a few observations (Table 1). Again, the increased frequency of small head circumference is seen in the group whose maternal exposure was 10–19 rad. At higher doses susceptibility during gestation seemed to begin a little later and last somewhat longer. Figure 2 shows that the most pronounced effect was in the most heavily exposed group (150 rad or more). Among those with the lowest exposure, 0–9 rad, cases unaccountably occurred regardless of the gestational age at exposure.

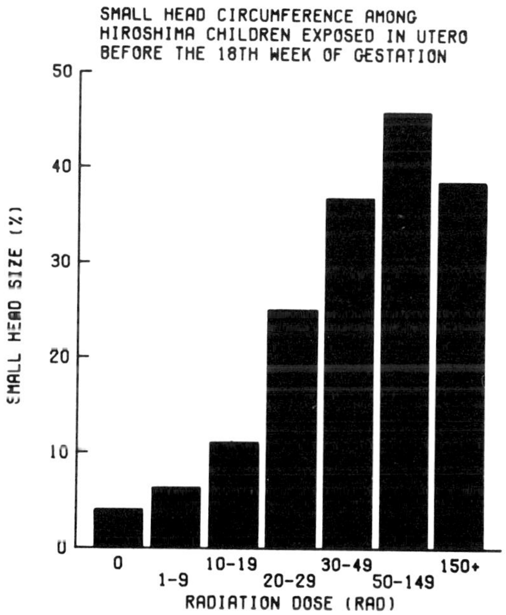

Fig. 1. Relation of dose to head circumference in Hiroshima children exposed in utero before the 18th week of gestation. Heads considered small were those with a circumference 2 or more standard deviations below the age- and sex-specific mean on at least 1 medical examination and 1 or more standard deviations below average at all other examinations during the ages (10-19 years) studied. (From Blot, '75.)

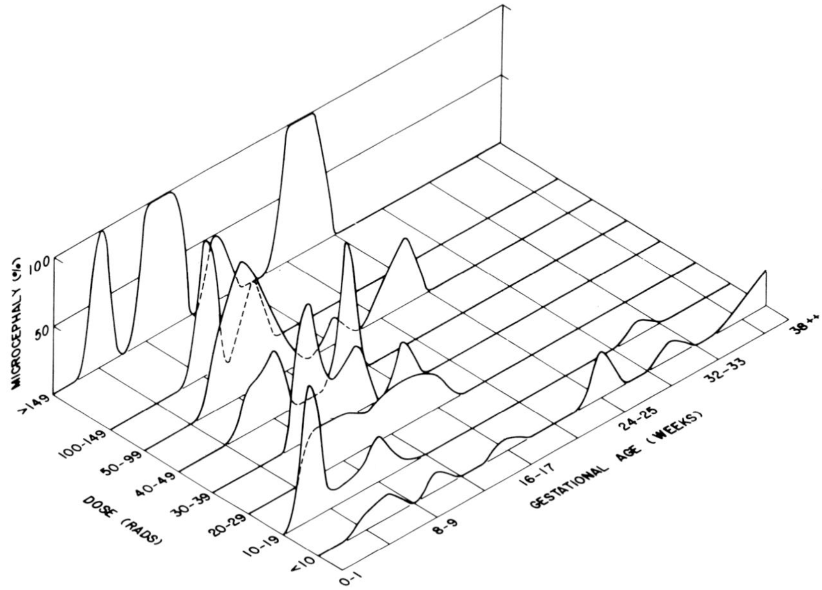

Fig. 2. Relation of dose to head circumference and gestational age among Hiroshima children exposed in utero to the atomic bomb.

TABLE 1. Frequency of small head circumference by dose and gestational age (Hiroshima)

Gestational age (weeks)	Dose (rad)								
	< 10	10-19	20-29	30-39	40-49	50-99	100-149	150 +	Total
0-1	0/2	—	0/1	—	—	0/1	—	—	0/4
2-3	0/3	1/1	0/1		0/1	—	—	0/1	1/7
4-5	1/9	1/8	0/3	—	—	—	0/1	1/1	3/22
6-7	1/6	1/7	1/3	—	1/3	2/4	—	—	6/23
8-9	0/5	2/6	1/3	1/1	1/2	3/3	1/1	4/4	13/25
10-11	1/8	1/11	1/4	1/3	0/1	2/3	—	2/2	8/32
12-13	0/4	0/3	1/3	1/2	—	1/4	1/2	0/3	4/21
14-15	0/9	0/8	1/3	—	1/1	0/1	—	1/2	3/24
16-17	1/12	0/11	1/4	1/3	0/1	1/5	—	0/1	4/37
18-19	0/4	0/1	0/1	—	0/1	0/3	—	—	0/10
20-21	0/6	0/3	0/2	—	—	1/4	0/1	2/2	3/18
22-23	0/5	0/6	0/1	—	0/1	1/2	0/1	1/1	2/17
24-25	1/3	0/4	0/5	—	—	0/2	0/1	0/1	1/16
26-27	0/5	0/3	0/1	—	0/1	0/4	0/1	—	0/15
28-29	0/4	0/3	0/3	—	—	0/2	—	—	0/12
30-31	1/8	1/9	—	0/2	0/1	—	0/1	0/2	2/23
32-33	0/9	0/2	—	—	0/1	0/5	0/1	—	0/18
34-35	0/1	0/6	0/1	—	—	0/2	0/2	—	0/12
36-37	1/8	0/3	0/3	0/4	0/1	—	—	—	1/19
38+	1/4	0/5	0/1	—	—	—	0/1	—	1/11
Total	8/115	7/100	6/43	4/15	3/15	11/45	2/13	11/20	52/355

In Nagasaki no effect was demonstrable under 150 rad. The number of intrauterine exposures there, though substantially fewer than in Hiroshima, was ample to show an effect comparable to that in Hiroshima, had there been one. Similar differences between the cities have been observed with regard to other radiation-induced disorders. The differences may be attributable to the dissimilar quality of the radiation in the 2 cities (20%

of that in Hiroshima was due to neutrons, as compared with a negligible percent in Nagasaki), or to an interaction in Hiroshima with other adverse influences on brain growth, such as malnutrition or severe illness during early life.

ADDENDUM

In May 1984 Otake and Schull published a reanalysis of the data on intrauterine exposures to the Japanese atomic bombs in relation to severe mental retardation. The evaluation was independent of small head size; that is, some of the children had severe mental retardation with normal head circumference. The results indicated that the doubling dose for severe mental retardation in the United States would be one rad absorbed dose. The estimate was based on linear extrapolation of a curve based on five affected among 112 with tissue doses of 1–49 rad, four affected among 11 with tissue doses of 50–99 rad and five affected among eight with doses of 100 or more rad. The short period of susceptibility matches the time in the human conceptus when cortical neurons proliferate and migrate from areas near the cerebral ventricles to the cortex. Otake and Schull stated that "fetal brain damage limited in time to the period 8–15 weeks postconception would be the result of either damage to cell production or cell migration (or both)." Cells killed before this time cause small head size without causing severe mental retardation because cerebral histogenesis is absent then, according to the authors. They do not believe that infection or malnutrition could have reduced the threshold for mental retardation due to radiation exposure. If such factors contributed to the effect, the observations made under conditions of stress and deprivation would not apply to risks in the practice of radiology. In any event, the International Commission on Radiological Protection concluded in 1984 that the new analysis did not alter its previous recommendations concerning radiologic exposures during pregnancy.

LITERATURE CITED

Blot, W.J. (1975) Growth and development following prenatal and childhood exposure to atomic radiation. J. Radiat. Res., *16*(Suppl.):82–88.

Blot, W.J., and R.W. Miller (1973) Mental retardation following in utero exposure to the atomic bombs of Hiroshima and Nagasaki. Radiology, *106:*617–619.

Goldstein, L., and D. Murphy (1929) Etiology of ill-health in children born after maternal pelvic irradiation. II. Defective children born after postconception pelvic irradiation. Am. J. Roentgen., *22:*322–331.

International Commission on Radiological Protection (1984) Statement from the 1983 meeting. Br. J. Radiol., *57:*415

Miller, R.W. (1956) Delayed effects occurring within the first decade after exposure of young individuals to the Hiroshima atomic bomb. Pediatrics, *18:*1–17.

Miller, R.W., and W.J. Blot (1972) Small head size following in utero exposure to atomic radiation. Lancet, *2:*784–787.

Milton, R.C., and T. Shohoji (1968) Tentative 1965 radiation dose estimation for atomic bomb survivors, Hiroshima and Nagasaki. ABCC Tech. Report, pp. 1–68.

Otake, M., and W.J. Schull (1984) In utero exposure to A-bomb radiation and mental retardation: A reassessment. Br. J. Radiol., *57:*409–414.

Plummer, G.W. (1952) Anomalies occurring in children exposed in utero to the atomic bomb in Hiroshima. Pediatrics, *10:*687–692.

Radiation Teratogenesis

ROBERT L. BRENT
Stein Research Center, Thomas Jefferson University, Philadelphia, Pennsylvania 19107

In spite of the fact that we have a great deal more to learn about radiation teratogenesis and teratogenesis in general, there have been many experiments and observations about the effects of radiation on the developing embryo. A complete review of this subject will not be presented, and the reader is referred to recent reviews on this subject (Brent, '70, '72, '76, '77, '82; Brent and Gorson, '72).

Prior to the blastocyst stage, the embryo is a multicellular organism with an insensitivity to the teratogenic and growth-retarding effects of radiation and the greatest degree of sensitivity to the lethal effects of irradiation (Russell, '50; Russell and Russell, '50; Brent and Bolden, '67a) (Figs. 1–3). During early organogenesis, the embryo is very sensitive to the *growth retarding, teratogenic and lethal* effects of irradiation, but has the ability to recover somewhat from the growth-retarding effects in the postpartum period. During the early fetal period, the fetus has diminished sensitivity to multiple organ teratogenesis, retains central nervous system sensitivity, is growth-retarded at term, but recovers poorly from the growth retardation in the postpartum period (Russell, '50, '56; Russell and Russell, '54; Rugh, '62). During the later fetal stages, the embryo is not grossly deformed by radiation but can respond with permanent cell depletion of various organs and tissues if the radiation exposure is high enough (Brent and Gorson, '72; Brent, '77). One can postulate many mechanisms for the effects of irradiation, which include cell death, mitotic delay, disturbances of cell migration, alteration in macromolecular structure, and many others. Until we know more about the mechanisms involved in embryopathology, it is difficult to determine which mechanisms are most important in the process of radiation-induced embryopathology. Furthermore, the same pathogenic mechanisms may not be primarily operative at all stages of gestation. Radiation-induced cell death may be minimally important at one stage of gestation because of the embryo's ability to replace the killed cells. At another stage of gestation, cell death may be a primary factor because the embryo has lost the ability to replace dead cells and that fetus may be permanently cell depleted.

Other radiation-induced effects that have been invoked to explain embryopathology are cytogenetic abnormalities and somatic mutation (Russell and Saylors, '63; Russell and Major, '57). Cytogenetic abnormalities may be responsible for preimplantation death in the irradiated mammalian zygote (Rugh, '65; Russell and Saylors, '63; Brent and Bolden, '67a), but point mutations are less likely to be a contributing factor to abnormal morphogenesis. Of course, neither phenomenon has been adequately studied at every stage of mammalian gestation.

Radiation effects may appear at once and result in cell death, embryonic death, or teratogenesis. Other effects may not be obvious immediately and can only be measured or ascertained in the postpartum or adult period. Neuronal depletion, infertility, tissue hypoplasia, neoplasia, or shortening of life span are phenomena whose significance can only be evaluated in the postpartum or adult organism (Hicks and D'Amato, '66; Murphree and Pace, '60; Brent and Gorson, '72; Brent and Bolden, '61, Brent, '70; Rugh and Wohlfromm, '64a, b; Cowen and Geller, '60).

The neurophysiological and behavior changes in adult organisms that have been irradiated in utero are the most difficult to evaluate. The difficulties arise for several reasons: 1) it is not easy to eliminate postnatal environmental effects as contributing factors; 2) reported findings are frequently not reproducible and are not dose-related; 3) behavioral changes may not be able to be correlated with the neuroanatomical changes, and 4) animal behavior tests may have minimal application to the human situation. This subject is reviewed by Furchtgott ('63) and Brent ('76). Except for the work of Piontkovskii ('58, '61), all behavioral studies of animals or humans exposed to radiation during gestation do not exhibit any measurable changes if the exposure is below 25 rads.

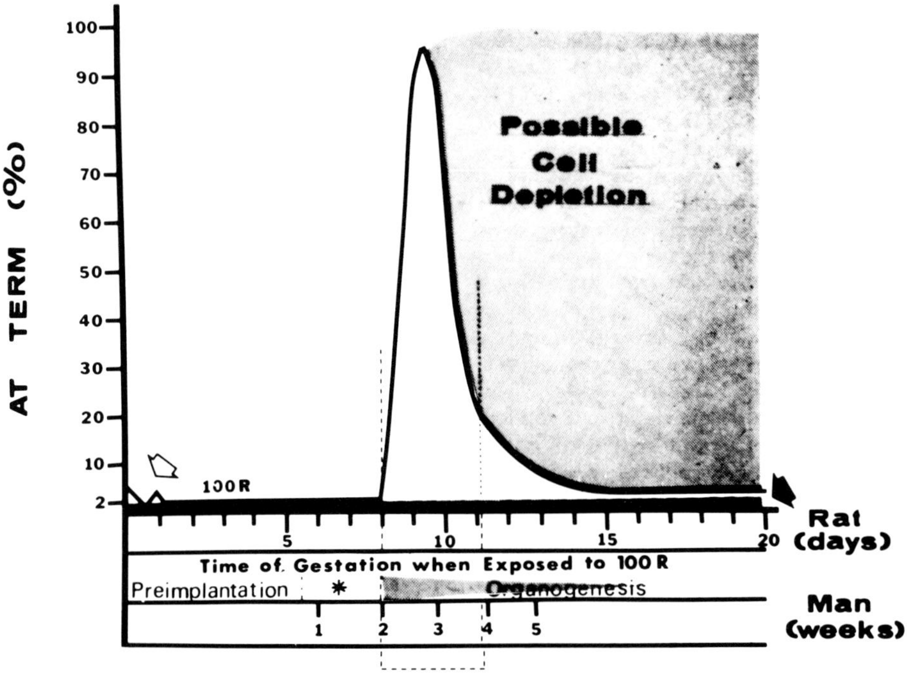

Fig. 1. This graph depicts the relative incidence of gross congenital malformations in the rat following an exposure of 100 R. The arrow on the right side of the ordinate points to the 2% control incidence of congenital malformations seen in this species. The incidence of malformations before the 9th day is the same as in the controls. The light arrow on the left side of the ordinate points to a slight increase in malformations on the 1st day. This was inserted because of the work of Russell in a particular strain of mice. A vary large increase in malformations occurs during the early organogenetic period. Note that this corresponds to the 3rd and 4th weeks of human pregnancy. This high incidence of gross malformations falls off rapidly as organogenesis diminishes. Note that organogenesis to some degree (CNS) continues to term. Also note that although gross malformations may not be produced during the late fetal stages with 100 R, an irreversible loss of cells occurs. The significance of these cell losses is under study. The asterisk (*) is placed at the stage of implantation to indicate that although malformations are not readily produced at this stage, growth retardation can be induced.

HUMAN RADIATION TERATOGENESIS

The classic effects of radiation on the developing mammal are *gross congenital malformations, intrauterine growth retardation, and embryonic death.* Each of these effects has a dose response relationship and a threshold exposure below which there is no difference between the irradiated and the control population. Since human pregnancies predominantly consist of a single embryo, it would be unusual to see the classical triad of effects, although it is conceivable that if the dose and timing were appropriate, a stillborn, growth-retarded, malformed embryo could result.

Growth retardation and central nervous system effects, such as microcephaly or eye malformations, are the cardinal manifestations of intrauterine radiation effects in the human. The occurrence of microcephaly is such a significant component of the effects of intrauterine radiation that a separate "Teratogen Update" has been written about this subject (Miller and Mulvihill, '76). The reports of Zappert ('26), Goldstein and Murphy ('29a, b), Glass ('44), Johnson ('38), Dekaban ('68), Miller ('69), Wood et al. ('67a, b), Plummer ('52), and Yamazaki et al. ('54) indicate that microcephaly is the commonest malformation observed in humans randomly exposed to high doses of radiation during pregnancy. In Goldstein and Murphy's reports, 19 of 75 irradiated embryos were microcephalic or hydrocephalic children, having received an estimated dose of greater than 100 rads as a minimum. Almost all the microcephalic children were mentally retarded. The following malformations were also reported: two children with hypoplastic genitalia, one child with cleft palate, one child with hypospadius, an abnormality of the large toe, and an ear abnormality. Many of the children had intrauterine growth retar-

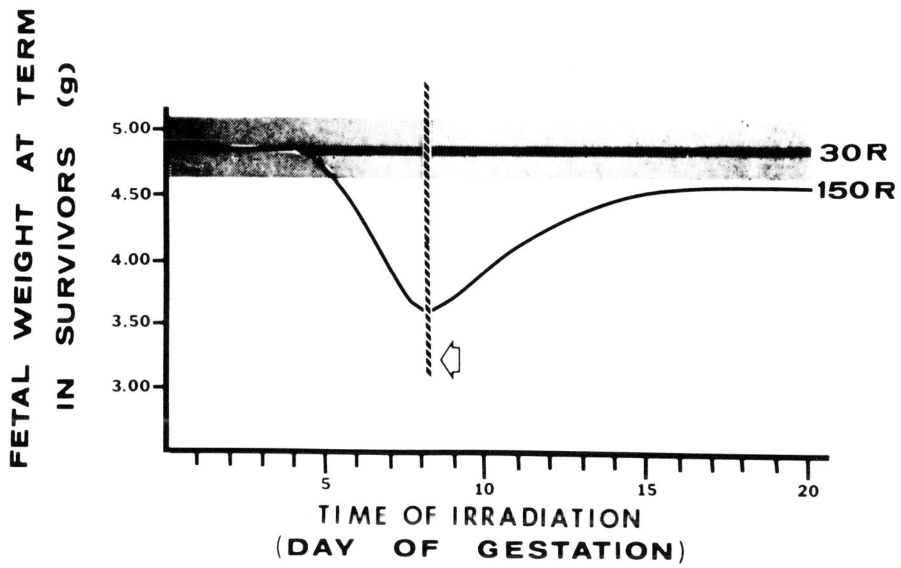

Fig. 2. The term fetal weight in the Wistar colony of rats in our laboratory averages 4.8 g on the 22nd day when delivered by cesarean section that morning. Note that 150 R causes growth retardation just after implantation but before the stage is sensitive to teratogenesis (arrow pointing to vertical line). From the time of implantation until term, 150 R produced some degree of growth retardation. Note that 30 R does not appear to produce significant deviations in growth, although it may be that all experimental groups are too small to show differences in weight at this low dose. The severity of term weight reduction does not correlate with the severity of growth retardation observed in adults irradiated in utero (Tables 4 and 5).

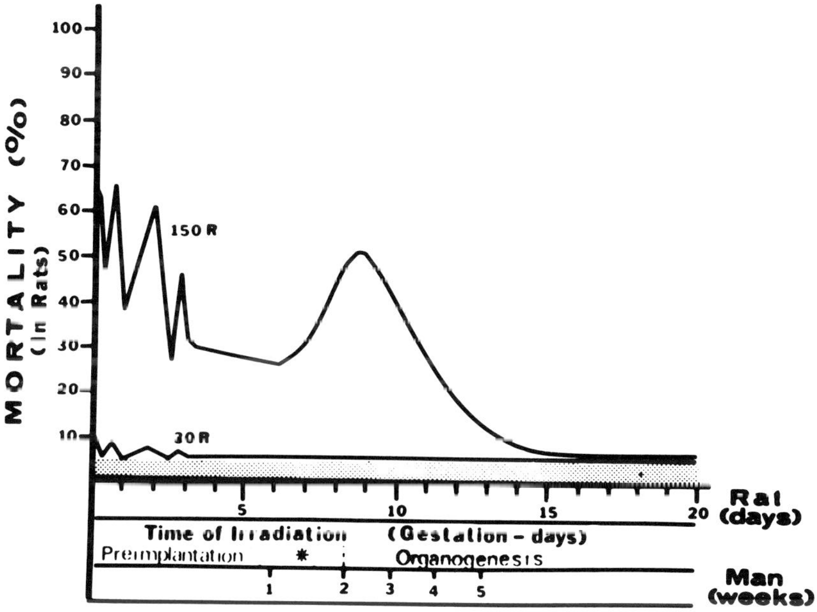

Fig. 3. The lethal effect of radiation in rats is greater on the 1st day. It appears that the LD/50 shifts at different times of the day during early gestation, possibly because the cells are dividing synchronously, therefore, the zygote will vary in its radiosensitivity, depending on the stage of the cell cycle. Note that the embryo becomes somewhat resistant in the implantation stage and then becomes sensitive to the lethal effect of radiation during early organogenesis. A 30 R dose apparently does increase the resorption rate when radiation takes place on the 1st day. The superimposition of this lethality curve for rats onto the human embryonic development timetable may not be appropriate and is for comparison purposes only, but it allows one to estimate at least roughly the stages at which the human embryo might be most readily killed by high doses of radiation.

dation and there were various abnormalities of the eyes, including microphthalmia, cataracts, strabismus, retinal degeneration, and optic atrophy. The unique finding was that no visceral, limb, or other malformations were ever found unless the child exhibited intrauterine growth retardation, microcephaly (congenital malformations of the brain), or readily apparent eye malformations. Dekaban reported that 22 infants that were exposed between the 3rd to 20th week of human gestation were microcephalic, mentally retarded, or both (Fig. 4). The estimated protracted exposure was 250 R, and all of the malformed infants exhibited growth retardation. The most frequent abnormalities were 1) small size at birth and stunted growth; 2) microcephaly; 3) mental retardation; 4) microphthalmia; 5) pigmentary changes in the retina; 6) genital and skeletal malformations, and 7) cataracts (Fig. 4). All of the embryos reported by Dekaban received hundreds of rads. The patients were treated with radiation for various reasons, including dysmenorrhea, metrorrhagia, myomata, arthritis or tuberculosis of the sacroiliac joint, and malignant tumors of the uterus or cervix. In several instances, radiation was initiated without knowing the patient was pregnant.

It is of interest to note that in one of the case reports (Murphy and Goldstein, '30) a typical campomelic dwarf was reported and the cause was attributed to radiation. High dose radiation was delivered from the 2nd to 5th month. This rare recessive syndrome was not described in 1930, and the authors were not in a position to recognize its possible genetic etiology (Maroteaux et al., '71).

Radiation-induced microcephaly, growth retardation, and microphthalmia are represented in Figures 5 and 6.

From a sample of 1,265 subjects exposed in utero at Hiroshima, 183 were analyzed by

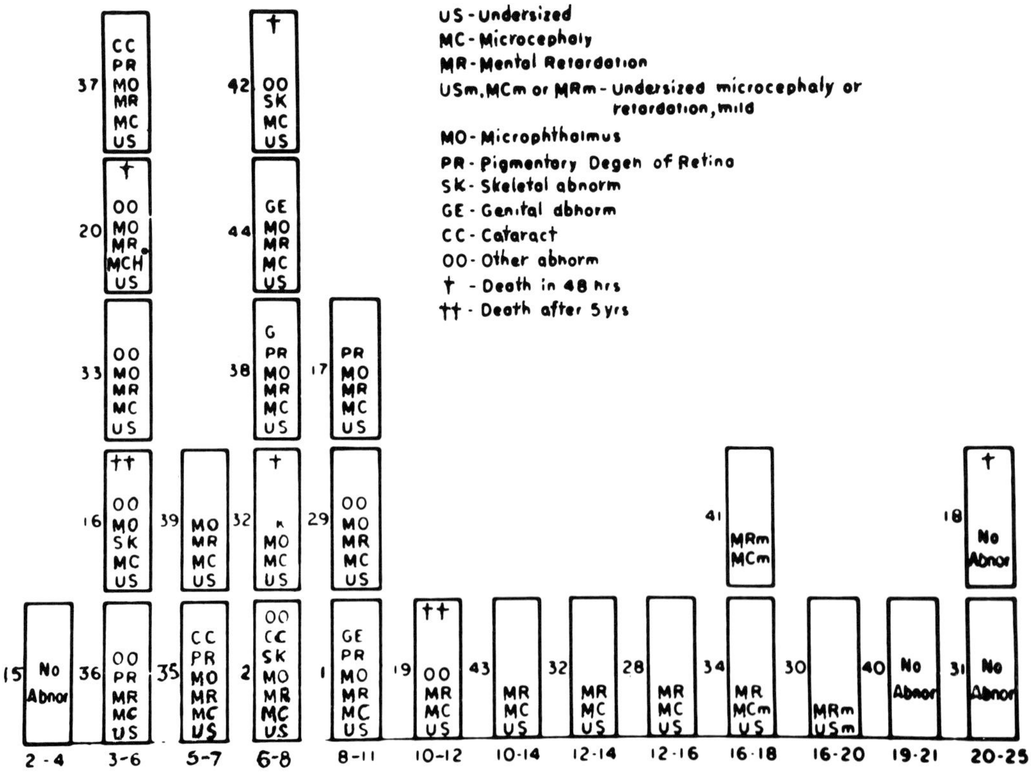

Fig. 4. The spectrum of malformations in 26 human infants in utero. Note that all infants receiving therapeutic doses of radiation were growth-retarded if they were irradiated between 3 and 20 weeks of gestation. Note that in no instance is there an associated malformation in structures other than the nervous system without either microcephaly or mental retardation (Dekaban, '68, with permission from the Journal of Nuclear Medicine).

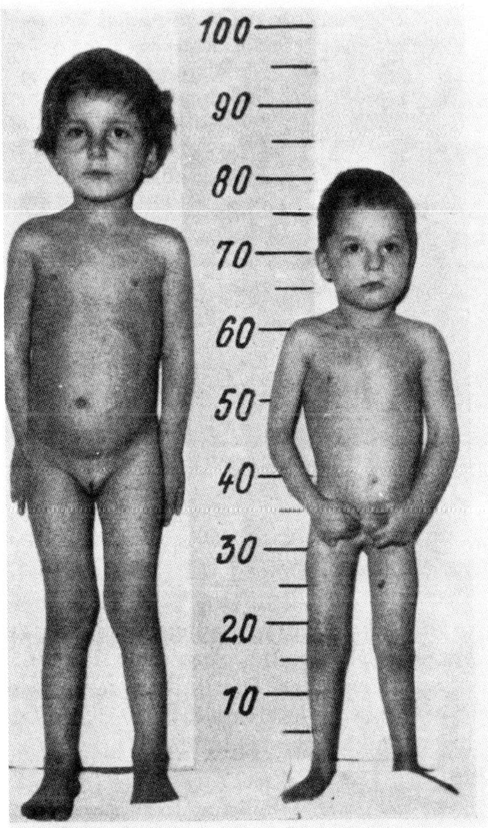

Fig. 5. The smaller child received in utero radiation during the 3rd to 4th month of gestation. The skin dose to the abdomen was 900 rads and was delivered for the purpose of sterilization of the mother because she had metatastic breast carcinoma. The child was full term but weighed only 1900 g. He had microcephaly and cerebral atrophy. Growth retardation persisted into childhood as evidenced by comparison with a child the same age who is in the 50th percentile. There was shortening of the left tibia and an exostosis on the right tibia. The eyes had decreased vessel size and pallor of the left disk. There was abnormal motor movements, weakness, and severe mental retardation.

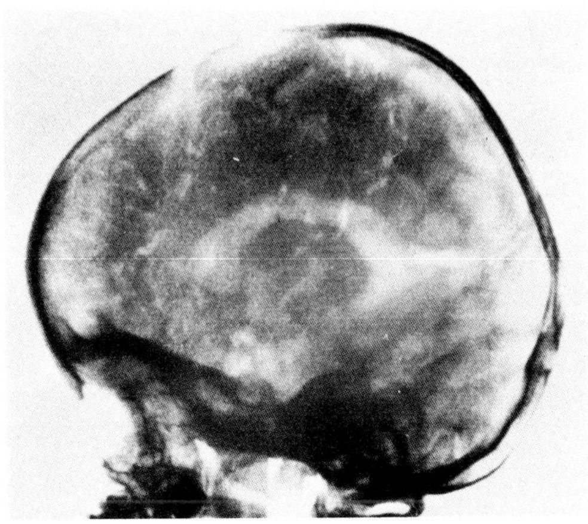

Fig. 6. Lateral view of the skull of the patient in Figure 5. The encephalogram revealed microcephaly and porencephaly. The mother received 900 rads of radiation to the abdomen. Based on the kilovoltage of the X-ray machine and the filtration, the estimated exposure to the embryo was 200–300 rads. The embryo could be as young as 9 weeks or as old as 20 weeks at the time of irradiation, based on the meager history that is available (Basic and Weber, '56).

Miller ('69) and Wood et al. ('67a, b). Seventy-eight of these fetuses were less than 16 weeks of age at the time of irradiation; 105 were 16 weeks or more. Of 78, 25 were microcephalic (head circumference more than two standard deviations below the mean), and 11 were mentally deficient. Of the 105, seven were microcephalic as defined, and four were mentally deficient. The incidence of microcephaly increased with increasing exposure. In 14 of the offspring with smaller than normal head circumference who were also mentally deficient, 10 were $\geqslant$ 2. S.D. below the mean height for age. In 16 children with small heads who were not mentally deficient, there was not a marked reduction in stature. Tables 1 and 2 summarize some of the characteristics of the patients exposed in utero before the 16th week of gestation (Miller, '69; Wood et al., '67b; Blot, '75). Severe mental retardation was not observed in any patients that received less than 50 rads while in utero (Blot and Miller, '73). In a summary of the microcephalic data, Blot ('75) noted that, while there was no increased risk for microcephaly in the population exposed in Nagasaki below 150 rads, there was an increased risk in the population exposed in Hiroshima at much lower doses. There were many differences between the results of the bomb explosion in the two cities that confound the ability to ascribe all pathological effects to irradiation. These confounding parameters may explain the differences between Hiroshima and Nagasaki.

Analysis of the human data reveals some interesting and important facts. Growth retardation, microcephaly, and mental retardation are predominant observable effects following acute exposures greater than 50 rads (low L.E.T. radiation). No report of a bonafide radiation-induced morphological malformation has been reported in a human that has not exhibited growth retardation or

TABLE 1. Frequency of small head circumference at ages 10–19 years according to city, gestational age, and radiation dose (Blot '75)

	Gestational age (weeks)					
	Hiroshima			Nagasaki		
Dose rad	0–17		18+	0–17		18+
Not in city or distally exposed	-	31/764	—	—	10/246	—
0–9	4(1)/63+		4/65+	0/1		0/9
10–19	6(1)/54		0/44	0/7		0/6
20–29	6/24		1/14	0/5		2/7
30–39	4/8		0.10	2/4		0/6
40–49	3/11		0/6	0/6		0/3
50–59	9(2)/20		2/24	0/9		0/11
100–149	2/4		0/10	0/2		1/5
150+	5(5)/13		1(1)/8+	8(3)/9		2(1)/9
Unknown	1/7		0/3	0/0		0/0
Total (in city)	40(9)/204		8(1)/184	10(3)/43		5(1)/56

Cases in parentheses give number with small head circumference and mental retardation. Plus (+) indicates one person with mental retardation without small head circumference.

TABLE 2. Number of cases and relative risk of mental retardation according to dose category (Blot '75)

	Hiroshima			Nagasaki		
Dose (rad)	Sample size	Cases[1]	Relative risk[2]	Sample size	Cases	Relative risk
Not in city or distally exposed	830	5 (2)	1.0 (1.0)	246	4 (2)	1.0 (1.0)
0–9	145	3 (1)	3.4 (3.8)	11	0	—
10–49	189	2 (1)	1.8 (1.5)	45	0	—
50–99	47	3 (1)	10.6 (11.8)	20	0	—
100–199	29	4 (1)	22.9 (28.6)	13	0	—
200–299	8	3	66.3 (104)	5	1 (1)	12.3
300	6	2	55.3 (92.2)	7	3	26.4 (52.7)

[1]Numbers in parentheses are numbers of cases (included in the totals) whose mental retardation was apparently due to causes other than intrauterine radiation.
[2]Numbers in parentheses are relative risks excluding cases whose mental retardation was apparently due to non-radiation causes.

a central nervous system abnormality. One might question why the central nervous system seems to be more sensitive in the human than in experimental animals in whom many organ systems are malformed by irradiation. The explanation for this apparent discrepancy is that the central nervous system maintains its sensitivity to radiation throughout gestation and into the neonatal period, while the other organ systems have much narrower periods when obvious morphological alterations can be produced (Brent, '70, '72, '76, '77) (Fig. 1). Secondly, the period of exquisite sensitivity to multiple system malformations is quite small in the human (2nd to 4th week) when compared to the rat (9th to 13th day). In the human, all organ systems can be readily malformed by high doses of radiation during 5% of pregnancy, while in the rat it can occur over 20% of pregnancy. Thirdly, human exposures have occurred at random during pregnancy and the exposure is controlled for purposes of therapeutic irradiation (100's of rads), or not controlled, as at Hiroshima and Nagasaki. Therefore, the exposures that occur in the human during the period of maximum sensitivity will be infrequent and/or will result in a high incidence of abortions, while the great majority of exposures will occur during the fetal stages when the central nervous system is unable to repair radiation-induced neuronal death. Thus, the nature of radiation effects in the human and the apparent discrepancies with animal data can be explained by the manner in which human populations have been exposed.

There are rare instances in which human embryos have been studied immediately after exposure to high doses of irradiation. Driscoll et al. ('63) were able to study the acute effects in two human fetuses exposed to radiation from radium with which their mothers were being treated for cancer of the cervix. The fetuses, 15 cm and 21 cm in crown-rump length, were examined 2 and 10 days after the beginning of irradiation, which lasted 48 hours in the first case and 4 days in the second. The crowns of the heads received about 800 R and 1600 R, respectively.

Destruction of primitive proliferative and migratory cells in the brains and of granulopoietic cells in the hematopoietic tissue occurred in both, but evidence of acute necrosis of lymphoid and mesenchymal cells was still visible only in the smaller fetus exposed for 48 hours. Mesenchyme cell necrosis extended as far as the kidney, where the dose may have been of the order of 50 to 100 rads in this fetus. In the larger fetus exposed for 4 days, more degenerating ova were seen than in comparable unirradiated subjects. These observatons provide a link between human laboratory animal data, suggesting that patterns of cellular radio-sensitivity in man are similar to those in other mammals (Hicks and D'Amato, '66).

Irradiation of the human fetus from diagnostic exposures below 5 rads have not been observed to cause congenital malformations or growth retardation (Nokkentred, '68; Tabuchi, '64; Tabuchi et al. '67; Kinlen and Acheson, '68; Vilumsen, '70), but all such epidemiological studies are not negative (Heinonen et al., '77; Jacobsen and Millimgaard, '68). These are extremely difficult studies to perform, and it appears that the animal data support the contention that gross congenital malformations will not be increased in a human pregnant population exposed to 5 rads or less. This contention is further strengthened by the fact that most human exposures to extensive diagnostic radiation studies are fractionated and/or protracted. This type of exposure is likely to be less effective in producing malformations than is an acute exposure (Brizzee and Brannon, '72; Brent, '71).

Although the animal and human data support the conclusion that no increase in the incidence of gross congenital malformations, intrauterine growth retardation, or abortion will occur with exposures below 5 rads, that does not mean that there are definitely no risks to the embryo exposed to lower doses of radiation. Whether there exists a linear or exponential dose-response relationship or a threshold exposure for genetic, carcinogenic, cell-depleting, and shortening-of-life-span effects has not been determined. In establishing maximum permissible levels for the embryo at low exposures, we can estimate the risk at 1 rad on the basis of a linear relationship (Table 3).

TABLE 3. Estimate of risks of 1 rad exposure (low L.E.T.) to the developing human embryo

Age (days)	Mutagenic effect[1,4,6]	Carcinogenic effect (Stewart, '73)[2] (Stewart et al., '56, '58) (Mole, '79)	Carcinogenic effect ABCC[3] Wood et al., '67c Kato, '71	Gross congenital malformations, death, growth retardation	Permanent cell depletion
1	No data	No data	No data		No effect[5]
14					
18	10^{-7} per locus	10^{-3}	8×10^{-6}	Same as controls	?
28					
50					
Late fetus to term					

[1]Based on an estimated doubling dose for mutagenesis of 100 rads. Assuming a linear dose response curve and no threshold for mutagenic effects.
[2]Stewart's data would indicate that the embryo is 100 times more sensitive to the carcinogenic effect of radiation than the adult. This is a controversial matter and others (Miller, '70; Jablon, '73; Brent '77; Diamond et al., '73) feel that this association may be other than a radiation effect.
[3]ABCC Atomic Bomb Casualty Commission Data on Carcinogenesis do not indicate that the embryo and fetus are at increased risk. The risk presented is the same carcinogenic risk attributed to adults, assuming maximal effect at low doses, namely, a linear dose response curve—and no threshold for carcinogenic effects.
[4]The mutagenic effects have not been studied in the preimplantation period.
[5]During the preimplantation period, the surviving embryos are not reduced in size even when the dose is very high although, at this stage, the embryo is very sensitive to the lethal effects of radiation. The estimate is assumed to be the adult risk, since there was no increased carcinogenic effect in the population of exposed fetuses in Hiroshima and Nagasaki.
[6]Estimate is assumed to be adult risk since there was no increased carcinogenic effect in the population of exposed fetuses.

COUNSELING PREGNANT WOMEN EXPOSED TO RADIATION AND ESTIMATING THE RISKS

Radiation effects in various mammalian embryos are more similar than the effects of most other teratogens or embryopathic agents because radiation has a direct effect on the developing embryo (Brent, '60; Brent and Bolden, '67a, b, '68, '61; Brent and McLaughlin, '60), and variations in placental transport and maternal metabolism do not significantly alter the results of irradiating the embryo. Thus, one can more readily transfer the results of radiation experiments with pregnant mammals to the human than with any other teratogen.

The biologic effects of embryonic radiation are summarized for exposures of 10 rad and 100 rad in Tables 4 and 5 for various species and different stages of gestation. Table 6 lists the estimated LD/50, minimum malforming dose, minimum lethal dose, minimum dose to produce growth retardation, and other parameters for the human embryo, based on extrapolations from animal data.

Table 7 lists the effects of low exposures to developing mammalian embryos. The data indicate that continuous exposures below 2,000 mrads per day have no effect on numerous parameters such as fertility, growth, mortality, or the incidence of congenital malformations.

In the human, diminished body growth, head size, and mental development have been observed after 50 rads to the mother during the earlier months of gestation, and some disturbances of growth may occur after as little as about 25 rads. Blot and Miller ('73) report that small head size was observed in children receiving 10 rads while in utero, but there was no mental retardation associated with this exposure and there were other important considerations. The groups were very small and there were other serious environmental

TABLE 4. A compilation of the effects of 10 rads or less acute radiation at various stages of gestation in rat and mouse[a]

	Stage of gestation (days)				
	Preimplantation	Implantation	Early organogenesis	Late organogenesis	Fetal stages
Mouse	0–4 1/2	4 1/2–6 1/2	6 1/2–8 1/2	8 1/2–12	12–18
Rat	0–5 1/2	5 1/2–8	8–10	10–13	13–22
Corresponding human gestation period	0–9	9–14	15–28	28–50	50–280
Lethality	+[b,c]	–	–	–	–
Growth retardation at term	–	–	–	–	–
Growth retardation as adult	–	–	–	–	–
Gross malformations[d] (aplasia, hyperplasia, absence or overgrowth of organs or tissues)	±	–	–	–	–
Cell depletions, minimal but measurable tissue hypoplasia	–	–	–	–	–
Sterility	–	–	–	–	–
Significant increase in germ cell mutations[e]	±	±	±	±	±
Cytogenetic abnormalities	–	–	–	–	–
Neuropathology	–	–	–	–	–
Tumor induction[e,f]	–	–	±	±	±
Behavior disorders[g]	–	–	–	–	–
Reduction in life-span[e]	–	–	–	–	–

[a]Dose fractionation or protraction effectively reduces the biologic result of all the pathologic effects reported in this Table.
[b](–) no observed effect; (±) questionable but reported or suggested effect; (+) demonstrated effect; (+ +) readily apparent effect; (+ + +) occurs in high incidence.
[c]At this stage the murine embryo is most sensitive to the lethal effects of irradiation. With 10 rads in the mouse, Rugh reports a slight decrease in litter size in the mouse (Brent, '77).
[d]Rugh reports exencephalia with 15 and 25 rad in a strain of mice with a 1% incidence of exencephalia. Others have not been able to repeat these results (Brent and Bolden, '67a).
[e]The potential for mutation induction exists in the embryonic term cells or their precursors. Several long-term studies indicate that considerably greater doses in mice and rats do not affect longevity, tumor incidence, incidence of congenital malformation, litter size, growth rate, fertility.
[f]Stewart and others have reported that 2 rad increases the incidence of malignancy by 50% in the offspring. See text for discussion.
[g]Piontkovskii reports behavioral changes in the rat after 1 rad daily irradiation. This work has not been reproduced. See text for discussion.

TABLE 5. A compilation of the effects of 100 rads acute radiation on embryonic development at various stages of gestation in rat and mouse [a]

	Stage of gestation (days)				
	Preimplantation	Implantation	Early organogenesis	Late organogenesis	Fetal stages
Mouse	0–4 1/2	4 1/2–6 1/2	6 1/2–8 1/2	8 1/2–12	12–18
Rat	0–5 1/2	5 1/2–8	8–10	10–13	13–22
Corresponding human gestation period	0–9	9–14	15–18	28–50	50–280
Lethality	+ + +[b,c]	+	+ +	±	–
Growth retardation at term	–	+	+ + +	+ +	+
Growth retardation as adult	–	+	+ +	+ + +	+ +
Gross malformations (aplasia, hypoplasia, absence or overgrowth of organs or tissues)	–	–	+ + +	±[d]	–[d]
Cell depletions, minimal but measurable tissue hypoplasia	–	–	±	+ +	+
Sterility	–	–	±	–	+ +[e]
Significant increase in germ cell mutations[f]	±	±	±	±	±
Cytogenetic abnormalities[g]	±			+	+
Cataracts	–	–	+	+	+
Neuropathology	–	–	+ + +	+ +	+
Tumor induction[h]	–	–	±	±	+
Behavior disorders[i]	–	–	+	+	±
Reduction of lifespan[j]	–	–	–	–	–

[a]Dose fractionation or protraction effectively reduced the biologic result of all the pathologic effects reported in this Table.
[b](–) no observed effect; (±) questionable but reported or suggested effect; (+) demonstrated effect; (+ +) readily apparent effect; (+ + +) occurs in high incidence.
[c]Russell reported that 200 rads increased the incidence of XO aneuploidy in 2–5% of offspring in mice with a spontaneous incidence of 1%. 100 rads kills substantial numbers of mouse and rat embryos at this state, but the survivors appear and develop normally.
[d]100 rads produces changes in the irradiated fetus which are subtle and necessitate detailed examination and comparison with comparable controls.
[e]The male gonad in the rat can be made extremely hypoplastic by irradiation in the fetal stages with 15 rads. In the mouse the newborn female is most sensitive to the sterilized effects of radiation. Much of this research on other animals cannot be applied to the human.
[f]The potential for mutation induction exists in embryonic germ cells or their precursors. The relative sensitivity of the embryonic germ cells when compared to adult germ cells is not known. Several long-term studies in animals do not indicate any exceptional differences.
[g]Footnote a refers to the aneuploidy produced in a strain of mice with a 1% incidence of spontaneous XO aneuploidy. Bloom has reported a much higher percentage of chromosome breaks in human embryos receiving 100–200 rads in utero than in adults receiving the same dose of irradiation. As yet, there have been no diseases associated with this increase in frequency of chromosome breaks.
[h]Animal experiments and the data from Hiroshima and Nagasaki do not support the concept that in utero irradiation is much more tumorigenic than extrauterine irradiation. On the other hand, Stewart and colleagues and many others report that irradiation from pelvimetry (2 rads) increases the incidence of leukemia and other tumors.
[i]A statistically significant increase in percentage of mental retardation occurs with this dose of radiation. On the other hand, normal intelligence has been found in children receiving much higher doses in utero.
[j]Animal experiments indicate that survivors of in utero irradiation have a life-span which is longer than groups of animals given the same dose of radiation during their extrauterine life and the same life expectancy as unirradiated controls.

TABLE 6. Estimation on the acute LD/50 dose, minimal malforming doses, cell depleting dose, and lethal doses for the human embryo based on compilation of mouse, rat, and human data

Age	Approximate minimal lethal dose, rads	Approximate LD/50 rads	Minimum dose recuperable growth retardation in adult, rads[1]	Minimal dose for recognizable gross malformation, rads	Minimum dose for induction of genetic, carcinogenic, and minimal cell depletion phenomena
Day 1	10	70–100	No effect	No effect	Unknown
Day 14	25	140	25	—	Unknown
Day 18	50	150	25–50	25	Unknown
Day 28	> 50	220	50	25	Unknown
Day 50	> 100	260	50	50	Unknown
Late fetus to term		300–400	50	> 50	Unknown

[1]Estimates for maximum dose effective in reducing body weight. Specific organs or measurements may be more or less sensitive.

TABLE 7. Reported effects of low exposures of radiation on the embryo when administered throughout pregnancy

	Organism	Source	Approximate exposure rate per minute (R)	Exposure per day	Exposure per pregnancy	Comments	Effects
Russell et al. ('59)	Mouse	^{137}Cs	0.0086	12.4 R	171 R	1st–18th day	None except shortened breeding period in female
Ronnback ('65)	Mouse	^{137}Cs		8.4 R	170 R	During gestation and in some instances 20 days postpartum	None
Vorisek ('65)	Rat	^{60}Co	0.0017	2.5 R	—	Daily during pregnancy	None
Stadler and Gowan ('64)	Mouse		0.0015	2.2 R		Continuous through 10 generations	None
Coppenger and Brown ('65)		^{60}Co	0.0014	2.0 R	—	Continuous through 11 generations	None
Konerman ('69)	Mice	^{60}Co	0.007 0.014	10 R 20 R 20 R	180 R 360 R	1st–18th day 1st–18th day	None
Wesley ('60)	Humans	Background		0.3mR	0.1 R	Variation in background radiation	Increased congenital malformation
Genrry et al. ('59)	Humans	Background		0.3mR	0.1 R	Variation in background radiation	Increased congenital malformation
Grahn and Kratchman ('63)	Humans	Background		0.3mR	0.1 R	Variation in background radiation	Background radiation level not a factor in incidence of congenital malformations
Segal et al. ('64)	Humans	Background		0.3mR	0.1 R	Background radiation	Background radiation level not a factor in incidence of congenital malformations
Kriegel and Langendorf ('64)	Mouse	X-ray		2.5 R 5 R 10 R 20 R		Acute dose given daily	No influences No influence No influence Malformations, resorptions, growth retardation
Piontkovskiy ('58, '61)	Rat	X-ray		1 R	20 R	Acute dose given daily	Functional changes in behavior and motor activity (questionable)
Laskey et al. ('73)	Rat	HTO	Continuous 0.01–10 uCi HTO ml of body water	0.003–3 rad/day	0.066–66	Tritiated water continuous exposure	Male testes reduced 10u Ci; no growth or reproductive impairment in F_1; F_2 generation had reduced weight

factors that could have contributed to disturbances of fetal growth. Even if one considers this effect to be etiologically related to radiation exposure, the total human data from Hiroshima and Nagasaki do not support a significant effect attributable to radiation in the groups that received below 10 rads in utero. In experiments with laboratory mammals, in which more precise observation of dose and stage of development is possible, doses as low as 25 rads have produced some impairment of neurologic function and behavior. Alterations in the morphologic development of some brain neurons and certain other cellular changes have been observed after as little as 10–20 rads in fetal and infant rats, but tests thus far have not revealed corresponding changes in function.

Innumerable developmental processes are sensitive to radiation, as to other environmental teratogenic agents, and each process has its individual threshold or dose-range below which radiation has no visible effect. In radiogenic microcephaly or impaired body growth, the development of the abnormality depends on the summation and interaction of the interruptions of a large number of processes characteristic of the stage of development, and there are threshold dose-ranges below which these effects are not observed. Furthermore, the embryo does have sophisticated recuperable powers which are present in all mammalian cells.

Based on this information, it would appear that the hazards of exposures in the range of diagnostic roentgenology (20 mrads–5000 mrads) present an extremely low risk to the embryo, when compared to the spontaneous mishaps that can befall the human embryo (Table 3). Approximately 30–50% of human embryos abort spontaneously. Human infants have a 2.75% malformation rate at term, which rises to approximately 6–8% once all malformations and genetic disease become manifest. In spite of the fact that doses of 1–3 rads can produce cellular effects and the fact that diagnostic exposure during pregnancy has been associated with malignancy in childhood, the *maximum* theoretical risk to the human embryos exposed to doses of 5 rads or less is extremely small (Table 3 and 6). In my experience, when the data and risks are explained to the patient, the family with a wanted pregnancy invariably continues with the pregnancy. The difficulty that frequently arises is that the radiation risk from diagnostic radiation is evaluated without considering the significant normal risks of pregnancy. Furthermore, many physicians approach the evaluation of a diagnostic radiation exposure with a cavalier attitude. The usual procedures in clinical medicine are ignored and opinion based on meager information is given the patient. Frequently, it reflects the physician's bias about radiation effects or his total ignorance of the fields of radiation biology. We have patient records in our files of scores of patients who have been told to have an abortion following a radiation exposure. In many instances the embryo received no measurable exposure. In most instances the exposure was well below 5 rads–and in several instances the physician's evaluation was so unsystematic that he was not aware that the patient was not pregnant at the time of the exposure. Why is it that a physician ignores the systematic approach of patient evaluation when confronted with a pregnant woman who has been exposed to radiation? Whatever the reason, there is a minimal systematic approach that every patient deserves. The following information should be obtained.

1. Stage of pregnancy of the exposure.
2. Menstrual history.
3. Previous pregnancy history.
4. History of congenital malformations.
5. Other potential harmful environmental factors that have occurred during this pregnancy.
6. Mother's and father's age.
7. Type of radiation study. Dates and number of studies performed.
8. Calculation of the embryonic exposures by a medical physicist or competent radiologist.
9. Status of this pregnancy: wanted, unwanted.
10. Evaluation of this information. Arriving at decision by both patient and counselor.
11. Placing in the medical record a summary of the information and the fact that patient has been informed that a normal pregnancy has a significant risk of having something go wrong and that the decision to continue the pregnancy does not mean that the counselor is guaranteeing the outcome of the pregnancy.

12. The use of amniocentesis and ultrasound to evaluate the fetus is an individual decision that would have to be made in each pregnancy.

Our experience has taught us that there are many variables involved in a radiation exposure to a pregnant or potentially pregnant woman. Therefore, it is impossible to provide a routine stereotyped response for each patient. The following examples are typical cases of radiation exposure that necessitated evaluation.

> A 27-year-old mother, gravida 3, para 2, abortus 0, called on Friday afternoon because she was 8 weeks pregnant and was scheduled for a therapeutic abortion on Monday morning. Her obstetrician and a pediatric genetic counselor had advised her to have a therapeutic abortion because at the time of conception she had several X-ray examinations of the abdomen, and they were concerned that the embryo would be malformed. No dosimetry had been performed and no evaluation initiated. It took about 10 minutes on the phone to determine that she became pregnant after the diagnostic radiation studies and that her two previous boys had minor problems (hemangioma and pyloric stenosis). We canceled the abortion and the mother delivered a normal, full-term girl. She was adequately warned that we could not guarantee the outcome of the pregnancy–that there are 27.5 serious malformations per 1,000 births–as a minimum. She had another determining factor in that she had a serious problem with varicose veins and planned a tubal ligation after either the abortion or the delivery.

The case history illustrates the minimal data that were collected by the physicians before counselling the patient. There was an added feature in this case. The paternal family was Catholic and the thought of an abortion was causing much dissention within the family.

> Mrs. John B., a 26-year old para 1, gravida 2, abortus 0 woman, had LMP on October 31, 1966. On November 18, she had the onset of a mild gastroenteritis with pain localized to the RUQ. Although the other symptoms of gastroenteritis disappeared, the pain persisted. Mrs. B. had just moved to this city with her husband and one child and this was the first time she had seen her new family physician. The pain persisted on and off for 10 days, and on November 28 and 29 she had a cholecystogram and an upper G.I. series. The diagnostic studies were negative and she was treated symptomatically for several days when the symptoms disappeared. On December 6, she realized that she had missed her menstrual period and a pregnancy test revealed that she was pregnant.

By the time our laboratory was called, several physicians had recommended therapeutic abortion and the woman was exhibiting significant anxiety. We requested that the local medical physicist estimate the dose to the embryo, and at the same time the number and position of the films and length and position of fluoroscopy were submitted to us. We calculated that the embryo had received approximately 1.1 rad over a period of 2 days. The physicists in their locale estimated the dose by performing dosimetry with a phantom and the equipment utilized for the actual procedure. He reported that the dose for the fractionated exposure was 1.4 rad. The recommendation to the family and physicians involved was that this dose of radiation would not result in embryonic death, embryonic growth retardation, or malformations, and that the woman could continue with the pregnancy. She chose to continue the pregnancy and delivered a 3,400 gm normal boy at 40 weeks of gestation.

Case histories similar to this are transmitted to our laboratory frequently. In most instances, the dose to the embryo is below 5 rads and frequently is below 1 rad. The variations in the approach of the physician in charge are dependent on many factors: (1) whether the pregnant woman is married, (2) whether the pregnancy was planned, (3) the mental status of the mother and/or father, (4) the abortion laws in that state, and (5) the knowledge of the physician regarding radiation hazards to the embryo.

Other case histories illustrate these problems.

> A 19-year-old unmarried secretary went to her physician because of abdominal pain. She told him her menstrual periods were regular and the pain was periumbilical and per-

sistent. An upper G.I. series was performed but was unsatisfactory because the young girl had eaten breakfast before the study. When the second study was performed, she mentioned that she was 2 weeks past her scheduled menstrual period and that she could be pregnant. The father of the child was married. The radiation therapist at the hospital recommended a therapeutic abortion because of radiation hazards to the embryo. The estimated dose to the embryo over a period of 3 days was 1.6 rad.

Our laboratory was called and informed of the case history and recommendation. Our conclusion was that this dose of radiation would not result in embryonic malformation, growth retardation, or death, and that the radiation hazard should not be used as the scapegoat to obtain a therapeutic abortion for "social" reasons. The laws of that state did not permit any therapeutic abortions, so the girl flew to another state where the therapeutic abortion was performed.

The spector of radiation hazards, we believe, should not be invoked to circumvent a social or legal problem. If the abortion laws are archaic or unfair, physicians should work together to change them. They should not create an implied serious radiation hazard problem, which is not justified by the facts, in order to solve social, psychological, or legal problems.

A 29-year-old housewife, para 0, gravida 1, abortus 0, presented in her 6th month of pregnancy with the history that she had been to her dentist the week before and one radiograph of her left upper first molar was made. She was anxious and very worried about the effect of radiation on her baby. She was reassured but called back six times asking new questions. The estimated dose to the embryo was practically 0 rads. She continued to be anxious and became more hyperactive. She delivered a 3,100 gm baby boy with a minimal syndactyly of the 4th and 5th finger of the left hand, but who otherwise was normal. A legal suit was almost instituted in this case.

It is surprising the number of cases that are evaluated or brought to trial in which the only radiation exposure of the mother pertains to the head, the neck or chest, and yet there is both clinical and basic science information that indicates that embryopathology is only a consequence of direct embryonic exposure. High doses of radiation to the mother, while shielding the embryo, result in offspring who have the same incidence of congenital malformations as control embryos (Brent, '60; Brent and McLaughlin, '60; Neifakh, '57).

Although it is our opinion that a dose of less than 10 rads to the implanted embryo does not result in a significant increase in the incidence of congenital malformations, growth retardation, or fetal death, possibly significant tumorigenic or genetic hazards cannot be ruled out. Even if one believed that the tumorigenic (leukemogenic) effects of radiation were real, let us examine how difficult it would be to utilize this informaton in counseling a patient who has received a dose of perhaps 2 rads during her pregnancy. According to Stewart, the risk of leukemia following this exposure in utero is 1:2,000 vs. 1:3,000 in exposed controls over a 10-year period (Table 8). If one were inclined to recommend therapeutic abortion for this embryo because the probability of developing leukemia is 50% greater than controls, one would perform abortions in 1,999 exposed non-leukemics for every leukemic "saved." It is one thing to avoid radiation because of a potential or conjectured hazard, but it is another matter to recommend therapeutic abortion on this basis. If a physician were inclined to accept this increased probability (1 in 2,000) as great enough risk to recommend therapeutic abortion, he would be placed in a serious dilemma, since there are other epidemiologic situations in which the risk of leukemia is greater. In fact, the hypothetical increment risk for 2 rads of in-utero radiation is 1 in 6,000 over a 10-year period. It is the combined control risk plus the increment risk that result in a 1 in 2,000 risk for these patients. If one examines Table 8, it is obvious that the risk of leukemia is greater in "unirradiated" siblings of leukemics (1 in 720) than in patients subjected to diagnostic radiation (1 in 2,000), according to Stewart's data.

Certainly, it would be untenable to hold the position that all future pregnancies of parents with one leukemic child should be

TABLE 8. Risk of leukemia in various groups with specific epidemiologic and pathologic characteristics in populations followed for 10 to 30 years

Group	Approximate risk	Increased risk over control population	Occurrence
Identical twin of leukemic twin	1/3	1,000	weeks to months
Irradiation-treated polycythemia vera	1/6	500	10–15 years
Bloom syndrome	1/8	375	< 30 years of age
Hiroshima survivors who were within 1,000 meters of the hypocenter	1/60	50	average 12 years
Down's syndrome	1/95	30	< 10 years of age
Irradiation-treated patients with ankylosing spondylitis	1/270	10	15 years
Siblings of leukemic children	1/720	4	to 10 years
Children exposed to pelvimetry in utero (gestational exposure)	1/2,000	1.5	< 10 years
US white children < 15 years of age	1/2,800	1	to 10 years

Modified from Iller ('70).

aborted. One can carry this argument to its ridiculous extreme by advocating that all pregnancies should be aborted, since the risk of malformation is approximately 40–60 per 1,000 deliveries, and this does not include the probability of postnatal diseases occurring in these offspring. Some may interpret this as a facetious discussion, but to the clinician and family it is not a game of probabilities. It is a medical problem involving an individual human pregnancy.

The physician will never be able to guarantee the outcome of a pregnancy. The basic logic of the practice of medicine will be undermined when some of its practitioners recommend therapeutic abortion for possible hazards with probabilities far below the expected incidence of disease and malformations in the embryo and infant. In all instances of counseling parents concerning the hazards to the embryo of a particular radiation exposure, the biologic knowledge is only one facet to be considered. The risk of radiation damage is based on the estimated dose and the stage of gestation. The reaction to this risk depends on the age of the parents, the number of children in the family, the religion and ethics of the family, and the options available to the family based on the regional laws regarding therapeutic interruptions of pregnancy. Information that is more difficult to acquire pertains to the emotional maturity of the family and whether the pregnancy was planned or unplanned.

There were many instances in the past in which a radiologist recommended a therapeutic abortion for a patient whose embryo received a fractionated dose of 0–5 rads during the 1st trimester of pregnancy, because of the possibility of having a malformed embryo. Frequently, this recommendation was made for unmarried women, primarily to assist them in eliminating unwanted pregnancies. It is this type of "good samaritan" recommendation that will reap retribution when that same radiologist attempts to defend himself against the contention that a series of diagnostic radiologic examinations caused a particular malformation.

EXPOSURE FROM RADIATION THERAPY

There is ample evidence to indicate that radiation therapy in the region of the abdomen can result in doses of radiation that will deleteriously affect the fetus. In such a case it is important to confer with either the radiotherapist or a qualified medical physicist in order to determine the total dose delivered to the embryo. If the fetus absorbs 50 rads or more at any time during gestation, there is a significant possibility that the fetus might be damaged. There are, of course, instances in which human fetuses exposed to greater doses have survived. (Dekaban, '68; Ronderos, '61) and appeared normal, but at this dose, the probability of central nervous system damage or other malformations is real and the parents should be so informed. If the dose observed by the embryo during the early organogenetic period amounts to several hundred rads, there is a reasonable possibility that the embryo may abort. As one proceeds into the 2nd and 3rd trimester, the chance of abortion and malformation declines, but irreparable damage to the central nervous system can occur.

When the radiation therapist fails to investigate the possibility of pregnancy or fails to record all the information regarding the pregnancy and the steps taken in arriving at a decision, he places himself in double jeopardy. He may be accused of poor medical practice in a suit over a malformed infant and thereby may be more likely to lose the case even when the radiation may not have been responsible for the abnormal embryonic development (Brent, '67).

Let us examine some representative cases.

> A 31-year-old woman was in her 6th month of pregnancy when her physician noted an enlarged lymph node in the anterior cervical region. A diagnosis of Hodgkin's disease was made and she received approximately 3,200 rads to the anterior cervical region and adjacent areas over a period of 4 weeks. The fetus was viable at the time of the diagnosis and the family wanted the baby. The dose of radiation to the fetus was less than 25 rads. The mother delivered a full-term baby who appeared to be normal.

In this case, the physician supported the wishes of the family.

> A 36-year-old woman, para 4, gravida 6, abortus 1, was 1 week past her menstrual period, which usually was regular. Examination revealed a moderate-sized lesion of the cervix. the pregnancy test was positive. A biopsy of the cervix revealed a carcinoma of the cervix that had invaded the muscle layer. A dilation and curetage was performed and the patient was treated with instillation of radium. In this case, the options were presented to the family before the biopsy and above-mentioned course was taken.

THE USE OF DIAGNOSTIC OR THERAPEUTIC RADIATION IN WOMEN OF REPRODUCTIVE AGE WHEN THE OVARIES OR UTERUS WILL BE EXPOSED

1. In a woman of reproductive age, it is important for the patient and physician to be aware of the pregnancy status of the patient before any type of abdominal X-ray exposure is planned. If the embryonic exposure will be 5 rads or less, the radiation risks to the embryo are miniscule when compared to the spontaneous risks. The patient will accept this information if it is offered as part of the preparation for the X-ray studies at a time that both the physician and patient are aware that a pregnancy exists.

The pregnancy status of the patient can be determined by several means: (a) the X-ray referral slip can request the L.M.P. and the PMP and whether the patient could possibly be pregnant; (b) if the patient is uncertain about her pregnancy status, a pregnancy test should be performed; (c) pregnancy tests could be performed on all hospital admissions of women of reproductive age.

2. Because the risks of 5 rad fetal irradiation are so small, the immediate medical care of the mother should take priority over the risks of diagnostic radiation exposure to the embryo. X-ray studies which are essential for optimal medical care of the mother and evaluation of medical problems that need to be diagnosed or treated should be postponed. Elective procedures, such as employment examinations or follow-up examinations, once a diagnosis has been made, need not be performed on a pregnant women even though the risk to the embryo is very small. If other procedures (ultrasound, etc.) can provide adequate information without exposing the embryo to ionizing radiation then, of course, they should be utilized. Of course, there is an initial period when a pregnancy test will be negative and the patient can be pregnant. Furthermore, the menstrual history will be of little use in this circumstance. The risks of 5 rads or less of radiation are extremely small during this period of gestation. The patient will benefit from knowing that the diagnostic study was indicated and should be performed, in spite of the fact that she might be pregnant.

3. In those instances in which *elective* X-ray studies need to be scheduled, it is difficult to know whether to schedule them during the first half of the menstrual cycle just before ovulation or during the second half of the menstrual cycle when most women will not be pregnant. The risk of diagnostic exposures to the oocyte of the preimplanted embryo is extremely small and there is no data on which to compare the relative risk of 5 rads to the oocyte or the preimplanted embryo (Brent, '70, '72; Brent and Gorson, '72). If the diagnostic study is performed in the first 14 days of the menstrual cycle, should

the patient be advised to defer conception for several months, based on the assumption that the deleterious effect of radiation to the ovaries decreases with increasing time between radiation exposure and a subsequent ovulation? The physician is in a dilemma because he is warning the patient about a very low risk phenomenon. On the other hand, avoiding conception for several months is not an insurmountable hardship. This potential hazard is quite speculative for the human as indicated by the NCRP ('71) report dealing with preconception radiation.

> It is not known whether the interval between irradiation of the gonads and conception has a marked effect on the frequency of congenital changes in human offspring, as has been demonstrated in the female mouse. Nevertheless, it may be advisable for patients receiving high doses to the gonads (over 25 rads) to wait for several months after such exposures before conceiving additional offspring.

Since the patients exposed during diagnostic radiologic procedures absorb considerably less than 25 rads, the recommendation made here may be unnecessary, but it involves no hardship to the patient or physician. Since both the NCRP and ICRP have recommended that elective radiologic examinations of the abdomen and pelvis be performed during the first part of the menstrual cycle to protect the zygote from possible but largely conjectural hazards, a recommendation to reduce another possible hazard by avoiding fertilization of recently irradiated ova perhaps should merit equal attention.

4. If a woman is exposed to greater than 5 rads of radiation and then is found to be pregnant, then a determination of the merits of continuing the pregnancy must be decided by the physician, patient, and radiation expert. A decision as to whether to terminate the pregnancy will depend on: (a) the non-radiation-related hazard of the pregnancy to the expectant mother; (b) the extent and type of radiation hazard to the embryo or fetus; (c) the ethnic and religious background of the family; (d) the laws of the state pertaining to legal abortion, and (e) any other relevant consideration. Usually, the radiation risk to the embryo or fetus will not be the predominating factor in arriving at a decision unless one is dealing with exposures in the therapeutic range.

If exposures below 5 rad do not measurably affect the exposed embryos, and others (Brent and Gorson, '72) recommend performing diagnostic procedures at any time of the menstrual cycle, if necessary, for the medical care of the patient, why spend so much effort and energy in determining the pregnancy status of the patient?

There are several reasons why the physician and patient should have the burden of determining the pregnancy status before an X-ray or nuclear medicine procedure is performed that will expose the uterus.

First, if the physician is *forced* to include the possibility of pregnancy in the differential diagnosis, a fraction of diagnostic studies may no longer be considered necessary. Early symptoms of pregnancy may mimic certain types of gastrointestinal or genito-urinary disease.

Second, if the physician and patient are both aware that pregnancy is a possibility and the procedure is still performed, it is much less likely that the patient will be upset if she proves to be pregnant.

Third, the careful evaluation of the reproductive status of women undergoing diagnostic procedures will prevent many unnecessary lawsuits. Many lawsuits are stimulated by the factor of surprise and won on the basis of the double jeopardy of the defendant (Brent, '67, '76, '75, '77). In some instances the jury is not concerned with cause and effect, but with the fact that something was not done properly by the physician. In this day and age, failure to adequately communicate can be interpreted as less than adequate medical care. Both these factors are eliminated if the patient's pregnancy status has been properly evaluated and the situation adequately discussed with the patient. Physicians are going to have to learn that practicing good technical medicine may not be enough in this litigation-prone society. Even more important, the patient will have more confidence if the decision to continue the pregnancy is made before the medical X-ray procedure is performed, since the necessity of the procedure would have been determined with the knowledge that the patient was pregnant.

In summary, this "Teratogen Update" reviews the effects of radiation on the developing mammalian embryo and, especially, the human embryo. Counseling the women of reproductive age who will be exposed to radiation or have been exposed to radiation is frequently performed by physicians in a cavalier fashion, without the benefit of knowing the radiation exposure or the risks. The patient deserves to be counseled about radiation hazards to the embryo by individuals who are both knowledgeable about the data that are available and willing to obtain the necessary information from the patient. Superficial evaluation of radiation exposures are a disservice to the patient and an example of poor medical care.

ACKNOWLEDGMENTS

This study was supported by NIH HD 19165 HD 7075, Foederer Foundation.

LITERATURE CITED

Basic, M., and D. Weber (1956) Uber intrauterine Fruchtschadingung durch Rongenstrahlen. Strahlentherapie, *99:*628.

Blot, W. (1975) Growth and development following prenatal and childhood exposure to atomic radiation. J. Radiat. Res., *16*, Supplement:82–88.

Blot, W.J., and R.W. Miller (1973) Mental retardation following in utero exposure to the atomic bomb of Hiroshima and Nagasaki. Radiol., *106:*617–619.

Brent, R.L. (1960) The indirect effect of irradiation on embryonic development. II. Irradiation of the placenta. Am. J. Dis. Child., *100:*103.

Brent, R.L. (1967) Medicolegal aspects of teratology. J. Pediat., *71:*288–298.

Brent, R.L. (1970) Effects of radiation on the foetus, newborn and child; in Fry, Grahn, Griem and Rust Late Effects of Radiation; pp. 23–60 (Taylor & Francis, London 1970).

Brent, R.L. (1971) The response of the 9 ½-day-old rat embryo to variations in exposure rate of 150 RX-irradiation. Radiat. Res., *45:*127–136.

Brent, R.L. (1972) Irradiation in pregnancy; in Sciarra Davis' Gynecology and Obstetrics; Vol. 2, pp. 1–32 (Harper & Row, New York).

Brent, R.L. (1975) Medicolegal aspects of teratology; in Biologic and Clinical Aspects of Malformations, Mead Johnson Symposium on Perinatal and Developmental medicine No. 7, Vail, CO; pp. 65–76.

Brent, R.L. (1976) Environmental factors: radiation; in Brent and Harris Prevention of Embryonic, Fetal and Perinatal Disease; Fogarty International Center Series on Preventive Medicine; Vol 3, pp 179–197 (DHEW Publication No. NIH 76-853, Bethesda, MD).

Brent, R.L. (1977) Radiations and other physical agents; in Wilson and Fraser Handbook of Teratology; Vol., 1, pp. 153–223 (Plenum Press, New York).

Brent, R.L. (1977) Litigation-produced pain, disease and suffering.: an experience with congenital malformation lawsuits. Teratology, *16:*1–13.

Brent, R.L. (1982) Teratogenic and carcinogenic effects of in utero irradiation; in Bolognese, Schwartz, Schneider: Perinatal Medicine: 2nd edition; pp. 85–105 (Williams and Wilkins, Baltimore, 1982).

Brent, R.L., and B.T. Bolden (1961) The long-term effects of low dosage embryonic irradiation. Radiat. Res., *14:*453–454.

Brent, R.L., and B.T. Bolden (1967a) The indirect effect of irradiation on embryonic development. III. The contribution of ovarian irradiation, uterine irradiation, oviduct irradiation and zygote irradiation to fetal mortality and growth retardation in the rat. Radiat. Res., *30:*759–773.

Brent, R.L., and B.T. Bolden (1967b) The indirect effect of irradiation on embryonic development. IV. The lethal effects of maternal irradiation on the first day of gestation in the rat. Proc. Soc. Exp. Biol. Med., *125:*709–712.

Brent, R.L., and B.T. Bolden (1968) Indirect effect of x-irradiation on embryonic development. V. Utilization of high doses of maternal irradiation on the first day of gestation. Radiat. Res., *36:*563–570.

Brent, R.L., and R.O. Gorson (1972) Radiation exposure in pregnancy; in Moseley, Baker, Gorson, Lalli, Latourette and Quinn Current Problems in Radiology; Vol. 2, pp. 1–48 (Year Book Medical Publishers, Chicago).

Brent, R.L., and M.M. McLaughlin (1960) The indirect effect of irradiation on embryonic development. I. Irradiation on embryonic development. I. Irradiation of the mother while shielding the embryonic site. Am. J. Dis. Child., *100:*9–102.

Brizzee, K.R., and R.B. Brannon (1972) Cell recovery in foetal brain after ionizing radiation. Int. J. Radiat. Biology, *21:*375–378.

Cowen, D., and L.M. Geller (1960) Long-term pathological effects of prenatal x-irradiation on the central nervous system of the rat. J. Neuropath. Exp. Neurol., *19:*488–527.

Coppenger, C.J., and S.O. Brown (1965) Postnatal manifestations in albino rats continuously irradiated during prenatal development. Tex. Rep. Biol. Med., *23:*45–55.

Dekaban, A.S. (1968) Abnormalities in children exposed to x-irradiation during various stages of gestation: tentative timetable of radiation injury to the human fetus. J. Nucl. Med., *9:*471–477.

Diamond, E.L., H. Schmerler, and A.M. Lilienfeld (1973) The relationship of intrauterine radiation to subsequent mortality and development of leukemia in children. A prospective study. Am. J. Epidem. *97:*283–313.

Driscoll, S.E., SP Hicks, E.H. Copenhaver, and C.L. Easterday (1963) Acute radiation injury in two human fetuses. Archs. Path., *76:*113–119.

Furchtgott, E. (1963) Behavioral effects of ionizing radiations, 1955–61. Psychol. Bull., *60:*157–199.

Gentry, J., E. Parkhurst, and G. Bulin (1959) An epidemiological study of congenital malformations in New York State. Am. J. Publ. Health *49:*497.

Glass, S.J. (1944) Dwarfism associated with microcephalic idiocy and renal rickets. J. Clin. Endocrinol., *4:*47–53.

Goldstein, L., and D.P. Murphy (1929a) Microcephalic idiocy following radium therapy for uterine cancer during pregnancy. Am. J. Obstet. Gynec. *18:*189–195, 281–283.

Goldstein, L., and D.P. Murphy (1929b) Etiology of ill health in children born after maternal pelvic irradiation. II. Defective children born after postconceptional maternal irradiation. Am. J. Roentg., *22:*322–331.

Grahan, D., and J. Kratchman (1963) Variation in neonatal death rate and birth weight in the United States and possible relations to environmental radiation, geology and altitude. Am. J. Hum. Genet., *15:*329–352.

Heinonen, O.P., D. Slone, and S. Shapiro (1977) Birth defects and drugs in pregnancy; p. 516 (Publishing Sciences Group, Littleton, MA).

Hicks, S.P., and C.J. D'Amato (1966) Effects of ionizing

radiations on mammalian development; in Woollam Advances in Teratology; Vol. 1, pp 196–250 (Logos Press, London).
Jablon, S. (1973) Comments Hlth. Phys., *24:*257–258.
Jacobsen, L., and L. Mellemgaard (1968) Anomalies of the eyes in descendants of women irradiated with small X-ray doses during fertility. Acta Ophthal., *46:*352–354.
Johnson, F.E. (1983) Injury of the child by roentgen ray during pregnancy. J. Ped., *13:*894–901.
Kato, H. (1971) Mortality in children exposed to the A-bombs while in utero. Am. J. Epidem., *93:*435–442.
Kinlen, L.J., and E.D. Acheson (1968) Diagnostic irradiation, congenital malformations and spontaneous abortion. Br. J. Radiol. *41:*648–654.
Konermann, G. (1969) Die Keimesentwicklung der Maus nach Einwirkung kontinuierlicher Co^{60}Gammabestrahlung wahrend der Blastogenese, der Orangenese und der Fetal periode. Strahlentherapie, *137:*451–466.
Kriegel, H., und H. Langendorff (1964) Die Wirkung einer fraktionierten Rontgenbestrahlung auf die Embrynalentwicklung der Maus. Strahlenterapie, *123:*429–437.
Laskey, J.W., J.L. Parrish, and D.F. Cahill (1973) Some effects of lifetime parental exposure to low levels of tritium on the F2 generation. Radiat. Res., *56:*171–179.
Maroteaux, P., J. Spranger, J.M. Opitz, J. Kucera, R.B. Lowry, N. Schimke, and S.M. Kagan (1971) Le syndrome campomelique. Presse Med., *22:*1157–1162.
Miller, R.W. (1969) Delayed radiation effects in atomic bomb survivors. Science, *166:*569–574.
Miller, R.W., and J.J. Mulvihill (1976) Small head size after atomic irradiation. Teratogen Update. Teratology, *14:*355–358.
Miller, R.W. (1970) Epidemiological conclusions from radiation toxicity studies; in Fry, Grahn, Griem and Rust Late Effects of Radiation (Taylor & Francis, London).
Mole, R.H. (1979) Radiaton effects on prenatal development and their radiological significance. British J. Radiol., *52:*89–101.
Murphree, R., and H. Pace (1960) The effects of prenatal radiation on postnatal development in rats. Radiat. Res. *12:*495–504.
Murphy, D.P., and L. Goldstein (1930) Micromelia in a child irradiated in utero. Surg. Gynec. Obs., *50:*79–80.
National Council on Radiation Protection and Measurements (1971) Basic Radiation Protection Criteria (NCRP Report No. 39, Washington, D.C.).
Neifakh, A.A. (1957) Role of the maternal organism in the irradiation illness of fetal mice. Dokl. Akad. Nauk. Biol. Sci. Sect. *116:*821–824.
Nokkentred, K. (1968) Effect of radiation upon the human fetus; p. 228 (Munksgaard, Copenhagen).
Piontkovskii, I.A. (1958) Certain properties of the higher nervous activity in adult animals irradiated prenatally by ionizing radiations. The problem of the effect of ionizing irradiation on offspring. Byull. Eksp. Biol. Med. (in Russian), *46:*77–80.
Piontkovskii, I.A., M.B. Goldberg, and O.E. Miklashevskii (1961) Some pecularities of the higher nervous activity in adult animals subjected antenatally to the action of ionizing radiation. Part III. Byull. Eksp. Biol. Med. (in Russian), *51:*24–31.
Plummer, G. (1952) Anomalies occurring in children exposed in utero to the atomic bomb in Hiroshima. Pediatrics, *10:*687–692.
Ronderos, A. (1961) Fetal tolerance to radiation. Radiology, *76:*454.
Ronnback, C. (1965) Effects of continuous irradiation during gestation and suckling period of mice. Acta Radiol. (Ther.), *3:*169–176.
Rugh, R. (1962) Major radiobiological concepts and ionizing radiation on the embryo and fetus; in Haley and Snider Response of the Nervous System to Ionizing Radiation; pp. 3–26 (Academic Press, New York).
Rugh, R. (1965) Effect of ionizing radiations, including radioisotopes on the placenta and embryo. Birth Defects, Orig. Article Series *1:*64–73.
Rugh, R., and M. Wohlfromm (1964a) X-irradiation sterilization of the premature female mouse. Atompraxis, *10:*511–518.
Rugh, R., and M. Wohlfromm (1964b) Can x-irradiation prior to sexual maturity affect the fertility of the male mammal (mouse)? Atompraxis, *10:*33–41.
Russell, L.B. (1950) X-ray induced developmental abnormalities in the mouse and their use in the analysis of embryological patterns. I. External and gross visceral changes. J. Exp. Zool., *114:*545–602.
Russell, L.B. (1956) X-ray induced developmental abnormalities in the mouse and their use in the analysis of embryological patterns. II. Abnormalities of the vertebral column and thorax. J. Exp. Zool., *131:*329–395.
Russell, L.B., and N.H. Major (1957) Radiation-induced presumed somatic mutations in the house mouse. Genetics, *42:*161–175.
Russell, L.B., and W.L. Russell (1950) The effects of radiation on the preimplantation stages of the mouse embryo. Anat. Res., *108:*521.
Russell, L.B., and W.L. Russell (1954) An analysis of the changing radiation response of the developing mouse embryo. J. Cell Comp. Physiol., *43:*103–149.
Russell, L.B., and C.L. Saylors (1963) The relative sensitivity of various germ-cell stages of the mouse to radiation-induced nondysjunction, chromosome losses and deficiencies; in Sobels Repair from Genetic Radiation; pp. 313–342 (Pergamon Press, New York).
Russell, L.B., S.K. Badgett, and C.L. Saylors (1959) Comparison of the effects of acute, continuous and fractionated irradiation during embryonic development; In: Buzzati-Traverso Special Suppl. Int. J. Radiation Biol., pp. 343–359. Immediate and Low Level Effects of Ionizing Radiation Conference held in Venice (Taylor & Francis, London).
Segall, A., B. MacMahon, and M. Hannigan (1964) Congenital malformations and background radiation in northern New England. J. Chron. Dis., *17:*915–932.
Stadler, J., and J.W. Gowen (1964) Observations on the effects of continuous irradiation over 10 generations on reproductivities of different strains of mice; in Carlson and Gassner Proceedings of an International Symposium on the Effects of Ionizing Radiation on Reproductive Systems (Pergamon Press, New York).
Stewart, A. (1973) The carcinogenic effects of low level radiation. A re-appraisal of epidemiologists methods and observations. Hlth. Phys., *24:*223–240.
Stewart, A., J. Webb, D. Giles, and D. Hewitt (1956) Malignant disease in childhood and diagnostic irradiation in utero. Lancet, *ii:*447.
Stewart, A., D. Webb, and D. Hewitt (1958) A survey of childhood malignancies. Br. Med. J., *i:*1495–1508.
Tabuchi, A. (1964) Fetal disorders due to ionizing radiation. Hiroshima J. Med. Sci. *13:*125–173.
Tabuchi, A., S Nakagawa, T. Hirai, H. Sato, I. Hori, M. Matsuda, K. Yano, K. Simada, and Y. Nakao (1967) Fetal hazards due to X-ray diagnosis during pregnancy. Hiroshima J. Med. Sci. *16:*49–66.
Vilumsen, A. (1970) Environmental factors in congen-

ital malformations. F.A.D.L.'s Forlag, Copenhagen.
Vorisek, P. (1965) Einfluss der kontinuierlichen intrauterinen Bestrahlung auf die perinatale Mortalitat der Frucht. Strahlentherapie, *127:*112–120.
Wesley, J.P. (1960) Background radiation as the cause of fetal congenital malformation. Int. J. Radiat. Biol. *2:*97–118.
Wood, J.W., K.G. Johnson, Y. Omori, S. Kawamoto, and R.J. Keehn (1967a) Mental retardation in children exposed in utero to the atomic bombs in Hiroshima and Nagasaki. Am. J. Publ. Hlth., *57:*1381–1390.
Wood, J.W., K.G. Johnson, and Y. Omori (1976b) In utero exposure to the Hiroshima atomic bomb. An evaluation of head size and mental retardation: twenty years later. Pediatrics, *39:*385–392.
Wood, J.W., R.J. Keehn, S. Kawamoto, and K.G. Johnson (1967c) The growth and development of children exposed in utero to the atomic bombs of Hiroshima and Nagasaki. Am. J. Publ. Hlth., *57:*1374–1380.
Yamazaki, J.M., S.W. Wright, and P.M. Wright (1954) Outcome of pregnancy in women exposed to atomic bomb in Nagasaki. Am. J. Dis. Child., *87:*448–463.
Zappert, J. (1926) Uber roentgenogene fetale Microcephalie. Mschr. Kinderheilk., *34:*490–493.

TERATOGEN UPDATE: ENVIRONMENTALLY INDUCED BIRTH DEFECT RISKS, PAGES 165–176 (1986)

Malformations in Infants of Diabetic Mothers

JAMES L. MILLS
Epidemiology and Biometry Research Program, National Institute of Child Health and Human Development, NIH, Bethesda, Maryland 20205

ABSTRACT Maternal insulin-dependent diabetes has long been associated with congenital malformations. As other causes of mortality and morbidity have been eliminated or reduced, malformations have become increasingly prominent. Although there is not universal agreement, the great majority of investigators find a two- to threefold increase in malformations in infants of insulin-dependent diabetic mothers. This increase is not seen in infants of gestational diabetics. It probably is not present in women whose diabetes can be controlled by diet or oral hypoglycemic agents. The risk does not appear to be primarily genetic since diabetic fathers do not have an increased number of malformed offspring. Most studies show a generalized increase in malformations involving multiple organ systems. Multiple malformations seem to be more common in diabetic than non-diabetic infants. Caudal regression has the strongest association with diabetes, occurring roughly 200 times more frequently in infants of diabetic mothers than in other infants. The teratogenic mechanism in diabetes is not known. Hyperglycemia may be important but human studies focusing on the period of organogenesis are lacking. Hypoglycemia has also been suggested based mainly on animal experiments. Insulin appears unlikely. Numerous other factors including vascular disease, hypoxia, ketone and amino acid abnormalities, glycosylation of proteins, or hormone imbalances could be teratogenic. None has been studied in sufficient detail to make a judgment. A large-scale prospective study is required to determine early fetal loss rates, correlate metabolic status during organogenesis with outcome, and assess the effect of diabetic control on malformation rates.

An association between diabetes mellitus in women and congenital malformations in their offspring has been suspected since the nineteenth century. In 1885, LoCorchó reported two infants of diabetic mothers with hydrocephalus. The prognosis for diabetic women prior to the discovery of insulin was poor, however, and few women delivered successfully. It was not until better control of hyperglycemia, close monitoring in the last months of pregnancy, and early delivery for fetal distress were instituted that salvage rates in diabetic pregnancies improved substantially. At this point, the full impact of congenital malformations was appreciated.

Until very recently better diabetic management had not resulted in a decrease in congenital malformations (Soler, '76). Now there is some preliminary evidence (Fuhrmann, '83) that malformation rates can be reduced by better control; however, rates have not fallen and malformations have now replaced respiratory distress syndrome as the leading cause of death in some diabetes centers (Soler, '76). This has stimulated investigators to examine the relationship between maternal diabetes and malformations.

EVIDENCE THAT INFANTS OF DIABETIC MOTHERS HAVE HIGHER MALFORMATION RATES

Evidence that infants of diabetic mothers have higher malformation rates has accumulated over the last several decades. Initially, centers reporting their experience with diabetic pregnancies noted high malformation rates in the infants of diabetic mothers. The author is aware of more than a dozen studies reporting malformation rates of 6% or more. Since malformations were not the primary focus of most of these studies, they were frequently uncontrolled and, hence, useful mainly to direct attention to the question of teratogenesis.

Numerous animal studies (to be discussed in detail later) were then performed to define the relationship between diabetes and malformations. Rats and mice made diabetic by alloxan or streptozotocin consistently produced more malformed offspring than expected. One recent experiment (Sadler, '79) took serum from diabetic rats and injected it into mouse embryo cultures. The injected (but not control) embryos developed a dose-related increase in malformations, suggesting that some diabetic factor, not the alloxan or streptozotocin, is teratogenic.

The definitive study relating diabetes to malformations in humans has not yet been reported. Before discussing specific studies comparing malformation rates in infants of diabetic mothers with control infants, it would be wise to consider some of their methodologic weaknesses. The diabetic group may not be representative of all diabetics. This is particularly true at university hospitals with referral populations, since those with more severe disease or complications are more likely to be referred. If, for example, vasculopathy were responsible for the increased malformation rate, the university hospitals would be likely to see a larger percentage of malformed infants, since those who have vascular disease are more likely to be cared for at a university hospital than those who do not. To overcome this problem, a population-based study in which all diabetic women from a given area are included would be needed.

The source of the control population is just as important as the source of the diabetic population. Control subjects chosen from a different area or bearing children at a different time may be totally inappropriate. To use an extreme example, suppose control subjects were chosen from a time and place where thalidomide was being used during pregnancy. The control population would show a large number of limb defects. If the diabetic group were from a non-thalidomide-exposed area or time period, they would not show the same thalidomide-induced defects. If diabetes produced limb defects, the association could be masked by the high rate in the control population. On the other hand, if the control group were contemporaneous, both groups would show the thalidomide effect and the diabetes effect would show up as an added risk.

Another advantage to contemporaneous control subjects is that diagnosis or definition of congenital malformations is more likely to be consistent. Ideally, the same person should examine all subjects using an agreed upon plan for diagnosing malformations. Agreement on what constitutes a malformation is important because, if cosmetic problems such as nevi or skin tags are counted as malformations in one group but not the other, inaccurate comparisons of rates will result.

The question of how malformations are ascertained is a particularly thorny one in studies of infants of diabetic mothers. Since these children are at high risk for respiratory distress syndrome, hypoglycemia, and hypocalcemia, it is not surprising that they receive a good deal of medical attention in the neonatal period. This attention could result in the discovery of malformations which would go unnoticed in the control population. The infants of diabetic mothers would then appear to have more malformations when, in fact, they merely had more complete ascertainment of their malformations. Fortunately, this is not as great a problem with major malformations as it is with minor malformations, since most (although not all) are readily diagnosable. All of those potential biases must be kept in mind when evaluating a report of malformations associated with diabetes.

Nonetheless, nearly all studies to date are consistent in finding a significantly increased risk for major malformations in the infants of diabetic mothers (Molsted-Pedersen et al., '64; Soler et al., '76; Chung and Myrianthopoulos, '75; Yssing, '75). Now let us review the evidence offered by some of the better studies.

Moltsed-Pedersen et al. ('64) examined 853 consecutive infants of diabetic mothers in Denmark and compared them to 1212 infants of nondiabetic mothers. As shown in Table 1, the frequency of major (including fatal) and total malformations was three times higher in the diabetic group. Fatal malformations and malformations involving several organ systems were approximately six times more frequent in the diabetics. All subjects came from the same departments of the hospital. Most of the infants of diabetic mothers were examined by the same person. Unfortunately, the control subjects were obtained over a six-month period while the diabetics spanned 37 years. Data were obtained retrospectively. This study is particularly note-

TABLE 1. Congenital malformations in 853 infants of diabetic mothers and 1,212 control infants (over 1000 gm)

		Number with congenital malformations		
	Total	Total	Major	Fatal
Infants of diabetic mothers	853	55 (6.4%)	44 (5.2%)	18 (2.1%)
Infants of nondiabetic mothers	1,212	26 (2.1%)	14 (1.2%)	4 (0.3%)

Pedersen et al., Lancet, 1964.

worthy because of the large number of diabetic pregnancies studied and because 791 of the subjects were insulin-dependent before pregnancy.

The Collaborative Perinatal Project (Chung and Myrianthopoulos, '75), a prospective study, also found that infants of insulin-dependent diabetic mothers were more likely to have malformations. They examined 48,437 infants, diagnosing malformations throughout the first year of life. White infants of insulin-dependent diabetic mothers had a 17.7% major malformation rate compared to 8.3% in nondiabetics. Black infants of insulin-dependent mothers showed a risk of 17.3 versus 8.5% for nondiabetics. The increased rate in the diabetic groups was statistically significant in both whites and blacks. The Collaborative Perinatal Project obtained subjects from 14 geographically dispersed institutions. Its strengths include the prospective approach, careful diagnosis of diabetes and malformations, and a very large, well-studied, normal control population. Because of the rarity of diabetes, the Collaborative Perinatal Project added patients not selected according to the protocol procedure from the Joslin Clinic to increase the sample size. While these subjects were not, strictly speaking, from the same population as the remainder, they were followed in the same fashion.

Kucera's ('71) analysis of the world's literature, while not as well designed as the Collaborative Perinatal Project, is interesting nonetheless. Combining all reported case series of infants of diabetic mothers, he found an overall malformation rate of 4.8%. He selected data from the World Health Organization for comparison. This control group showed a malformation rate of 1.65% (see Table 2). The value of this study lies in its summary of reports of all types of malformations. Since the World Health Organization data also specify type of malformation, it is possible to look at specific malformations, albeit crudely, with this report. Despite the major limitations of this method (the use of literature reports for rates and different definitions of malformations), this report is consistent with other studies showing that diabetic women are two to three times more likely to produce malformed infants.

Whereas numerous other studies have also found higher malformation rates in infants of diabetic mothers, one well-performed study did not. Farquhar ('59, '69) reported that infants of diabetic mothers in Edinburgh did not show higher malformation rates than other infants. The reason for this discrepancy is not clear from Farquhar's data; he does not specify actual malformations seen. He does note, however, that the diabetic group had more severe malformations. This is con-

TABLE 2. Summary of the world literature on malformations in infants of diabetic mothers (1930–1964)

	Total	Number with malformations	Percentage with malformations
Infants of diabetic mothers	7,101	340	4.8
W.H.O. world survey of malformation rates in "normals"	431,764	7,124	1.65

Kucera, J. Reprod. Med., 1971.

sistent with others' observations that it is in major malformations rather than minor that the increase is found. Farquhar's work not withstanding, it is generally accepted that infants of insulin-dependent diabetic mothers have malformation rates two to three times higher than normal, and that major malformations account for most of the increase.

WHO IS AT RISK?

As the increased risk of malformations became evident, investigators turned their attention to determining which diabetics were at risk.

An obvious question was, do diabetic fathers have more malformed children? This question has important etiologic implications because a link between various HLA types and insulin-dependent diabetes has been established in many different populations. If this "diabetes-associated gene" were responsible for the higher malformation rate, infants of diabetic fathers would be likely to show an increase as well. Bennett and associates ('79) have reviewed the evidence from their own studies of Pima Indians and from the Collaborative Perinatal Project. As shown in Table 3, diabetic (and prediabetic) fathers do not produce more malformed children than nondiabetics. This suggests that the teratogenic effect of diabetes is not a result of genetic factors related to diabetes-associated genes. It does not, however, rule out the possibility that women with the genetic marker for diabetes might have an increased susceptibility to some potentially teratogenic metabolic derangement such as hyperglycemia.

Although the increased risk for producing malformed infants lies with the diabetic mother, not the diabetic father, it does not appear that women with all types of diabetes are at equal risk.

There is very little to suggest that "prediabetic" women are at increased risk of producing malformed infants. Only two highly controversial studies have found an increased risk of malformations in the "prediabetic" woman. In one study, 34.3% of women with normal carbohydrate tolerance during pregnancy who delivered malformed infants had developed diabetes 25 years later. Only 1% of control women were found to have diabetes (Navarette et al., '70). A second investigator (Hagbard, '58) found an increased incidence of malformations in infants delivered up to 20 years before clinically apparent maternal diabetes. These reports suggest that the "prediabetic" woman may already be at increased risk before she develops diabetes. There are, however, compelling reasons to question these findings. Selection bias may be a problem in this type study. A prevalence of diabetes 30 times higher in the case group than in the control group suggests either a very strong exposure effect (which in this case has not been confirmed) or a major selection bias. Without additional information on how diabetic and control women were selected for study and how malformations were searched out, these studies cannot be accepted. In fact, it is reasonable to conclude that the "prediabetic" woman is not at risk, since if she were, the woman who actually develops diabetes during pregnancy should certainly show an increased risk. This, as we shall see, does not appear to be the case.

Malformation rates in infants of gestational diabetic women (White Class A) have been published by many centers (Soler et al., '76; Chung and Myrianthopoulos, '75; Bennett et al., '79; Day and Insley, '76; Karlson and Kjellmer, '72). There is general agreement that malformation rates are not increased. The findings of the Collaborative Perinatal Project are typical. Among 392 gestational diabetics, the malformation rates

TABLE 3. Incidence of malformations and paternal diabetes

	Number of pregnancies	Malformations			Significance
		Number	Percentage		
Collaborative perinatal project					
Nondiabetic father	51,803	4,298	8.28		P > 0.05
Diabetic father	253	23	9.09		
Pima Indians					
Nondiabetic father	395	13	3.3		
Prediabetic father	197	7	3.6	3.7 (prediabetic and diabetic combined)	P > 0.05
Diabetic father	44	2	4.5		

Bennett, Pregnancy Metabolism Diabetes and the Fetus, 1979.

were 15.3% for whites and 13.7% for blacks. The corresponding rates for nondiabetics were 14.6 and 17.0%, respectively. The differences were not significant. This study is very strong on several counts. The number of diabetics and normal controls is large. It is prospective, making good documentation of gestational diabetes possible, and all participants were carefully screened for malformations. This study clearly demonstrates that those who do not have diabetes prior to pregnancy are not at increased risk for producing malformed infants.

Among women who already have diabetes at the time of conception, those who are non-insulin-dependent must be considered separately. Data on women treated with oral hypoglycemic agents are not clear-cut. The Birmingham Maternity Hospital Series (Day and Insley, '76) showed that 31 women treated by diet or hypoglycemic agents at the time of conception had no more malformed infants than control women. Since the percentage receiving oral hypoglycemic agents is not given, it is impossible to tell whether an increased risk in those on hypoglycemic agents was diluted out by a larger number in the diet group. The Collaborative Perinatal Project (Heinonen et al., '77) examined the risk of malformations in offspring of 21 women receiving oral hypoglycemic agents. Their survival and race-standardized relative risk was 1.10, not significantly different from nondiabetic women. On the other hand, Soler et al ('76) reported that the offspring of 46 women receiving oral hypoglycemics in the first trimester had an 8.7% malformation rate. This was similar to the insulin-dependent diabetics' rate (8.1%) in their center. The authors estimated the rate among nondiabetics to be only 1.7%. They acknowledged that the rate among nondiabetics did not come from the same source and was not strictly comparable. They maintained, however, that their results suggested an increased risk for non-insulin-dependent diabetics receiving oral hypoglycemic agents.

It is difficult to draw any conclusions from these studies. The number of subjects in each is small, making their rates unstable. While most of the evidence suggests that women treated with oral hypoglycemic agents do not produce more malformed infants, the evidence is not conclusive.

As noted previously, the evidence that insulin-dependent diabetic women produce more malformed infants is very strong. Investigators have examined factors such as duration of disease and age of onset in insulin-dependent women to determine how they influence malformation rates. White Class, which is based on age of onset, duration of disease, and presence of complications, correlates well with malformation rates. Those with earliest onset, longest duration, and with complications have the highest risk according to most authors (Molsted-Pedersen et al., '64; Soler et al., '76; Karlson and Kjellmer, '72). Day and Insley ('76) are an exception. They found no correlation between malformations and age of onset, duration of diabetes, vascular complications, maternal age, or parity. It is likely that their failure to find an association is due to the small number of cases examined. It is reasonable that early onset and long duration of diabetes would be associated with higher malformation rates, since early onset and long duration would generally result in a more abnormal maternal milieu during pregnancy. Diabetic complications, particularly vascular, could be a reflection of this metabolic disorder as well as a direct mechanism for teratogenesis. Later, we shall consider how specific aspects of the disturbed metabolic environment and complications relate to malformations.

WHAT TYPES OF MALFORMATIONS ARE ASSOCIATED WITH DIABETES?

Multiple organ systems are susceptible to the teratogenic effects of diabetes. All studies of congenital anomalies in infants of diabetic mothers have shown cardiovascular, genitourinary, musculoskeletal, and other malformations. No single study has contained enough cases to determine whether or not the risk for each specific defect is significantly increased. The number of subjects required would be enormous. Kucera ('71) tried to estimate relative risks based on cases reported in the literature. His estimates are derived from malformation rates in published series of diabetic pregnancies (1945–1965) and from additional data obtained directly from the authors. He reviewed 7101 pregnancies, of which 340 produced malformed offspring. This is a rough estimate of relative risk because reported series may not be a good choice of a denominator for mothers at risk and because his comparison group, World Health Organization "normals," does not come from the same population. Keeping these limitations in mind, it is interesting that he found that abnormalities of the skeleton, kidneys, heart, gastrointestinal system, and genitalia all occurred significantly more frequently in infants of diabetic mothers. An estimate of the risk ratio for infants of diabetic mothers calculated from Kucera's data is shown in Table 4. Thus, the teratogenic action of diabetes is generalized.

It is also apparent that the teratogenic effect occurs early in gestation. The malformations Kucera found to be significantly more frequent were examined by the author and his associates (Mills et al., '79), using a developmental morphologic approach. This method is based on the knowledge of when organ development occurs and on the assumption that malformations of an organ cannot occur after the organ has been completely differentiated. Thus, for each anomaly, a time was assigned before which the defect must have occurred. As shown in Table 5 all the anomalies occur before the seventh week of gestation.

The developmental morphologic approach has been validated by Baker et al. ('81) in

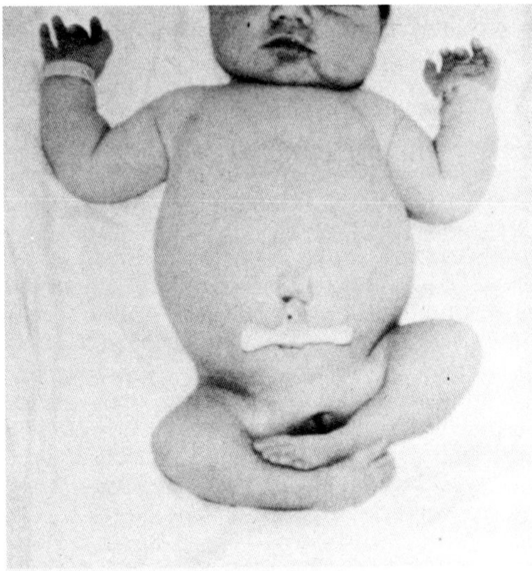

Fig. 1. See legend below.

TABLE 4. Congenital anomalies most often seen in infants of diabetic mothers with risk ratios

Anomaly	Risk ratio
Caudal regression	252
Situs inversus	84
Ureter duplex	23
Renal agenesis	6
Cardiac anomalies (TGA, VSD, ASD)	4
Anencephalus	3

Mills, Diabetes, 1979.

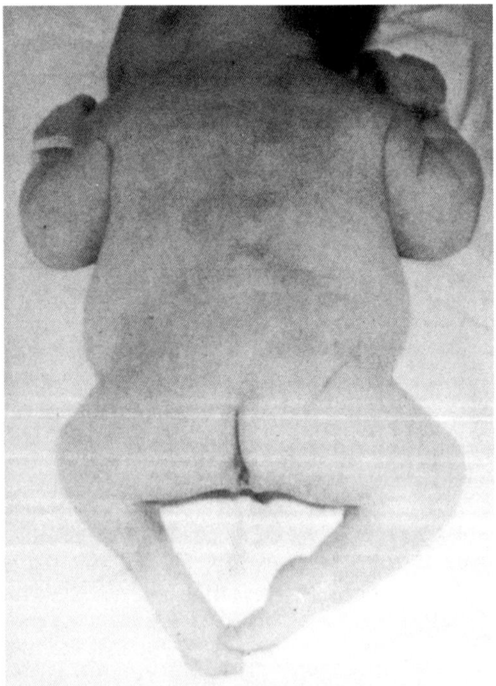

TABLE 5. Latest date at which common anomalies in infants of diabetic mothers could occur

Anomaly	Gestational age after ovulation in weeks
Caudal regression	3
Situs inversus	4
Ureter duplex	5
Renal agenesis	5
Cardiac anomalies	
TGA	5
VSD	6
ASD	6
Anencephalus	4

Mills, Diabetes, 1979.

Figs. 1–2. Infant with caudal regression syndrome: Sacral dysgenesis and shortening of the femorae. (Photographs courtesy of Lewis Holmes, M.D.).

rats. By making rats diabetic at different times and treating some but not all, they demonstrated that only uncontrolled diabetes during organogenesis produced lumbosacral defects.

While infants of diabetic mothers are at risk for a wide variety of malformations, one syndrome seems particularly strongly associated with diabetes. Caudal regression is a condition in which agenesis or hypoplasia of the femorae occurs in conjunction with agenesis of the lower vertebrae (see Figs. 1 and 2). It is very rare in the general population. In Kucera's ('71) review of the literature, he found 9 cases in 7101 infants of diabetic mothers. Comparing the incidence with data from the World Health Organization, he concluded that the relative risk of caudal regression syndrome in infants of diabetic mothers was over 200. This estimate is unstable, yet it seems conservative in comparison with Pedersen's ('77) relative risk estimate of 600 based on 4 cases in his series.

As previously stated, the number of subjects available is too small to estimate the relative risk of most specific anomalies in the infant of the diabetic mother. Data from the Collaborative Perinatal Project (Mitchell et al., '71) did, however, provide an estimate of relative risk of congenital heart disease. Infants of diabetic mothers had an incidence of 25.4 per 1000 compared to 8.1 per 1000 in infants of normal mothers (relative risk 3.1). Defects of the great vessels and septal defects accounted for virtually all cases. These findings are particularly important. They came from a prospective study where the special attention paid to diabetic pregnancies would not have biased the results, since all infants were screened for congenital heart disease.

While the relative risk of caudal regression is many times higher than the relative risk of cardiac anomalies, the magnitude of the problem is actually much greater for cardiac anomalies because their incidence rate is so much higher. One infant in 40 will have congenital heart disease, whereas, even using the highest estimate, only 1 in 350 will have caudal regression (Pedersen, '77).

In summary, there is good evidence that maternal diabetes is associated with a wide range of malformations in the offspring. Multiple malformations are common in infants of diabetic mothers. While no single syndrome is specific for diabetes, caudal regression occurs far more often than in the general population.

POSSIBLE TERATOGENIC MECHANISMS IN DIABETES

The search for a teratogenic agent in diabetes is complicated by the fact that diabetes is not simply a disorder of carbohydrate regulation. Diabetes is responsible for a loss of normal homeostasis not only of carbohydrate but of fat and protein metabolism as well. Vascular complications may lead to additional metabolic changes such as hypoxia or impaired renal clearance of toxins. In short, there are multiple factors in the disordered milieu of the pregnant diabetic which could be teratogenic.

In addition to considering all the metabolic changes in diabetes, care must be taken to relate these events to the appropriate period during gestation. Unfortunately, most studies to date have not addressed this problem. Either because the investigators did not appreciate how early in pregnancy organogenesis occurs, or because the women did not come to medical attention early enough, few studies have examined diabetic control during the critical period. Because of this, most evidence on possible teratogenic agents comes from retrospective analysis or from animal studies.

A number of animal studies have suggested that hyperglycemia could be teratogenic. Mice made diabetic with alloxan produced offspring with abnormally high malformation rates (Watanabe and Ingalls, '63). Rats given alloxan or streptozotocin to make them diabetic had three times as many malformed offspring as control animals (Deuchar, '77). These studies could be criticized on the grounds that the alloxan or streptozotocin could have caused the malformations. However, Horii and associates ('66) reduced the increased malformation rate produced by alloxan in mice to baseline by treating the mice with insulin, strong evidence that it was the uncontrolled diabetes which was responsible. Since insulin corrects a number of metabolic abnormalities in diabetes, not just hyperglycemia, this experiment does not establish hyperglycemia as the teratogenic agent. It does indicate that appropriate treatment, including the prevention of hyperglycemia, might reduce the risk of congenital malformations.

Until recently, most human studies compared hyperglycemia and other measures of diabetic control in the third trimester with malformations, an inappropriate comparison. Within the last few years, several studies have begun to examine the relationship between diabetic events in the first trimester and congenital anomalies.

Fuhrmann and co-workers ('83) reported that a group of 128 diabetic women who began intensive medical management before conception produced only one malformed infant (0.8%) among them. By comparison, 292 women who began treatment after 8 weeks gestation produced 22 malformed infants (7.5%). The women who enrolled prior to conception had lower mean daily glucose levels during weeks 5 to 7 than the later entrants did at registration (weeks 8 to 14). Other risk factors for producing a malformed infant noted by the authors (White Class, maternal age, previous bad pregnancy outcomes) did not favor the early entrants and, thus, could not explain the difference in outcomes. While it was not stated whether the infants were examined blindly or in a standard fashion, the malformations reported would probably have been diagnosed by routine examination. Except for the unavoidable bias that women who are more motivated (i.e., go to a doctor before conception) tend to have better outcomes, it would appear that good control during organogenesis was the cause of the improved results. Unfortunately, this study provides little information on metabolic events during organogenesis. Other than the fact that 118 of 128 early entrants had mean daily glucoses under 130 mg/dl from weeks 5 to 7, there is no information linking outcomes to metabolic status. While the authors document that those entering after 8 weeks of gestation had higher mean daily glucose levels, they do not discuss how glucose level at entry related to malformations. This omission is probably deliberate since most of the malformations had presumably occurred before the eighth week, but it makes it impossible to relate bad outcomes to specific metabolic events during organogenesis.

It is possible to look at diabetic control retrospectively by measuring hemoglobin A_{1c}. Since hemoglobin A_{1c} represents an integrated measure of blood glucose over the preceding weeks, elevation of hemoglobin A_{1c} in the second or third month of pregnancy is a fair indicator of hyperglycemia during organogenesis.

Miller and co-workers ('81) examined 116 infants of insulin-dependent diabetic women, 15 with major anomalies. Hemoglobin A_{1c} levels drawn on the mothers before the fourteenth week of gestation were strongly correlated with malformation rates. The malformation rate in infants whose mothers' hemoglobin A_{1c} had been 8.5 or less was 3.4%; the malformation rate in infants whose mothers' hemoglobin A_{1c} had been over 8.5 was a remarkable 22.4%. A hemoglobin A_{1c} determination sometime before the fourteenth week of pregnancy hardly tells us all we would like to know about the diabetic state during organogenesis. Indeed, it may reflect hyperglycemic episodes occurring after the critical period. Nonetheless, it is an important first step toward relating diabetic events during organogenesis to malformations.

A second, more modest study also found an association between high hemoglobin A_{1c} and malformations. Leslie and associates ('78) found that three of five insulin-dependent diabetic mothers with elevated hemoglobin A_{1c} levels at presentation for prenatal care had malformed infants. None of 18 babies born to diabetic mothers with hemoglobin A_{1c} in the range reflecting good diabetic control had malformations. Unfortunately, this paper does not provide enough detail to relate the hemoglobin A_{1c} determinations to organogenesis. "Presentation" may have occurred far enough beyond the critical period that the hemoglobin A_{1c} measurements are not relevant.

Both of these studies offer suggestive evidence that diabetic control is important in preventing malformations. It is not, however, possible to say that hyperglycemia is responsible for the malformations associated with high hemoglobin A_{1c}. While elevated hemoglobin A_{1c} certainly indicates past hyperglycemia, it tells us nothing about other events which could also have been present, such as ketosis or rapid fluctuations in blood sugar level.

Hypoglycemia is another state which has been said to cause malformations. Malformations have been reported in animals when their mothers were made hypoglycemic during pregnancy either by insulin or fasting (Duraiswami, '50; Smithberg and Runner, '63; Kalter and Warkany, '59). It appears that hypoglycemia rather than insulin was the likely cause, both because the same effect was produced by fasting and because the malformation rate was reduced when insulin and adequate food to prevent hypoglycemia were administered simultaneously (Hannah and Moore, '71).

Data on hypoglycemia in pregnant human beings are scarce. Malformations have been reported in infants whose mothers received insulin-shock treatment during pregnancy (Wickes, '54; Impastato et al., '64). The number of cases is, however, very small. It is very likely that these cases represent nothing more than coincidental occurrence of malformations in women receiving shock therapy.

Weak evidence against hypoglycemia as a teratogen comes from two sources. Rowland and his colleagues ('73) obtained a history of hypoglycemia during pregnancy nearly four times as often from diabetic women with normal infants as from diabetic women whose offspring had congenital heart disease. Most of these women had not come to medical attention until after the critical period of gestation, and it is not clear whether questions about hypoglycemia were related to the period of organogenesis. Molsted-Pedersen et al. ('64) reported that only 8 of 55 mothers with malformed infants had noted insulin reactions in the first trimester. They concluded that hypoglycemia could not, therefore, be an important cause of malformations. Here again, it is not clear that questions about hypoglycemia were directed to the appropriate period. In any such retrospective study, patient recall is a serious problem; moreover, some hypoglycemic reactions (particularly during sleep) go totally unrecognized.

Since congenital malformations occur most frequently in infants of insulin-dependent diabetic women, it is not surprising that insulin has been proposed as a teratogen. Early evidence supporting this contention came from animal studies. Injecting chicken eggs (Landauer, '45) with insulin caused "rumplessness," a condition tantalizingly like caudal regression. It was soon discovered, however, that this was not unique to insulin. In fact, merely shaking the egg could produce the same result (Landauer, '45). As noted previously, insulin produced malformations in other animals as well, but the role of insulin was put in doubt when it was found that if glucose was given simultaneously the malformation rate returned to normal. In addition, diabetic mice treated with insulin had fewer malformations than those whose diabetes remained untreated.

Developmental morphologic dating provided additional evidence that insulin is not responsible for malformations. The malformations, as noted previously, occur before the seventh week of gestation. Beta cells have been reported to differentiate in the fetus at 10.5 weeks (Like and Orci, '72). Maternal insulin does not cross the placenta at 16 to 20 weeks (Adam et al., '69) or at term (Kalhan et al., '75). Unless maternal insulin can reach the embryo earlier in gestation, there is no insulin exposure during the critical period.

Many other abnormalities of the diabetic milieu have been mentioned as possible teratogens. The apparent association between White Class and malformation rates has generated several hypotheses. Women in White Classes D and F (those women with vascular disease) have the highest malformation rates, leading to speculation that vascular disease could be teratogenic. Whether it is vascular disease per se or some concomitant of it remains to be determined. Hypoxia, also associated with poor White Class and vascular disease, has been considered a possible teratogen. There are no data in humans to support or refute this theory.

Still other metabolic abnormalities created by diabetes could cause malformations. Maternal ketonuria has been associated with reduced I.Q. in infants of diabetic mothers (Churchill et al., '69; Stehbens et al., '77), raising speculation that ketones might interfere with normal development. Proteins may be glycosylated in the presence of high glucose concentration (as in hemoglobin A_{1c}). This could result in abnormal structural proteins in the fetus. Abnormal protein synthesis might also result from a lack of glucogenic amino acids or an overabundance of branched-chain amino acids as is seen in poorly controlled diabetes (Felig et al., '70).

As anyone who has cared for diabetic patients well knows, diabetes changes much more than carbohydrate, insulin, fat, and protein metabolism. It has an enormous impact on the patient's life style as well. Some of the changes in life style dictated by diabetes and its management ought to be considered in our discussion of teratogenesis. Diabetic women are advised to restrict their diets, generally in terms of caloric intake and free sugars. At the same time, they may be encouraged to use artificial sweeteners. They are often told to eat, sleep, and exercise on schedule. It is not difficult to imagine that some of these changes in life style might be teratogenic, nor is it difficult to see how complex the search for a teratogenic mechanism in diabetes could become given all these additional factors. Fortunately, one piece of evidence clarifies the situation. As noted previously, women with non-insulin-dependent diabetes do not produce more malformed infants than normal women. They do experience most of the changes in life style that insulin-dependent diabetics undergo. This suggests that the teratogenic effect of diabetes is not related to these changes; if it were, both groups should show a similar effect.

Studies linking HLA types, DR 3 and DR 4 in particular, to diabetes have stimulated interest in a possible link between genetic factors and malformations. Since infants of diabetic fathers are not at increased risk, it appears that HLA-related factors are not primary determinants. There may, however, be a link between genetic factors, e.g., HLA types, and susceptibility of the conceptus to metabolic insults. Preliminary reports (Koppe et al., '83; Simpson et al., '83) have been inconclusive because of small numbers, but the question is being addressed by the NICHD Diabetes in Early Pregnancy Study (Mills et al., '83) as well.

Finally, the possibility that diabetes-induced changes in other endocrine systems might influence fetal development needs to be considered. Jovanovic and co-workers ('80) were able to study diabetic women before the tenth week of gestation. Women whose diabetes was not well controlled had estradiol, prolactin, and human chorionic gonadotropin levels below the range associated with normal pregnancy. In their small sample, there were no major malformations in any of the offspring. To say for certain that these subtle endocrine changes are not deleterious will require a larger study. Jovanovic's work shows that other endocrine organs may be affected by diabetes during pregnancy.

FUTURE INVESTIGATIONS

One important area which remains unexplored is early fetal losses in diabetic pregnancy. Is the early loss rate higher in diabetics than nondiabetics? If so, is the increase due to higher malformation rates? Conversely, could the rate be lower due to failure of diabetic women to abort malformed fetuses? If this is the case, it might explain the excess malformation rate among live births.

Both the question of early fetal losses and the question of teratogenic factors in diabetic pregnancies could best be addressed by a prospective controlled study beginning before pregnancy. Due to the rarity of malformations, a large sample size would be required. The National Institute of Child Health and Human Development is currently performing a collaborative study to examine the problems of malformations in infants of diabetic mothers. In addition, the study will attempt to assess the role of good diabetic control during organogenesis in reducing malformations.

Malformations associated with maternal diabetes mellitus present an unusual opportunity to the teratologist. If insulin can be excluded as the teratogen, some endogenous factor created by the diabetic state must then be teratogenic. What is even more remarkable is the possibility that appropriate medical management can eliminate the risk.

The physician who must advise diabetic women about the risk of having a malformed infant faces a difficult task. He or she can say with confidence that only diabetics who are insulin-dependent during organogenesis are at increased risk (although the situation is not clear in those on oral hypoglycemics). Gestational diabetics and diabetic fathers are not at risk. The relative risk for malformations is roughly three, and major malformations, not minor, account for the increase. Nonetheless, the diabetic women should be reassured that approximately nine out of ten infants of diabetic mothers are not malformed. The physician's difficulty begins when the relationship between malformations and diabetic control is considered. Clearly, control very early in pregnancy is the issue. Many women will not be aware that they are pregnant and, hence, not pay particular attention to their diabetic control. Several recent reports have suggested that good control may prevent malformations (Miller et al., '81; Fuhrmann et al., '83) but this requires confirmation. For the present, the best course to follow would be 1) to recommend that women get into good control before getting pregnant since the risk of hypoglycemia seems small compared to the risk of poor control; 2) not to recommend interrupting the pregnancy purely on the basis of poor early pregnancy control but to inform women of the reported association between poor control and malformations; and 3) to offer women prenatal diagnosis to help identify congenital anomalies.

ACKNOWLEDGMENTS

The author wishes to thank Drs. Heinz Berendes, Carl Keller, and Michele Forman for their insightful suggestions and Mrs. Beverly Trainor for preparing the manuscript.

LITERATURE CITED

Adam, P., K. Teramo, N. Raiha, D. Gitlin, and R. Schwartz (1969) Human fetal insulin metabolism early in gestation. Diabetes, *18:*409–415.

Baker, L., J.M. Egler, S.H. Klein, and A.S. Goldman (1981) Meticulous control of diabetes during organogenesis prevents lumbosacral defects in rats. Diabetes, *30:*955–959.

Bennett, P.H., C. Webner and M. Miller (1979) Pregnancy, Metabolism, Diabetes and the Fetus. Exerpta Medica, New York.

Chung, C.S., and N.C. Myrianthopoulos (1975) Factors affecting risks of congenital malformations. II Effect of maternal diabetes. Birth Defects Series, Vol. XI, No. 10.

Churchill, J.A., H.W. Berendes and J. Nemore (1969) Neuropsychological deficits in children of diabetic mothers: A report from the collaborative study of cerebral palsy. Amer. J. Obstet. Gynecol., *105:*257–268.

Day, R., and J. Insley (1976) Maternal diabetes and congenital malformations. Arch. Dis. Child., *51:*935–938.

Deuchar, E.M. (1977) Embryonic malformations in rats resulting from maternal diabetes: Preliminary observations. J. Embryol. Exp. Morphol., *41:*93–99.

Duraiswami, P. (1950) Insulin-induced skeletal anomalies in developing chickens. Brit. Med. J., *2:*384–390.

Farquhar, J.W. (1959) The child of the diabetic woman. Arch. Dis. Child., *34:*76–96.

Farquhar, J.W. (1969) Prognosis for babies born to diabetic mothers in Edinburgh. Arch. Dis. Child., *44:*36–47.

Felig, P., E. Marliss, J.L. Ohman and G.F. Cahill (1970) Plasmo amino acid levels in diabetic ketoacidosis. Diabetes, *19:*727–729.

Fuhrmann, K., H. Reiher, K. Semmler, F. Fischer, M. Fischer, and E. Glockner (1983) Prevention of congenital malformations in infants of insulin-dependent diabetic mothers. Diabetes Care, *6:*219–223.

Hagbard, L. (1958) The "pre diabetic" period from an obstetric point of view. Acta Obstet. Gynecol. Scand., *37:*497–518.

Hannah, R.S., and K.L. Moore (1971) Effects of fasting and insulin on skeletal development in rats. Teratology, *4:*135–139.

Heinonen, O.P., D. Slone and S. Shapiro (1977) Birth Defects and Drugs in Pregnancy. Publishing Sciences Group, Inc., Littleton, MA.

Horii, N., G. Watanabe and T.H. Ingalls (1966) Experimental diabetes in pregnant mice. Prevention of congenital malformations in offspring by insulin. Diabetes, *15:*194–203.

Impastato, D.J., A.R. Gabriel and H.H. Lardaro (1964) Electric and insulin shock therapy during pregnancy. Dis. Nerv. Sys., *25:*542–546.

Jovanovic, L., C.M. Peterson, B.B., Saxena, Y.M. Dawood and C.D. Saudek (1980) Feasibility of maintaining normal glucose profiles in insulin-dependent pregnant diabetic women. Amer. J. Med., *68:*105–112.

Kalhan, S., R. Schwartz and P. Adam (1975) Placental barrier to human insulin I^{125} in insulin-dependent diabetic mothers. J. Clin. Endocrinol. Metabol., *40:*139–142.

Kalter, H., and J. Warkany (1959) Experimental production of congenital malformations in mammals by metabolic procedure. Physiol. Rev., *39:*69–115.

Karlson, K., and I. Kjellmer (1972) The outcome of diabetic pregnancies in relation to the mother's blood sugar level. Amer. J. Obstet. Gynecol., *112:*213–220.

Koppe, J.G., M.E. Smorenberg-Schoorl, E.M. van den Berg-Loonen, and J.L. Mills (1983) Diabetes, congenital malformations, and HLA-types. In: Intensive Care in the Newborn, Volume 4. L. Stern, H. Bard, and B. Friis-Hansen, eds. Masson Publishing, New York.

Kucera, J. (1971) Rate and type of congenital anomalies among offspring of diabetic women. J. Reprod. Med., *7:*61–70.

Landauer, W. (1945) Rumplessness of chicken embryos produced by the injection of insulin and other chemicals. J. Exp. Zool., *98:*65–77.

LeCorché, E. (1885) Du diabete dans ses rapports avec la vie uterine. La menstruation et la grossesse. Ann. Gynecol. Obstet., *24:*257.

Leslie, R.D.G., D.A. Pyke, P.N. John and J.M. White (1978) Hemoglobin A_1 in diabetic pregnancy. Lancet, *2:*958–959.

Like, A., and L. Orci (1972) Embryogenesis of the human pancreatic islets: A light and electron microscopic study. Diabetes, *21:*511–534.

Miller, E.M., J.W. Hare, J.R. Cloherty, P.J. Dunn, R.E. Gleason, J.S. Soeldner and J.L. Kitzmiller (1981) Major congenital anomalies and elevated hemoglobin A_{1c} in early weeks of diabetic pregnancy. N. Eng. J. Med., *304:*1331–1334.

Mills, J.L., L. Baker and A.S. Goldman (1979) Malformations in infants of diabetic mothers occur before the seventh gestational week. Diabetes, *28:*292–293.

Mills, J.L., A.R. Fishl, R.H. Knopp, C.L. Ober, L.G. Jovanovic, B.F. Polk, and The Diabetes in Early Pregnancy Study (1983) Malformations in infants of diabetic mothers: Problems in study design. Prev. Med., *12:*274–286.

Mitchell, S.C., A.H. Sellmann, M.C. Westphal and J. Park (1971) Etiologic correlates in a study of congenital heart disease in 56,109 births. Amer. J. Cardio., *28:*653–657.

Molsted-Pedersen, L., I. Tygstrup and J. Pedersen (1964) Congenital malformations in newborn infants of diabetic women. Lancet, *1:*1124–1126.

Navarette, V.N., C.E. Rojas, C.R. Alger and H.E. Paniagua (1970) Subsequent diabetes in mothers delivered of a malformed infant. Lancet, *2:*993–995.

Pedersen, J. (1977) The Pregnant Diabetic and Her Newborn. Munksgaard, Copenhagen, p. 194.

Rowland, T.W., J.P. Hubbell and A.S. Nadas (1973) Congenital heart disease in infants of diabetic mothers. J. Pediatr., *83:*815–820.

Sadler, T.W. (1979) Effects of maternal diabetes on early embryogenesis: The teratogenic potential of diabetic serum. Teratology *21:*339–347.

Simpson, J.L., S. Elias, A.O. Martin, M.S. Palmer, E.S. Ogata, and R.A. Radvany (1983) Diabetes in pregnancy, Northwestern University series (1977–1981) I. Prospective study of anomalies in offspring of mothers with diabetes mellitus. Am. J. Obstet. Gynecol., *146:*263–270.

Smithberg, M., and M.N. Runner (1963) Teratogenic effects of hypoglycemic treatments in inbred strains of mice. Amer. J. Anat., *113:*479–489.

Soler, N.G. (1976) Perinatal Medicine. Fifth European Congress of Perinatology. Almqvist and Wiksell Int., Stockholm.

Soler, N., C. Walsh and J. Malins (1976) Congenital malformations in newborn infants of diabetic mothers. Q.J. Med., *178:*303–313.
Stehbens, J.A., G.L. Baker and M. Kitchell (1977) Outcome at ages 1, 3, and 5 years of children born to diabetic women. Amer. J. Obstet. Gynecol., *127:*408–413.
Watanabe, G., and T.H. Ingalls (1963) Congenital malformations in the offspring of alloxan diabetic mice. Diabetes, *12:*66–72.
Wickes, I.G. (1954) Fetal defects following insulin coma in early pregnancy. Brit. Med. J., *2:*1029–1030.
Yssing, M. (1975) Long term prognosis of children born to mothers diabetic when pregnant. In: Early Diabetes in Early Life. R.A. Camerini-Davalos and H.S. Cole, eds., Academic Press, New York.

Iodine Deficiency

JOSEF WARKANY
Children's Hospital Research Foundation, Cincinnati, Ohio 45229

This deficiency was once one of the most important and widespread teratogens that caused a disease picture of dwarfism, neuromuscular disturbances, deafness, and mental retardation. It occurred, and still occurs, in endemic form; it is called "endemic cretinism" and is associated with endemic goiter. The disorder prevailed in many regions of the world where the soil and water were poor in iodine and isolation prevented importation of foodstuffs from the outside. Owing to isolation of affected populations, valid prevalence figures could not be obtained worldwide, but it was estimated that about 25 years ago there were still 200 million people affected by endemic goiter and there existed hundred thousands of cretins (Kelly and Snedden, '60). There has been a continuous decrease of this condition as iodine in one form or another reached the deficient areas, but it still exists in some parts of the world (Warkany, '71).

Endemic goiter cannot be called a congenital malformation unless it is present in a newborn baby, which is quite rare. Generally, it is an acquired anomaly, and it has been noted and described since ancient times. Langer ('60) has written a fascinating history of goiter, which mentions that in a Chinese treatise on herbs and roots written about 4,700 years ago, the seaweed sargassum was recommended as an efficacious remedy for goiter. When in 1811 the element iodine was discovered by the French chemist Courtois in the ashes of seaweed (which had been for millenia a treatment for goiter), Coindet in 1820 introduced iodine itself as a remedy for goiter. The results were not satisfactory since the doses used were more than a thousand times larger than daily optimal doses. By the middle of the 19th century the iodine-deficiency theory was already conceived, and to prove it, iodine determinations in water and food were made in areas of endemic goiter. Although some deficiencies were found and published, the results were not generally accepted until more recent times, when the methods of chemical determination of iodine were sufficiently refined to achieve credibility.

Much of the work and research was done in Switzerland, where the present concept of the origin, prevention, and treatment was conceived by a number of physicians who helped to eradicate endemic goiter and cretinism in their homeland. Based on the knowledge that the thyroid gland contained much iodine and that iodine is excreted and lost daily in small amounts, it was concluded that the human body needs replenishment from the outside to keep its thyroid gland supplied for formation of its hormones (Hunziker, '24). A similar theory was developed by Marine and Kimball ('17) in the United States; like their Swiss colleagues, they recommended goiter prophylaxis by "minimal doses" of iodine, since in the absence of iodine supplementation, the thyroid gland responds by enlargement and goiter formation.

A regional association of goiter and *cretinism* has been known since ancient times. Goitrous persons were often described as stupid, and fools were depicted with goiters. But treatises dealing with goiter and cretinism did not appear before the 16th century, when several books appeared in Switzerland that described the simplemindedness, immense tongue, and the struma that occurred in persons of certain Alpine valleys (Langer, '60). Subsequently, much was written about these anomalies as related conditions, but it was recognized that endemic goiter was much more widespread than cretinism. It was thought that goiter was the "father" of cretinism and that the latter appeared only if several generations had been affected by severe goiter. Most authors asserted that there was no cretinism without goiter of the mother; but, of course, not all goitrous women had cretin children. In the United States goiter was endemic in all states bordering on the Great Lakes; westward through North Dakota, Montana, Idaho, Oregon, Washington; and in other regions; but endemic cretinism was not observed (Kelly and Snedden, '60). Cases of sporadic cretinism (congenital thyroid aplasia or congenital myxedema) have been seen in North American goiter areas and have been mistaken for endemic cretins. It should be realized that sporadic athyrotic cretinism was not recognized and was not distinguished from endemic cretinism until the second half of the 19th century. These cases are relatively rare in endemic areas but do exist in goiter-free regions. They are not dependent on iodine deficiency.

In a typical situation in an area of endemia, a goitrous mother and a goitrous father have several children with various degrees of thyroid deficiency. Some of the children have goiter but are otherwise free of complications; others are retarded in growth, are deaf-mute, and mentally retarded. Intermediate forms occur (half-cretins). Although many of the goitrous persons are able to work and can take care of themselves and their houses, the general mental development of the population is depressed, and school achievements are below those of non-affected children. There were reports from some Swiss and Austrian villages where 10% to 20% of the children could not progress in regular schools because of mental subnormality and deaf-mutism. In some children cretinism could not be recognized at birth, whereas in more severe cases a saddle nose, large tongue, goiter, swelling of the skin, pallor, and umbilical hernia permitted an early diagnosis.

In contrast to athyrotic cretins, endemic cretins always have some thyroid tissue at birth that may be hyperplastic or show signs of atrophy and sclerosis. In most endemic cretins physical and mental retardation becomes manifest within the first 2 years. Growth, dentition, ossification, walking, and talking are delayed. In general, growth is better in goitrous cretins than in those with atrophic thyroids. Neuromuscular deficiencies consist of anomalies of gait and posture.

In India a "nervous cretinism" was described that was characterized by spasticity, cerebral dysplasia, increased tendon reflexes, tremors, and loss of cutaneous sensibility (McCarrison, '08), but in the Alps this type was rare. Everywhere deafness and deafmutism were specific symptoms of endemic cretinism, while they were not present in the sporadic form.

Changes have been found in the middle ear and some degenerative signs have been noted in the inner ear. These changes cannot be corrected by iodine and thyroid treatment after birth and are thought to be of prenatal origin. Mental development is delayed and incomplete. All degrees from mediocrity to idiocy occur. Cretins are slow, cautious, and lack initiative. As a rule, goitrous cretins learn better than those with atrophic thyroids. Mildly affected patients are employed in agriculture or handicrafts; a few can read and write, but they forget these achievements when they leave school. More affected cretins cannot do regular work and are barely capable of communicating with their relatives. Full-cretins do not talk and are bound to the house or institutions, where they live a vegetative existence. They do not develop sexually and do not procreate. Half-cretins mature slowly and females can have children. Matings with normal and cretinoid persons do occur and in endemic regions many degrees of subnormality can coexist.

The dependence of cretinism on maternal goiter has been mentioned: the key question was how and when the future cretins were damaged. The fact that neither thyroid nor iodine treatment after birth could render an endemic cretin normal indicated that the harm was done in utero and that attention must be given to the mother's disease. Thus, treatment of the maternal goiter was often tried, but it was found that this did not guarantee normal offspring. However, if young girls in endemic areas received iodized salt or other iodine preventives early, they grew up goiter-free, and when they reached reproductive age they had normal children. Thus it seemed that eradication of cretinism was a two-generation problem. More recently it was shown by Hetzel ('70) that endemic cretinism can be prevented in one generation if iodine is brought to the embryo in the first weeks of gestation. This was shown in Papua and New Guinea, where women with endemic goiter were treated with single intramuscular injections of iodized oil. This was the treatment of choice there because regular intake of iodized salt or iodine tablets was not possible in the highland villages. The injections with iodized oil reduced the incidence of goiter in these regions, and, most important, cretinism was prevented if the injections were given prior to conception (Pharoah et al., '71). This leads to the conclusion that severe iodine deficiency in the mother and in the embryo produces neurological and aural damage during fetal development.

With few exceptions (Greenwald, '46), it is now generally recognized that iodine deficiency is the cause of endemic goiter and cretinism. It is true that there exist accessory factors: positive dietary goitrogens that contribute to goiter formation by interfering with synthesis of thyroid hormones. Cabbage and other vegetables of the genus *Brassica* have goitrogenic properties. There may be other accessory factors at work in certain areas, such as infections and water pollution (McCarrison, '08); but iodine deficiency is the main cause, and iodine supplementation is the best preventive.

The regional iodine lack in soil, water, and food has been explained by the action of glaciers during the quaternary ice age. In Switzerland and in North America, there was good correlation between previous glaciation and distribution of endemic goiter. The ice masses, melting water, and fluvioglacial gravel carried iodine-containing soil toward the oceans (Merke, '67). Seawater and sea sponges are relatively rich in iodine, and both have been recommended against goiter since ancient time (Langer, '60). The present prevention of iodine deficiency by iodized salt has a long and fascinating history (Warkany, '71). In the United States one part of iodide per 10,000 parts of salt is used, but in Switzerland one part of potassium iodide per 100,000 parts of salt is given, reflecting the fear and reluctance that existed regarding the general distribution of this element in the past.

In summary: Iodine deficiency was and is an important teratogen because it is the main cause of endemic cretinism. It damages embryos in utero during early gestation and is best prevented by administration to the mother of ample amounts of iodine before conception. Goiter of the mother, once thought to be the cause of endemic cretinism, is now considered a parallel phenomenon and an indicator of regional iodine deficiency. The existence on earth of regional iodine deficiencies is best explained by previous glaciation, which led, by melting of huge ice sheets, to erosion of the iodine-containing soil and to its transportation toward the sea, leaving behind areas deprived of iodine.

In addition to cosmic iodine deficiency, some cases are drug-induced. In the treatment of maternal thyrotoxicosis, thiouracil and its derivatives can damage a fetus. Abortion, stillbirth, or birth of a goitrous child can result. In the last case spontaneous recovery is possible, but sometimes cyanosis and dyspnea may require thyroidectomy (Bongiovanni et al., '56). Protracted treatment of women with iodides can lead to thyroid enlargement.

Iodides are sometimes prescribed for asthma, and in case of pregnancy, congenital goiter may be present in the child. Such a goiter can disappear spontaneously, but fatal cases have occurred. Radioactive iodine administered to women in the treatment of cancer or thyrotoxicosis after the eighth week of pregnancy can damage the thyroid of the fetus. Hypothyroidism or absence of thyroid tissue can be found in the child (Warkany, '71). In addition to the effect on the thyroid, several case reports have associated these drugs with the production of congenital malformation of other organs (Schardein, '76).

LITERATURE CITED

Bongiovanni, A.M., W.R. Eberlein, P.Z. Thomas, and W.B. Anderson (1956) Sporadic goiter of the newborn. J. Clin. Endocrinol. Metab., *16:*146–152.

Greenwald, I. (1946) Is endemic goiter due to lack of iodine? J. Clin. Endocrinol., *6:*708–741.

Hetzel, B.S. (1970) The control of iodine deficiency. Med. J. Aust., *2:*615–622.

Hunziker, H. (1924) Die Prophylaxe der Grossen Schilddrüse. E. Bircher Akt., Bern u. Leipzig.

Kelly, F.C., and W.W. Snedden (1960) Prevalence and geographical distribution of endemic goiter. In: Endemic Goiter. World Health Organization, Geneva, pp. 27–233.

Langer, P. (1960) History of goitre. In: Endemic Goiter. World Health Organization, Geneva, pp. 9–25.

Marine, D., and O.P. Kimball (1917) Prevention of simple goiter. J. Lab. Clin. Med. *3:*40–48.

McCarrison, R. (1908) Observations on endemic cretinism in the Central and Gilgit valleys. Lancet, *II:*1275–1280.

McCarrison, R. (1909) Further research on the etiology of endemic goiter. Quart. J. Med., *2:*279–287.

Merke, F. (1967) Weitere Belege Für die Eiszeit als primordiale Ursache des endemischen Kropfes: Eiszeit und Kropf im Wallis. Schweiz. Med. Wochenschr., *97:*131–140.

Pharoah, P.O.D., I.H. Buttfield, and B.S. Hetzel (1971) Neurological damage to the fetus resulting from severe iodine deficiency during pregnancy. Lancet, *1:*308.

Schardein, J.L. (1976) Drugs as Teratogens. CRC Press, Inc., Cleveland.

Warkany, J. (1971) Congenital Malformations. Notes and Comments. Year Book Medical Publishers, Inc., Chicago.

Hyperthermia

JOSEF WARKANY
Children's Hospital Research Foundation, Cincinnati, Ohio 45229

Hyperthermia is considered a human teratogen by some observers, whereas others doubt that its role as a cause of congenital malformations has been established in man. There are several problems involved in this controversy that will be analyzed in the following pages. When I was asked several years ago to contribute case reports pertaining to this question, I declined because I could not think of any situations in which a maternal fever could be separated from possible underlying causes such as infections, traumas, toxins, or other accidents. Much has been written about this topic since, but there still exist differences of opinion that need clarification.

EXPERIMENTAL HYPERTHERMIA AND CONGENITAL MALFORMATIONS

The influence of high temperatures on nonmammalian embryos has been demonstrated many times in the past. In the 19th century it was particularly Dareste (1877) who used overheating for the production of malformations in fowl. In the 20th century it was shown that mammalian embryos were also damaged by maternal hyperthermia so that death or occasionally microphthalmia in the offspring occurred (Hsu '48). The fact that rubella and other maternal infections could result in congenital malformations in children raised the questions of fever versus viruses as teratogens so that as early as 1957 Brinsmade and Rübsaamen undertook experiments in which an "unspecific" fever was tested for teratogenicity in *rabbits*. When milk injections between the 6th and 9th day of pregnancy were used to produce fever, many embryos examined 12 weeks later showed hemorrhages in the skin, meninges, and eyes, in some fetuses there were encephaloceles or changes in the brain, liver, and intestine. The question was reopened when Edwards ('67) used guinea pigs for teratologic experiments. Normal guinea pigs have a gestation time of 68.5 days and rectal temperatures of 39.4°C (102.9°F). In experiments, pregnant guinea pigs were placed in incubators that raised their rectal temperatures to about 43.3°C (110°F). After 1 hour of treatment, repeated on 8 consecutive days, a high incidence of abortions or malformations in the newborns occurred. Microencephaly, defects of the abdominal wall, failure of incisor teeth to erupt, cataract, and anomalies of the extremities were noted. Those heated in early pregnancy (18–25 days) generally had more severe defects of the brain and musculo-skeletal system than those heated in mid- or late gestation.

Two years later Edwards ('69a, '69b) published again on the same subject with emphasis on hyperthermia in early gestation. The mean maximum temperature elevation was 3.6°C above normal. There was little effect of hyperthermia treatment during days 4–11 of pregnancy, but after treatment on days 18 to 25, developmental anomalies in the newborn were common (Edwards '69a). Mean brain weight was reduced and microencephaly increased most after hyperthermia during days 15–32.

As mentioned before, fever treatment of pregnant *rats* was practiced in 1948 by Hsu and also described by Skreb and Frank in 1963. Edwards ('68) exposed pregnant rats for 40 to 60 minutes in incubators that raised deep body temperatures from 38.1°C to 42.7°C. Fetal resorption, growth retardation, microphthalmia, anencephaly, and palatal and limb defects were observed. Arora et al. ('79) described fetal and placental responses to artificially induced hyperthermia. Exposures were to temperatures of 43°C to 44°C in various stages of pregnancy. Microencephaly, microphthalmia and skeletal defects were obtained in 2.4 to 6.7% of the offspring in early treatment groups. The placentas usually were larger and heavier in treated rats than in controls.

Detailed experiments were done by Webster et al. ('85) to establish an early embryonic period that is particularly sensitive to hyperthermia. Microphthalmia, encephalocele, and other head defects were induced particularly during the gastrulation process, the critical period being 9 days, 6 hours to 10 days gestational age. Germain et al., ('85), determined in convincing experiments in rats the relation between duration and degree of hyperthermia and the induction of malformations of the head. Rats at gastrulation stage were partially immersed in a water bath until their core temperatures were elevated to from 40.5°C to 43.5°C. Various durations of each of these temperatures were tested for potential teratogenicity. Experimental and control rats were killed on day 17, 18, or 19 of gestation and the fetuses were examined for malformations. A single elevation of 5.0° or 4.5°C needed only a very short ("spike") duration to be teratogenic; 4.0°C was teratogenic after 5 minutes; 3.5°C after 10 minutes; 3.0°C after 20 minutes and 2.5°C after 1 hour. But an elevation of 2.0°C was not teratogenic even after 8 hours exposure. With all effective temperatures microphthalmia was most common; facial clefting and maxillary hypoplasia were also frequent. The threshold for teratogenicity was 1 hour exposure to 2.5°C temperature elevation. An illustration in the paper of Germain et al. shows a litter of seven 18-day fetuses, with devastating effects after a temperature elevation of 3.5° C for 30 minutes during gastrulation. Encephaloceles, severe facial clefts, anophthalmia, and maxillary hypoplasia are illustrated.

For hyperthermia experiments in mice, the reader is referred to Webster and Edwards ('84). Differences in strains, sex, and neural tube development were particularly analyzed in this species.

Hamsters have been used in hyperthermia experiments (Kilham and Ferm, '76; Umpierre and Dukelow, '77). Various degrees of temperature elevation and various durations of exposure were used. Among malformation observed, exencephalies and encephaloceles seemed to be characteristic for this species.

It has long been known (Yeates, '58) that pregnant *ewes* exposed to high environmental temperatures produced dwarf lambs that were distinct from light-weight lambs attributable to maternal malnutrition. To ascertain the mechanism of high-temperature dwarfing, Ryle and Morris ('61) placed sheep in a hot room for 8–9 hours per day during the last two-thirds of pregnancy; the room reached its maximum temperature of 40.6°C in about 2–3 hours. Light and food were the same in experimental sheep as in controls. The mean body weights of "hot-room-dwarfs" were 2 kg and those of control 4 kg. Examination of glandular tissues of the dwarfed lambs showed that their anterior pituitaries and their adrenals weighed relatively more than those of the controls, but the pituitary cell sizes of the dwarfs were reduced. The thyroids of the experimental lambs were apparently not affected. Teratologic effects of hyperthermia in bonnet *monkeys* (Macaca radiata) were reported by Hendrickx et al. ('79). Seventeen monkeys were exposed in a forced-draft incubator for a duration of 1, 3, 4 or 8 days between 21 and 46 days of gestation. On each day the core temperature of the pregnant animal was elevated 2.4°C to 5.4°C above the temperature recorded before heat exposure. The teratogenic period was from 23 to 30 days gestation following temperature elevation from 2.4°C to 4.1°C. No distinct pattern of malformations was observed, although skeletal and umbilical cord malformations (single umbilical artery) were most common. There were also some placental changes associated with some abnormal fetuses. The authors thought that the anomalies produced by hyperthermia in bonnet monkeys resembled those in other mammalian species after similar treatment.

SOME MECHANISMS OF HYPERTHERMIA

A number of attempts have been made to investigate mechanisms involved in teratogenic hyperthermia. Cockroft and New ('78) explanted 9 1/2-day-old-rat embryos and placed them into rotating bottles that contained rat serum; the effects of temperatures ranging from 38 to 41°C were studied. Embryos cultured at 40.5°C were retarded and many of them were abnormal, showing microcephaly and edema of the pericardium. Mirkes ('85) exposed rat embryos (8–12 somites) cultured in vitro to elevated temperatures (41–43°C) for varying lengths of time. When observed on day 11 after exposure to 43°C for 15 minutes, malformations could be noted. Exposures to lower temperatures had to be more extended to produce malformations (microcephaly or microphthalmia). The minimum effective duration of temperature at 42°C was 60 minutes; at 41°C it was 4 hours. Histologic examination of damaged embryos showed that necrotic debris was most prevalent in the neuroepithelium. Heat shock has long been used by geneticists to produce phenocopies in drosophila and many other organisms. German ('84) proposed that the heat-shock response in mammalian embryos during critical periods is comparable to that of lower organisms in which established programs of activation (and inactivation) of genetic loci are disturbed so that malformations result. The precise period during gestation when the response is induced determines the types of abnormalities. Edwards et al. ('74) found mitotic cell death and delay of mitotic activity in guinea pig embryos following brief maternal hyperthermia. Histologic preparations of embryos showed clumping of nuclear chromatin and subsequent death of cells at about the stage of mitosis. Affected cells were particularly numerous in the central nervous system. Billinson ('70), looking in rats for a mechanism elicited by thermal stress, found increased secretion of serotonin. Premature delivery occurred when these values were excessively high. With lower levels of serotonin output, low birthweight litters were produced. Nilsen ('84) demonstrated vascular abnormalities due to hyperthermia in chick embryos. The embryos were exposed to temperatures 3°C and 4°C above normal (38°C) from the beginning of incubation and examined with microangiography in vivo. Following hyperthermia, various abnormalities in the heart, ventral aortae, aortic arches, omphalomesenteric arteries, and the distal dorsal aortae occurred. There were also significant microvascular changes in the heart, in the lateral and caudal parts of the embryos, and in the yolk sac. Visualization of vascular abnormalities by microangiography is a useful and beautiful method available to students of hyperthermia in chicks. After a basic study of thermal injury of hamster cells in culture at various temperatures, Johnson and Pavelec ('72) concluded that at normal body temperature (37°C) over 0.2% of cells are irreversibly lost from the proliferating population each hour as a result of heat injury due to physiologic temperatures.

Because of the interest in hyperthermia as a teratogen many more studies of the mechanism involved can be expected in the future. They could contribute to a better understanding of teratologic effects of hyperthermia in animals and man.

HYPERTHERMIA OF WOMEN AND CONGENITAL MALFORMATIONS

The fact that it has been clearly demonstrated that hyperthermia can be a teratogen in experimental animals suggests that it can cause malformations in human embryos also. Yet, this suggestion has not been generally accepted. There are many publications that report that women who had elevated temperatures in early pregnancy gave birth to children or fetuses with malformations, but as mentioned before, it is difficult to separate in these cases the fever and the cause of the fever as malforming agents.

Edwards ('72) pointed to reports on teratologic effects of influenza accompanied by fever (e.g., Coffey and Jessop, '63), which, however, have not been confirmed by all writers (e.g., Leck et al., '69). Inconsistencies in these reports concerning types of malformations could be accounted for, according to Edwards ('72), by variations in the time of pregnancy when the fever occurred. The peak in February and March noted in the frequency of malformations in Finland (Hakosalo and Saxen, '71) indicated that the mothers of affected children were going through the sensitive stages of pregnancy (3–9 weeks) in summer. Edwards thought that sauna bathing might also be suspected as a possible cause of abortions, stillbirths and malformations. A few years later, D.W. Smith and his associates raised the question of maternal hyperthermia as a possible cause of anencephaly (Miller et al, '78). In seven of 63 pregnancies (11%) ending in the birth of anencephalic infants, a history of maternal hyperthermia (38.9°C to 40.0°C) near the presumed time of anterior neural-groove closure was given. Five cases involved different illnesses; in two cases the hyperthemia episodes were possibly a consequence of sauna bathing. In two control groups the frequencies of hyperthermia at corresponding periods of gestation were 0% and 0.1%. In addition, there was a note on an unusual outbreak of anencephaly in Yakima, Washington, where over a period of 9 months seven anencephalic infants were born (a rate of 5.2 per 1,000 live births). Two of six women gave histories of illnesses with high fever during the period of neural groove closure and one woman had taken sauna baths three times weekly during early pregnancy. It is understandable that these observations suggested to the authors that hyperthermia, whether secondary to infections or to sauna bathing may be a cause of anencephaly. The Seattle group then extended their studies to the histories of 43 women who had given birth to children with myelomeningocele; three of these (7%) recalled infectious illnesses with high fever at the time of posterior neural tube closure. In a control group no similar incidences were reported (Chance and Smith, '78). After an epidemiological study, Layde et al. ('80) also reported an association of spina bifida with maternal fever during the first trimester of pregnancy. Occipital encephalocele and early gestational hyperthermia were noted by Fisher and Smith ('81). But different anomalies — severe mental deficiency, seizures, hypotonia, microphthalmia, midface hypoplasia, and distal limb defects — were associated with high maternal fever at 4–6 weeks gestation (Smith et al., '78) or at 4–14 weeks gestation (Pleet et al., '81). No serious problems of morphogenesis were observed after hyperthermia during the latter half of gestation (Pleet et al., '81).

To test for possible teratogenicity of maternal fever, Fraser and Skelton ('78) selected 479 charts from the Montreal Children's Hospital in which the proband had one or more congenital malformations, cerebral palsy, mental retardation, or convulsive disorder and there was a statement on the occurrence, or non-occurrence, of a maternal febrile disorder. In 36 cases a fever occurred in the first 5 months of gestation. Of the many anomalies listed, microphthalmia showed a highly significant excess of cases in which fever was reported over those with no recorded fever. These findings supported the hypothesis that maternal fever (or some associated factor) in early pregnancy can increase the probability of a developmental disorder. Spraggett and Fraser ('82) reviewed 1,668 records of mothers referred because they had a child with a congenital defect. Each record was assessed for a recorded statement regarding fever episodes. The malformations with the highest frequency of recorded fever during the first 5 months of pregnancy were hypospadias, congenital heart disorders, and microphthalmia, one of the malformations implicated in previous studies. The etiologies of hyperthermia varied, suggesting that hyperthermia or related medications was the teratogenic factor rather than the infectious agent that provoked it. Shiota ('82), using human embryology data from Japan, ascertained retrospectively that febrile illnesses in mothers of embryos with exencephaly had been reported significantly more often than in mothers of normal, holoprosencephalic and spina bifida (without exencephaly) embryos.

A report by Superneau and Wertelecki ('85) is of interest because they described two children of mothers who had febrile illnesses at about the 10th week of gestation and a phenotype (oromandibular and limb anomalies) that resembeled defects induced by hyperthermia in guinea pigs (Edwards, '67) and rats (Edwards, '68). In both cases the pregnancies were complicated by many other possible teratogenic factors that cannot be clearly segregated from the maternal febrile incidents so that the role of hyperthermia remains speculative.

Thus, there is an abundance of case reports that seem to support the hypothesis that maternal fever can cause malformations in human fetuses according to the time of gestation. Yet, not all writers agree that this hypothesis has been proven.

An editorial in the British Medical Journal (1978) asked: "Is hyperthermia a teratogen?" While admitting that many studies in different species of animals have shown that induction of maternal hyperthermia can have a teratologic effect on the fetus, the editors felt it is still not known whether human congenital malformations ever have this cause. The teratogenicity of Asian influenza was not established. The work of Fraser and Skelton ('78) did not imply that microphthalmia develops as a result of maternal hyperthermia, since many other factors may be relevant. The argument of sauna baths as a teratogen is not established, since in Finland, where saunas are taken frequently, the incidence of microphthalmia is not higher than in countries where saunas are not used. The editors concluded that there is no convincing evidence to implicate hyperthermia per se as a human teratogen.

In the same year an editorial in the Lancet ('78) dealt with hyperthermia and the neural tube, referring to two Seattle studies that suggested a possible association between fever in early pregnancy and neurologic abnormality, especially anencephaly. Although the editors welcomed new ideas on the causes of human malformations, they thought the evidence concerning hyperthermia tenuous. Consideration of sauna bathing was ingenious, but the argument does not hold since the incidence of anencephaly in Finland is among the lowest in the world. They recommend caution in using hyperthermia as an explanation of neural tube defects and warn that "the prognosis for hyperthermia may be as bad as it was for blighted potatoes."

For other reasons, W.H. James ('78) expressed doubt because there have been no short-term anecephaly epidemics recorded. Kleinebrecht et al. ('79), working on a prospective study, found no correlation of congenital malformations with influenza, febrile illness, and other previously suspected causes. Their conclusions were cautious. They thought that "it seems unlikely that fever is a strong factor in congenital malformations, but it may have a part in a multifactorial model of human congenital anomalies." The Seattle group (Clarren et al., '79) cooperated with Myrianthopoulos of the National Institute of Health in a kind of prospective evaluation of data from the Collaborative Perinatal Project (CPP), in which 165 women had reported a first trimester illness with at least one documented temperature elevation to 38.9°C or higher. An additional 13 women reported a first trimester illness with "high fever." The results of this study were at variance with retrospective observations cited before: no offspring were identified who phenotypically resembled those patients who in previous retrospective studies were reported as victims of hyperthermic teratogenesis. This failure was apparently disappointing. To uphold the hypothesis of hyperthermia as a teratogen several "explanations" were proffered: 1) hyperthermia in early gestation might lead to early abortion so that important cases would not have been enrolled in the CPP since gravid women usually entered the study in midgestation – this could be the reason for the very low reported incidence of first trimester fevers; 2) the sample size of 178 pregnancies may have been too small to show any subtle effects of hyperthermia present; 3) nearly all reported first trimester fevers were brief episodes of high fever with intermittent temperature spikes over a 1- to 3-day period. Clarren et al. contended that this pattern of hyperthermia was quite different from that usually reported in retrospective cases, in which there was generally a prolonged hyperthermic period. They thought that a brief spike of high fever may not be adequate to produce permanent teratologic effects. It must be left to the reader to decide whether he/she considers the negative results of this prospective study explained by these arguments. Actually, the number of women from the CPP study — 178 — was much larger than that used in many positive animal experiments (Edwards, '67, '68; Kilham and Ferm, '76; Hendrickx et al., '79). And Germain et al, ('85) have pointed out that single elevations of temperature as "spikes" could be teratogenic. It seems better to list the results of the CPP study as negative than to explain them by laborious and cumbersome arguments, although it must be admitted that in humans a morphologic event takes longer than in rats. To separate hyperthermia from possible underlying disease processes, "pure" heat sources such as sauna baths and hot tub baths were considered early (Edwards, '72; Miller et al., '78), but in Finland where sauna baths are an essential component of every day life, the incidence of neural tube defects is among the lowest reported (Rapola et al., '82). Uhari et al. ('79) established that in Finland the great majority of women visit saunas during early pregnanacy and they are exposed to a temperature of 70 to 80°C for 10 to 20 minutes. Saxen et al. ('82) interviewed mothers of 100 consecutive cases of defects of the central nervous system and of 202 cases of orofacial defects, and compared them with time-area matched controls for their sauna habits. Ninety-eight percent of pregnant women had visited saunas regularly and yet the incidence of the CNS defects in Finland is among the lowest reported. No differences in sauna habits were observed between the case and control mothers. It was concluded that the relatively mild, temporal hyperthermia caused by the saunas should not be considered hazardous for the developing embryo.

In the U.S.A. Harvey et al. ('81) studied the length of time a woman must stay in a sauna or in a hot tub before her temperature reaches 38.9°C. Non-pregnant women became uncomfortable before they reached temperatures which are considered teratogenic in animal pregnancy. None of the women were able to remain in the sauna long enough for their temperatures to read 39.9 degrees C. As in Finland, tolerable temperatures seemed below those that might cause a problem for a developing embryo or fetus. Thus, it is not justified to cite sauna baths as a well-established source of maternal hyperthermia and of teratogenesis.

Summarizing, one can state that many reports on hyperthermia of women with malformed children have been published. Yet proof of causal connection has not been possible. Although in experimental animals such causation cannot be doubted, transfer to human situations is not permissible. This is not due to special biological properties of humans, but due to the fact that healthy pregnant women have not been subjected to conditions comparable to those used in animal experiments. Teratogenicity of excessive maternal temperatures demonstrated in animals should alert physicians and counselors to consider this possiblity for women also and to advise them to avoid situations in which their fetuses could be overheated and injured. On the other hand, an uncritical assumption that maternal fever readily explains human malformations should be warned against, since this could cover up the true causation and delay possible prevention. To mistake symptoms for causes is a well-known pitfall in teratology.

LITERATURE CITED

Arora, K.L., B.J. Cohen, and A.R. Beaudoin (1979) Fetal and placental responses to artificially induced hyperthermia in rats. Teratology, *19:*251–259.

Billinson, M.R. (1970) Prematurity and low birthweight litters: A mechanism elicited by thermal stress. Am. J. Obstet. Gynecol., *108:*970–974.

Brinsmade, A.B. and H. Rübsaamen (1957) Zur teratogenetischen Wirkung von unspezifischem Fieber auf den sich entwickelnden Kaninchenembryo. Beiträge zur Pathologischen Anatomie und zur Allgemeinen Pathologic, *117:*154–164.

Chance, P.F. and D.W. Smith (1978) Hyperthermia and memingomyelocele and anencephaly. Lancet, *1:*769–770.

Clarren, S.K., D.W. Smith, M.A.S. Harvey, R.H. Ward, and N.C. Myrianthopoulos (1979) Hyperthermia: A prospective evaluation of a possible teratogenic agent in man. J. Pediatr., *95:*81–84.

Cockroft, D.L. and D.A.T. New (1978) Abnormalities induced in cultured rat embryos by hyperthermia. Teratology, *17:*277–284.

Coffey, V.P. and W.J.E. Jessop (1963) Maternal influenza and congential deformities. A follow-up study. Lancet, *1:*748–751.

Dareste, C. (1877) Recherches sur la Production Artificielle des Monstruosites, ou Essais de Teratogenie Experimentale. Reinwald, Paris.

Editorial. Is hyperthermia a teratogen? (1978) Br. Med. J., *2:*1586–1587.

Editorial. Hyperthermia and the neural tube (1978) Lancet, *2:*560–561.

Edwards, M.J. (1967) Congenital defects in guinea pigs. Arch Pathol., *84:*42–48.

Edwards, M.J. (1968) Congenital malformations in the rat following induced hyperthermia during gestation. Teratology, *1:*173–178.

Edwards, M.J. (1969a) Congenital defects in guinea pigs: Fetal resorptions, abortions and malformations following induced hyperthermia during early gestation. Teratology, *2:*313–328.

Edwards, M.J. (1969b) Congenital defects in guinea pigs: Prenatal retardation of brain growth of guinea pigs following hyperthermia during gestaton. Teratology, *2:*329–336.

Edwards, M.J. (1972) Influenza, hyperthermia and congenital malformations. Lancet, *1:*320–321.

Edwards, M.J., R. Mulley, S. Ring, and R.A. Wanner (1974) Mitotic cell death and delay in mitotic activity in guinea pig embryos following brief maternal hyperthermia. J. Embryol. Exp. Morphol., *32:*593–602.

Fisher, N.L. and D.W. Smith (1981) Occipital encephalocele and early gestational hyperthermia. Pediatr., *68:*480–483.

Fraser, F.C. and J. Skelton (1978) Possible teratogenicity of maternal fever. Lancet, *2:*634.

Germain, M.A., W.S. Webster, and M.J. Edwards (1985) Hyperthermia as a teratogen: Parameters determining hyperthermia-induced head defects in the rat. Teratology, *31:*265–272.

German, James (1984) Embryonic stress hypothesis of teratogenesis. Am. J. Med., *76:*293–301.

Hakosalo, J. and L. Saxen (1971) Influenza epidemic and congenital malformations. Lancet, *2:*1346–1347.

Harvey, M.A.S., McRorie, and D.W. Smith (1981) Suggested limits to the use of hot tubs and sauna by pregnant women. Can. Med. Assoc. J., *125:*50–54.

Hendrickx, A.G., G.W. Stone, R.V. Henrickson, and K. Matayoshi (1979) Teratogenic effects of hyperthermia in the bonnet monkey (Macaca radiata). Teratology, *19:*177–182.

Hsu, C.Y. (1948) Influence of temperature on development of rat embryos. Anat. Rec., *100:*79–90.

James, W.H. (1978) Hyperthermia and meningomyelocele and anencephaly (letter). Lancet, *1:*770.

Johnson, H.A. and M. Pavelec (1972) Thermal injury due to normal body temperature. Am. J. Pathol., *66:*557–564.

Kilham, L. and V.H. Ferm (1976) Exencephaly in fetal hamsters following exposure to hyperthermia. Teratology, *14:*323–326.

Kleinebrecht, J., H. Michaelis, J. Michaelis, and S. Koller (1979) Fever in pregnancy and congenital anomalies. Lancet, *1:*1403–1404.

Layde, P.M., L.D. Edmonds, and J.D. Erikson (1980) Maternal fever and neural tube defects. Teratology *21:*105–108.

Leck, I., S. Hay, J.J. Witte, and J.C. Greene (1969) Malformations recorded on birth certificates folowing A2 influenza epidemics. Public Health Rep., *84:*971–977.

Miller, P., D.W. Smith, and T.H. Shepard (1978) Maternal hyperthermia as a possible cause of anencephaly. Lancet, *1:*519–520.

Mirkes, P.E. (1985) Effects of acute exposure to elevated temperatures on rat embryo growth and development in vitro. Teratology, *32:*259–266.

Nilsen, N.O. (1984) Vascular abnormalities due to hyperthermia in chick embryos. Teratology, *30:*237–251.

Pleet, H., J.M. Graham, Jr., and D.W. Smith (1981) Central nervous system and facial defects associated with maternal hyperthermia at 4 to 14 weeks. Pediatrics, *67:*785–789.

Rapola, J., L. Saxen, and G. Granroth (1982) Anencephaly and the sauna. Lancet, *1:*1162.

Ryle, M. and L.R. Morris (1961) Some quantitative studies on tissues of lambs dwarfed by high temperatures during gestation. Aust. J. Exp. Biol. Med. Sci., *39:*79–92.

Saxen, L., P.C. Holmberg, M. Nurminen, and E. Kuosma (1982) Sauna and congenital defects. Teratology, *25:*309–313.

Shiota, K. (1982) Neural tube defects and maternal hyperthermia in early pregnancy: Epidemiology in a human embryonic population. Am. J. Med. Genet., *12:*281–288.

Skreb, N. and Z. Frank (1963) Developmental abnormalities in the rat induced by heat shock. J. Embryol. Exp. Morphol., *11:*445–457.

Smith, D.W., S.K. Clarren, and M.A.S. Harvey (1978) Hyperthermia as a possible teratogenic agent. J. Pediatr., *92:*878–883.

Spragget, K. and F.C. Fraser (1982) Teratogenicity of maternal fever in women — a retrospective study. Teratology, *25:*78A.

Superneau, D.W. and W. Wertelecki (1985) Similarity of effects — experimental hyperthermia as a teratogen and maternal febrile illness associated with oromandibular and limb defects. Am. J. Med. Genet., *21:*575–580.

Uhari, M., A. Mustonen, and K. Konvalainen (1979) Sauna habits of Finnish women during pregnancy. Br. Med. J., *1:*1216.

Umpierre, C.C. and W.R. Dukelow (1977) Environment heat stress effects in the hamster. Teratology, *16:*155–158.

Webster, W.S. and M.J. Edwards (1984) Hyperthermia and the induction of neural tube defects in mice. Teratology, *29:*417–425.

Webster, W.S., M.A. Germain, and M.J. Edwards (1985) The induction of microphthalmia, encephalocele and other head defects following hyperthermia during the gastrulation process in the rat. Teratology, *31:*73–82.

Yeates, N.T.M. (1958) Fetal dwarfism in sheep: An effect of high atmospheric temperatures during gestation. J. Agric. Sci., *51:*84–89.

TERATOGEN UPDATE: ENVIRONMENTALLY INDUCED BIRTH DEFECT RISKS, PAGES 189–197 (1986)

The Complexities of Solving the Problem of Human Malformations

ROBERT L. BRENT
Departments of Pediatrics, Radiology, and Anatomy, Jefferson Medical College, Philadelphia, Pennsylvania 19107

Although congenital malformations and mental retardation were reported in the earliest recordings of history, teratology did not become a modern science until the middle of the 20th century (Warkany, '77). Malformed and retarded offspring have been the focus of ridicule and superstition for thousands of years. It was the development of modern genetics that influenced scientists and physicians during the first half of the 20th century, since it provided a simple explanation for the etiology of human malformations.

With the discovery and rediscovery in the 1930s and 1940s that environmental factors could also cause congenital malformations, the expansion of experimental teratology began (Warkany and Schraffenberger, '43; Hale, '37). During the evolution of experimental teratology and clinical teratology the emphasis was on discovering human teratogens and expanding the basic scientific foundation of experimental teratology. Teratology was quite isolated in the mid-20th century for the following reasons: 1) there was little impact of teratological research on clinical medicine and minimal interaction of teratologists with society; 2) there was only a small group of scientists and physicians interested in the problem of congenital malformations; and 3) although congenital malformations were considered a serious and debilitating group of diseases, they were also considered to be untreatable and unpreventable and were dwarfed by the morbidity and mortality from the infectious diseases.

With the founding of the Teratology Society and the occurrence of the thalidomide tragedy, the field of teratology was no longer isolated from the mainstream of science and clinical medicine. Progress in medicine in the past 20 years has resulted in improvement in the prevention and treatment of congenital malformations. Experimental teratologists have been joined by epidemiologists, clinicians, geneticists, and obstetricians with specific interests in the problem of congenital malformations. Regulatory agencies, politicians, lawyers, unions, and the lay public have all become interested in the problem of congenital malformations.

With all these complicated interactions, the teratologist faces a far different world today. Although some of the problems have been solved, new problems have arisen. The sophistication of the field and the accompanying notoriety create new problems to solve, while the unsolved problems of the past remain.

All of the problems and controversies listed in Table 1 will not be discussed in this paper. A few have been selected for more detailed discussion.

EPIDEMIOLOGY

We are fortunate that congenital malformation surveillance is continuing to expand, but the field could benefit from more resources.

The marked variability of reporting congenital malformations must be addressed. At the present time it is impossible to compare the statistics of one country with another or one group with another. The advantages of a uniform system are exemplified by the reliable and consistent reporting from the Congenital Malformations Surveillance branch of the Centers for Disease Control in Atlanta, GA ('80).

The third problem that has not been solved, and may never be solved, is the high frequency of the random association of frequently used medications and the occurrence of congenital malformations (Brent, '81). In a review dealing with the alleged teratogenicity of Bendectin, Holmes ('82) bemoaned the fact that limited epidemiological resources were continuing to be utilized on a drug that already had a dozen negative epidemiological studies, when many other drugs are not being studied at all.

ETIOLOGY OF CONGENITAL MALFORMATIONS

Various authors have estimated the etiology of human congenital malformations

TABLE 1. Problems and controversies of teratology in 1982

A. EPIDEMIOLOGY
   1. More resources for surveillance.
   2. World-wide variability of reporting.
   3. Evaluation of the simultaneous occurrence of a common disease (congenital malformations) and a common exposure.
B. ETIOLOGY
   What contributes to the 65% of congenital malformations that do not have a definite etiology?
   1. Polygenic factors.
   2. Multifactorial factors.
   3. Synergism.
   4. Intrinsic spontaneous errors of development.
C. MECHANISMS OF TERATOGENESIS
   1. Threshold dose reponse relationship.
D. PREVENTION AND TREATMENT
   1. Regulation of drug and chemical exposure.
   2. Protection of women in the working place.
   3. Surgical and medical therapy for the fetus.
   4. Surgical and medical therapy for the neonate.
   5. Eugenics.
   6. Genetic counseling.
   7. Therapeutic abortion.
E. EDUCATION AND MISEDUCATION
   1. Miseducation of physicians, lawyers, and the public concerning the etiology of human congenital malformation.
   2. Lack of appreciation by the epidemiologist, experimental teratologist, clinical teratologist, and geneticist of each other's expertise and ability to answer some of the unanswerable questions about congenital malformations.
F. RELATIONSHIP OF BIOMEDICAL EXPERTS
   1. In the field of congenital malformations with political and social issues.
   ECONOMIC, MEDICAL AND EMOTIONAL BURDEN

(Wilson, '73; Holmes '82; Heinonen et al., '77; Brent, '76, '82 [Table 2]). It is interesting that most analyses concluded that a definite etiology for 60 to 70% of human malformations is unknown. All agree that drugs and chemicals account for a very small percentage of malformations. At the conclusion of the 50,000-patient collaborative perinatal project, Heinonen et al. ('77) concluded that there was "no common drug analagous to thalidomide." They suggested that drugs with less potent teratogenic potential are of concern because their effects can go undetected. But they found their results "generally reassuring." Their results say in a very sophisticated manner that we will never be able to prove with the certainty of laboratory experiments that a drug is absolutely safe in the human population. That degree of risk reduction is not available for any potential environmental hazard.

The unknown category has several hypothetical models that have both experimental and clinical evidence in their favor. There are many congenital malformations that occur sporadically, such as Poland syndrome; they also exhibit familial occurrence. This common phenomenon for rare syndromes raises the question as to whether there are multiple etiologies for many syndromes or whether complicated genetic transmission is responsible for a large percentage of human

TABLE 2. Relative contributions of various causes to the frequency of human malformations

Etiology	Percent of malformed live births
Cytogenic	5
Mendelian inheritance Spontaneous mutations	15–20
Unknown	65–70
Polygenic	
Multifactorial	
Synergism	
Spontaneous errors of development	
Environmental (exposure of the embryo)	
Maternal infections (rubella, toxoplasmosis, herpes simplex, C.I.D., syphilis, etc).	3
Maternal disease states (diabetes, phenylketonuria, endocrinopathies and endocrine tumors, alcoholism, smoking, nutritional problems)	4
Problems of constraint	2
Drugs, chemicals, irradiation, hyperthermia	<1

malformations. No one can deny the great importance of genetics to this problem. McKusick ('75) reports the dramatic explosion in genetic information in the past 20 years. According to McKusick, the number of catalogued genetic diseases has increased six-fold between 1958 and 1975—from 412 to 2,336. It is true that *new* diseases with classical Mendelian inheritance will not account for the unknown group, since they will obviously be extremely rare, but new genetic and embryologic concepts may explain a substantial portion of the unknown group of malformations.

There may be confusion between the terms *polygenic* and *multifactorial.* If one assumed that the diseases with an increased recurrence risk are *polygenic* that is, solely due to two or more genetic loci, then mathematical models can be established for this group of malformations (neural tube defects, pyloric stenosis, cleft lip and palate, congenital dislocation of the hip, and certain congenital heart diseases). If one assumed that a polygenic disease was due to a homozygous recessive state at two loci, then the probability that parents who were heterozygote for both loci will deliver an infant that is homozygous recessive for all four loci is 6.25%. Thus, the mathematics are consistent with the reported recurrent risk of polygenic disease at approximately 5%. The problem is that the epidemiological and clinical data partially refute a purely genetic explanation for these malformations, since there should not be discordance for these malformations in identical twins, and there are many case reports in the literature of diseases with an increased recurrent risk that have been reported in only one of two identical twins. Thus, some other influence must be modulating the genome.

The *multifactorial/threshold* hypothesis (Wright, '34; Fraser and Fainstat, '51; Fraser, '77) is consistent with experimental and even some clinical observations because it includes several alternatives: namely, multiple loci genetic disease and/or the interaction of intrinsic and extrinsic environmental factors with a continuum of genetic characteristics. Although there are experimental models to support the hypothesis, we are not certain which factors are important in producing this group of malformations in the human. The modulating factors may be: 1) variations in placental blood flow, placental transport, or site of implantation; 2) maternal disease states; 3) infections; 4) drugs and chemicals; 5) all the other known environmental factors; or 6) simply "chance."

For those interested in an erudite discussion of the multifactorial/threshold hypothesis one should read Fraser's ('77) analysis.

A third suggestion is that some malformations are due to a multiplicity of environmental factors that might be acting synergistically. Although there are experimental models for apparent synergism, Fraser ('77) warns that if one believes that environmentally produced malformations have a threshold, then additive effects of teratogens could easily be misinterpreted to be synergistic. In the human situation it is extremely difficult to evaluate this hypothesis. The hypothesis is anxiety-provoking in itself, because it suggests that several non-teratogenic factors may, under certain circumstances, result in a malformation. The difficulty with the theory is that it is occasionally utilized, even when the exposure of the alleged teratogenic agents are several orders of magnitude below the threshold dose and no biochemical or physiological effects can be produced with the combination of agents.

Another explanation for the etiology of this large group of malformations is that they are due to *intrinsic spontaneous errors of development* (Brent, '64, '76) — "biologic errors inherent in the reproductive and developmental process, similar to the concept of spontaneous mutations." Some have referred to this as developmental noise (Adams and Niswander, '67). This pessimistic viewpoint suggests that even if the environment were optimal, embryopathology would occur because the reproductive and developmental processes have a built-in probability of going awry. If this interpretation is correct, then embryopathology can never be reduced to zero, unless we developed a technique that prevented abnormal embryos from reaching term. Nature does eliminate most abnormal embryos spontaneously (Nishimura and Yamamura, '69) and it is very likely that by the year 2,000, biomedical science will have available electronic, biochemical, and genetic techniques to evaluate the status of every human embryo at very early stages of gestation. What society will do with this information is yet to be determined, since the controversy over the appropriateness and/or the appropriate use of therapeutic interruption of pregnancy has not been resolved in many societies (Brent, '76).

We have now spent many decades with these several hypotheses in an attempt to explain the etiology of a large group of human malformations. Although we have more information and some of these hypotheses appear more likely to be correct, we must recognize the tremendous inertia that exists in the field of teratology with regard to these hypotheses. We may have to await a breakthrough in genetics, developmental biology, and/or biochemistry in order to determine the etiology of many malformations. It is also possible that the information is available and we have been too complacent about the status quo.

MECHANISMS OF TERATOGENESIS

Although most teratologists agree that teratogenesis resulting from environmental agents has a threshold below which an exposure would not result in an increase in malformations, one occasionally sees in print that all exposures to potential teratogens present a risk to the embryo (Epstein, '79). Frequently mutagenesis, carcinogenesis, and teratogenesis are linked together as though all of three had similar mechanisms and risks. In reality mutagenesis and carcinogenesis caused by environmental agents are considered to be stochastic phenomena and therefore, although the risk decreases with exposure, the *risk*, from a theoretical standpoint, *never disappears*. It is therefore important to differentiate between stochastic and threshold phenomena (Table 3).

While it is true that mutagens may be teratogenic, they do not produce malformations in the developing embryo by producing a mutation, which might lead to a clone of cells that results in malformation. Exposures to mutagens (X-ray, chemical mutagens) that may produce a significant number of somatic mutations will simultaneously produce multicellular and organ cytotoxic effects that result in embryotoxicity. Therefore an exposure of 1 Gy (100 rads) to the rat embryo on the tenth day of development will kill cells at a rate that is several orders of magnitude greater than its capacity to produce mutations in surviving cells. Furthermore, once the dose drops below a certain exposure, the incidence of cytotoxic effects is identical to the non-exposed embryos. This supports the threshold hypothesis and also emphasizes the fact that the embryo, although sensitive to cytotoxic agents, also has sophisticated recuperative mechanisms, especially when the

TABLE 3. Relationship of diseases produced by environmental agents and the risk of occurrence

Relationship	Pathology	Site	Diseases	Risk	Definition
Stochastic phenomenon	Damage to a single cell may result in disease	DNA	Cancer mutation	Exists at all exposures, although at low exposures, the risk is below the spontaneous risk	The *incidence* of the disease increases with exposure but the severity and the nature of the disease in the patient remain the same
Threshold phenomena	Multicellular injury	Great variation in etiology affecting many cell and organ processes	Malformations, growth retardation, death	Completely disappears below a certain threshold dose	Both the *severity* and *incidence* of the disease increase with higher exposures

exposure is low or administered at a low dose rate (Brent, '71).

There is one time during embryogenesis when the embryo may respond in stochastic fashion (Brent, '80); namely, at the time of fertilization. In this circumstance the risk of cell death to the one cell embryo might be stochastic in nature. One can readily recognize that the regulations and methodology of drug and chemical regulation for protecting the public should have a much different approach depending on whether one is dealing with a threshold or stochastic phenomena.

PREVENTION AND TREATMENT

Only one topic in this area will be discussed, namely, the regulation of drug and chemical exposure. Most of the new drugs approved by the FDA since 1964 contain a disclaimer in the accompanying package insert: "This drug has not been proven safe for pregnant women." Thus a woman and her embryo present a special and extremely difficult problem where medications are concerned. The responsibility of the FDA is enormous and its task extremely difficult. The possibility of approving a drug with the teratogenic effects of thalidomide is a realistic fear. Since the thalidomide tragedy, changes in regulations have made for drug labelling inconsistencies that create problems for the practicing obstetricians and others who care for women of reproductive age.

Some drugs that were in use before the 1966 regulations were adopted continue to be marketed without any change in labelling. Acetylsalicylic acid, vitamin A, and vitamin D bear no restriction for use in pregnancy, even though all three are teratogenic in rodent experiments. Drugs introduced after 1966, as well as some pre-1966 agents, are accompanied by a disclaimer. Meclizine and aurothioglucose are "contraindicated" in pregnancy because the drugs were "teratogenic in rats." Yet lithium carbonate, also a potent teratogen in rats, may be used in pregnancy if "in the opinion of the physician the potential benefits outweigh the possible hazards."

The FDA often uses animal data in a simplistic, sometimes even erroneous, fashion. Experimental teratologists have known for a long time that predicting human teratogenicity from animal experiments is a very difficult if not impossible task (Brent, '64, '72, '80). The fact that a drug is a teratogen in an animal species should be only one of many criteria for deciding if it can or should be used by pregnant women. The dose, the species, and the malformation produced are all considerations. Many drugs produce malformations when administered at 10,100 or 1,000 times the usual therapeutic dose. The antihistamines, such as meclizine, produce cleft palate in mice and rats at very high exposures. However, these large doses result in teratogenesis by reducing the animal's food and water intake (Szabo and Brent, '74, '75; Brent and Szabo, '75). Force feeding reverses the teratogenic process. Drugs that produce sedation, appetite suppression, or diarrhea may have a teratogenic effect that has little applicability to the human situation. The fact that cleft palate in the mouse or rat is the only teratogenic effect produced by very high doses of a compound may call into question the validity of the animal model.

To improve the information supplied to practicing physicians, the FDA has established five categories (A, B, C, D, and X) to indicate a particular drug's potential for causing birth defects (FDA, '79; Anon., '79).

Category A applies to drugs for which well-controlled studies in women fail to demonstrate a risk to the fetus. The bulletin states, "Although such studies can never entirely exclude a risk, a reasonable presumption can be made that when such drugs are used during pregnancy, the possibility of fetal harm is remote. However, as with other drugs, they should be used during pregnancy only when clearly needed."

Category B indicates that either "animal studies have not demonstrated a fetal risk but there are no adequate studies in women, or animal studies have uncovered some risk that has not been confirmed in controlled studies in women."

Category C means that "studies in animals have revealed adverse effects on the fetus and there are no adequate controlled studies in women, or studies in women and animals are not available."

Category D includes drugs whose potential benefits may be acceptable even though experience shows they are associated with birth defects (propylthiouracil for thyroid disease; streptomycin for tuberculosis; phenytoin sodium for epilepsy). Such drugs are for use in a life-threatening situation or serious disease for which safer drugs cannot be used or are ineffective. "If a category D drug is given to a pregnant woman, or if the patient becomes pregnant while taking it, the physician should inform her of the potential risk to the fetus."

Category X includes drugs contraindicated for use during pregnancy, because fetal abnormalities have been demonstrated in animal or human studies and potential risks clearly outweigh potential benefits. "FDA recommends that the physician advise the pregnant patient of the potential hazard if she intentionally or inadvertently uses the drug."

The wording of this classification is an improvement over the previous blanket disclaimer for new drugs, but it still has serious failings. Its attitude toward animal studies is too simplistic. Although it is important to know about the embryotoxic effects, it is more important to know whether these occur within the therapeutic range and what types of embryopathology are produced. Who is to make the determination that "the potential risk of a drug clearly outweighs potential benefits?" Vitamins A and D and acetylsalicylic acid fall into this category.

The package inserts and commentaries in the FDA Bulletin do not provide the information the physician needs in order to answer questions raised by patients when they learn they are pregnant. Is the risk of taking a medication during pregnancy great enough to warrant considering an interruption of pregnancy? This is not a hypothetical question. I believe that, where possible, the inappropriateness of interrupting a pregnancy should be indicated. Most drugs would fall into a category that would permit the following suggested labelling:

> "The embryotoxic risks of this drug have been evaluated with human epidemiologic studies and animal studies, or have been evaluated only with animal teratology studies, since no adequate human epidemiologic studies are available. The risk of spontaneous malformations is much greater than any risks of the drug that could be hypothesized from the available information. Therefore, following exposure during pregnancy, a therapeutic interruption of pregnancy is not warranted on the basis of this risk." (Brent, '82).

When the risk is considerable, the following statement is suggested:

> "The embryotoxic risks of methotrexate have been evaluated by human and animal teratologic studies. An inadvertant or therapeutic exposure during pregnancy imposes an increased risk substantially greater than the spontaneous risk" (Brent, '82).

The material in package inserts creates a second problem by implying that most drugs given in the therapeutic range are embryotoxic, since they "have not been proven safe for pregnant women." When epidemiologic studies report positive associations, the reader frequently concludes that the association is causal. In the ever-increasing number of allegations that various drugs produce human malformations, the wording in the package insert is used as evidence that the drug is embryotoxic. Even the disclaimer has been used to support the allegation that a drug is teratogenic in humans. It is evident that the FDA's labelling policy thus serves to instigate and aid non-meritorious lawsuits that involve congential malformations. If the present climate of litigation continues in the U.S.A., *there may come a day when the financial burden of litigation will force the pharmaceutical industry to contraindicate all drugs for pregnant women.*

The package insert frequently mentions that the drug crosses the *placental barrier*. In choosing between heparin and warfarin, this information is helpful, but for most other drugs it is useless. Most drugs cross the placental barrier. That does not mean a drug is embryotoxic. Furthermore, the fact that a drug does not cross the placenta does not prove that it is safe. This information is frequently misinterpreted by physicians. It certainly has been misinterpreted in negligence lawsuits.

The package insert also indicates that, in certain instances, it is up to the clinician to weigh the risks and benefits of a particular medication for a pregnant patient. This places an unrealistic and unfair burden on the practicing physician. if the risk is nonexistent or very small and the medication of benefit, then the package insert should state that fact. We need to know more about the quantitative aspects of potential risks than we are learning from the package inserts.

The lack of information and fear of another thalidomide has created a population of "therapeutic orphans" in this country (Shirkey, '68). What can be done to improve the situation? Much has been written about this problem, but no viable solution has been suggested. (Mirkin, '80; Ryan et al., '81). Ethically and scientifically, it would be impossible to administer drugs to pregnant women to determine whether they are embryotoxic. Even hundreds of exposures might not be enough to demonstrate lack of teratogenicity, since most malformations are not drug related (Table 2). Our present system—testing drugs for teratogenicity in animals and then for efficacy and toxicity in non-pregnant adults—is a good beginning. But that is not enough.

In 1964 I wrote, "At the present time, the most reliable method of protecting the public from all harmful effects of drugs is through clinical surveillance programs" (Brent, '64). That principle is still true today. The reports and leadership of the Congenital Malformation Surveillance Branch of the Centers for Disease Control (CDC), created in 1968, have been extremely helpful in providing information for several regions of the country (Anon. '80). *Competent, sophisticated surveillance should be a high priority health goal.*

It is difficult to mount a coordinated effort to protect the embryo, because the responsibility falls on many agencies and groups. If a cooperative effort could be developed among the FDA, the pharmaceutical industry, the CDC, the practicing physicians, the lay public, and the professionals interested in congenital malformations (obstetricians, pediatricians, teratologists, geneticists, and epidemiologists), many of our present difficulties could be eliminated.

Since no method of drug or animal testing could possibly permit the pharmaceutical industry or the FDA to label a drug as completely safe for an embryo or fetus, I believe a new approach is necessary (Brent, '80,'80a). A committee should be formed consisting of representatives from the FDA, obstetrics, the Teratology Society, the Congential Malformation Surveillance Branch of the CDC, and various experts in epidemiology, genetics, perinatology, and pediatrics. The committee would be responsible for creating a drug formulary for both women of reproductive age and pregnant women (Table 4).

TABLE 4. Suggestions for improving the regulation of drugs used for women of reproductive age

1. Create a formulary for pregnant women.
2. Drastically change the method of drug labeling.
3. Initiate a massive education program about the causes of congenital malformations.
4. Expand congenital malformation surveillance programs.

One of the difficulties in monitoring the association of birth defects with various drugs is the vast number of drugs available. Restricting the number of drugs that can be used in this population would simplify both labelling and monitoring. The responsibility for choosing these drugs should rest primarily with obstetricians, but with appropriate consultation from the pharmaceutical industry, teratologists, epidemiologists, geneticists, and the FDA.

The Bendectin saga is a very good example of the usefulness of restricting the number of drugs. After meclizine was contraindicated because it produced cleft palate in mice, Bendectin was literally the only antinausea medication available by prescription for pregnant women. Because the drug was so widely used, there have been 11 epidemiologic studies, indicating that Bendectin has no measurable teratogenic effect (Holmes, '83).

There are a number of suggestions that could *improve the present method of regulating drugs* (Table 4).

Our present method of *drug labelling* should include a rational protocol for estimating teratogenic potential. Any protocol for evaluating the allegation of human teratogenicity must include all the human epidemiological information, appropriate animal studies, and basic science embryological and teratological dogma (Brent, '78, Wilson and Brent, '81). It is of interest how many scientists conclude that one positive finding in one epidemiological study is enough to conclude that the agent being evaluated is a human teratogen. It should be obvious that any epidemiological study that tests the association of 40 malformations with a drug exposure may find a positive association for two malformations at the $p < .05$ level of significance just by chance. That is why these chance associations are not found in studies that attempt confirmation, unless the finding is a true association. Even in this instance an association and causality are not synonomous.

It should also include a statement concerning the risk of inadvertent exposure or planned therapy in pregnant women. This statement should include advice for or against therapeutic abortion, when appropriate. The use of terms like "crosses the placental barrier" should be clarified or eliminated; they stimulate allegations of drug-induced teratogenicity, as do the disclaimer statements. The whole concept of risk versus benefit has to be reevaluated, once an appropriate system for estimating risk has been adopted.

We need a *massive educational program* to correct the erroneous impression held by many physicians, and by large segments of the press, the public, and the judicial system, that most congenital malformations are caused by drugs and chemicals. This should be a combined effort of the professional societies and the appropriate federal agencies. At the same time, physicians should restrict the medications that pregnant women use to a small group of necessary drugs. It should be routine to inform patients of the risk pregnancy imposes when prescribing a potentially dangerous drug. The risk or safety of medications administered during pregnancy should also be discussed.

We should *expand the CDC monitoring programs* so that more pregnancies are monitored and a more detailed evaluation is done. The combination of a restricted formulary for pregnant women and improved surveillance should provide a more effective monitoring system. Such a system would enable us to allay anxiety or confirm embryotoxicity.

Without these changes, the practicing physician and pharmaceutical industry will continue to carry an unfair portion of the responsibility for treating women of reproductive age. The regulatory agencies have to share some of this responsibility by recognizing that there are better ways to safeguard the developing fetus than creating therapeutic orphans.

EDUCATION AND MISEDUCATION

There is widespread belief that many congenital malformations and abortions are caused by drugs and chemicals in the environment (Sholtz et al., '76). This belief has been popularized in the lay press and even by some physicians. The magnitude of the problem is represented in the United States by the exponential rise in negligence litigation involving malformed children (Brent, '67, '77a, '82). The vast majority of these lawsuits are non-meritorious. Recent examples of lawsuits include malformed infants whose parents allege that the following environmental factors were responsible for the child's malformation: 1) animal flea collar; 2) mimeograph machine; 3) paint restoration materials; 4) electronic surveillance; 5) routine pest control; and 6) vaginal spermicides.

Most of these lawsuits would never be initiated if it were not for the fact that some scientists are willing to state with a "reasonable degree of certainty" that the child's malformation was due to the exposure in question. This type of irresponsible behavior is frequently due to the fact that a scientific expert has never been taught what his proper role should be. Many of these experts function as partisans, rather than scholars (Brent, '82a). The solution to this serious problem rests with the scientific community, but so far organized science and medicine have ignored the problem of the irresponsible expert witness and the not-so-knowledgeable scientist.

SUMMARY

A number of controversies and unsolved problems in teratology have been listed in Table 1.

While we have solved some problems of teratology new ones have appeared. Teratology was an isolated clinical and research field 30 years ago and today it has immense visibility. The deliberations of teratology are no longer limited to the classroom, the clinic, and the laboratory.

Other facets of society are now affected by our field. Yet the scientific community has not met its responsibility in providing accurate information to the public and the courts. Misinformation appears to be a major problem and in reality has created major health problems when none existed. It is of interest that the three major *litogens* (alleged teratogens that stimulate malpractice suits) (Holmes, '83)—diagnostic radiation, Bendectin, and progestins (non-genital malformations)—have no measurable teratogenic risk in humans.

Teratology needs input from many fields. It may be more difficult to convince the multifaceted group of scientists and clinicians that teratology needs their expertise beyond the boundaries of the laboratory and clinic.

ACKNOWLEDGMENTS

The Stein Research Center Developmental Biology Laboratories are supported by NIH HL 7497, HD 18396, HD 19165, HD 7075, HD 18167; the Foederer Foundation, and the Harry Bock Charities.

LITERATURE CITED

Adams, M.S., and Niswander, J.D. (1967) Developmental noise and a congenital malformation. Genet. Res., *10*:313.

Anon. (1979) Pregnancy Labeling. FDA Drug Bull., *9*:23.

Anon. (1980) Congenital Malformations Surveillance Report. The Center for Disease Control, Atlanta, Georgia.

Brent, R.L. (1964) Drug testing in animals for teratogenic effects: Thalidomide in the pregnant rat. J. Pediatr., *64*:762.
Brent, R.L. (1967) Medicolegal aspects of teratology. J. Pediatr., *71*:288–298.
Brent, R.L. (1972) Protecting the public from teratogenic and mutagenic hazards. J. Clin. Pharmacol., *12*:61.
Brent, R.L. and Szabo, K.T. (1975) Nutritional supplementation of the pregnant mouse as a method of reducing the incidence of drug induced cleft palate. Pediatr. Res., *9*:358.
Brent, R.L. (1971) Response of the 9-1/2 day-old rat embryo to variations in dose rate of 150R X-irradiation. Radiat. Res., *45*:127.
Brent, R.L. (1976) Environmental factors: Miscellaneous. In: The Prevention of Embryonic Fetal and Perinatal Disease, R.L. Brent and M. Harris, ed. DHEW Publication (NIH) No. 76-853.
Brent, R.L. (1977 and 1977a) Litigation produced pain, disease, and suffering in experience with congenital malformation lawsuits. Teratology, *16*:1.
Brent, R.L. (1978) Methods of evaluating alleged human teratogens. Teratology, *17*:183.
Brent, R.L. (1980) Radiation teratogenesis. Teratology, *21*:281.
Brent, R.L. (1980) Radiation-induced embryonic and fetal loss from conception to birth. In: Human Embryonic and Fetal Death, I.H. Porter and E.B. Hook, eds. Academic Press, New York, pp 177-183.
Brent, R.L. (1980a) The prediction of human diseases from laboratory and animal tests for teratogenicity, carcinogenicity and mutagenicity. In: Controversies in Therapeutics, L. Lasagna, ed. W.B. Saunders, Philadelphia, pp. 134–150.
Brent, R.L. (1981) Drugs as teratogens. The Bendectin saga, another American tragedy. Teratology *23*:28A.
Brent, R.L. (1982) Drugs and pregnancy. Are the insert warnings too dire? Contemp. Obstet. and Gynecol., *20*:42.
Brent, R.L. (1982a) The irresponsible expert witness. Pediatrics, *70*:–762.
Epstein, S.S. (1979) The Politics of Cancer. Anchor Press, New York.
FDA talk paper on Bendectin: T79, October 1, 1979.
Fraser, F.C. and T.D. Fainstat (1951) The production of congenital defects in the offspring of pregnant mice treated with cortisone. A progress report. Pediatrics, *8*:527.
Fraser, F.C. (1977) Relationship of animal studies to man. In: Handbook of Teratology, Vol. 1. J.G. Wilson and F.C. Fraser, eds. Plenum Press, New York.
Hale, F. (1937) The relation of maternal vitamin A deficiency to microphthalmia in pigs. Tex. State J. Med., *33*:37.
Heinonen, O.P., D. Slone, and S. Schapiro (1977) Birth Defects and Drugs in Pregnancy, Publishing Sciences Group, Littleton, Mass., p. 516.
Holmes, L.B. (1982) Personal communication.
Holmes, L.B. (1983) Bendectin update. Teratology, *27*:277–281.
McKusick, V.A. (1975) Mendelian Inheritance in Man. 4th edition, Johns Hopkins University Press, Baltimore, Md.
Mirkin, B, (1980) Evaluation of drugs in children and pregnant women: An ineluctable conundrum. Trends in Pharmacological Sciences. Elsevier/North Holland Biomedical Press, November 1980, pp. 1–3.
Nishimura, H. and H. Yamamura (1969) Comparison between man and some other mammals of normal and abnormal developmental processes. In: Methods for Teratological Studies in Experimental Animals and Man. H. Nishimura and J.R. Miller, eds. Igaku Shoin, Lt., pp. 223–240.
Ryan, K.G., J.V. Brady, R.D. Cooke et al. (1981) Research on the fetus. Report and Recommendations of the National Commission for the Protection of Human Subjects of Biomedical and Behavioral Research. DHEW Publication No. 05, 76-127. Reprinted in: Biomedical Ethics. T.A., Mappes and J.S. Zambaty, eds. McGraw-Hill, New York.
Shirkey, H. (1968) Editorial Comment: Therapeutic Orphans. J. Pediatr., *72*:119.
Sholtz, R., H. Goldstein, and H.M. Wallace (1976) Incidence and impact of fetal and perinatal disease. In: The Prevention of Embryonic, Fetal and Perinatal Disease. R.L. Brent and M. Harris, eds. DHEW Publication (NIH) No. 76–853.
Szabo, K.T. and R.L. Brent (1974) Species differences in experimental teratogenesis by tranquilizing agents. Lancet, *1*:565.
Szabo, K.T. and R.L. Brent (1975) Reduction of drug induced cleft palate in mice. Lancet, *1*:1296.
Warkany, J. and E. Schraffenberger (1943) Congential malformations induced in rats by maternal nutritional deficiency. *V* Effects of a purified diet lacking riboflavin. Proc. Soc. Exp. Biol. Med., *54*:92.
Warkany, J. (1977) History of Teratology. In: Handbook of Teratology Vol 1. pp. 3–45. J.G. Wilson and F.C. Fraser, eds. Plenum Press, New York.
Wilson, J.G. (1973) Environment and Birth Defects. Academic Press, New York.
Wilson, J.G., and R.L. Brent (1981) Are female sex hormones teratogenic? Am. J. Obstet. Gynecol., *141* 567.
Wright, S. (1934) The results of crosses between inbred strains of guinea pigs, differing in number of digits. Genetics, *19*:537.

Methods of Evaluating the Alleged Teratogenicity of Environmental Agents

ROBERT L. BRENT
Departments of Pediatrics, Radiology, and Anatomy, Jefferson Medical College, Philadelphia, Pennsylvania 19107

The analysis of whether an environmental agent is a teratogen can take two approaches. First, does the agent (chemical, drug, etc) have the ability to produce malformations in the exposed human population? This is the general thesis. Second, in a single patient, what is the likelihood that a particular environmental agent was responsible for the occurrence of a malformation or groups of malformations?

There is a wide spectrum of approaches to the evaluation of potential or alleged teratogens. One cannot assume that all drugs and chemicals are teratogens until proved safe, since it is impossible to prove definitely that a drug or chemical is safe in all circumstances (Brent, '82; Wilson and Brent, '81). Also, one may conclude that only minimal data are needed to restrict the use of a drug that has embryotoxic potential. The same data that may be used to restrict the use of a drug or chemical may be insufficient to implicate the agent as a teratogen or to support the allegation that an exposure caused a malformation in an individual human being.

CLASSIFICATION

Criteria have been established by regulatory agencies to classify drugs according to their potential teratogenicity. The US Food and Drug Administration regulations have evolved in order to prevent a teratogen from being marketed for human use [FDA Drug Bill 1979]. These criteria utilize, when available, epidemiological studies and animal studies. Each new drug is classified with regard to its potential teratogenicity, based on the following characteristics.

Category A applies to drugs for which well-controlled studies in women fail to demonstrate a risk to the fetus. The bulletin states, "Although such studies can never entirely exclude a risk, a reasonable presumption can be made that when such drugs are used during pregnancy, the possibility of fetal harm is remote. However, as with other drugs, they should be used during pregnancy only when clearly needed."

Category B indicates either that "animal studies have not demonstrated a fetal risk but there are no adequate studies in women, or animal studies have uncovered some risk that has not been confirmed in controlled studies in women."

Category C means that "studies in animals have revealed adverse effects on the fetus and there are not adequate controlled studies in women, or studies in women and animals are not available."

Category D includes drugs whose potential benefits may be acceptable even though experience shows they are associated with birth defects (propylthiouracil for severe thyroid disease; streptomycin for severe tuberculosis; phenytoin for severe epilepsy). Such drugs are for use in a life-treatening situation or serious disease for which safer drugs cannot be used or are ineffective. "If a category D drug is given to a pregnant woman, or if the patient becomes pregnant while taking it, the physician should inform her of the potential risk to the fetus."

Category X includes drugs contraindicated for use during pregnancy because fetal abnormalities have been demonstrated in animal or human studies and potential risks clearly outweigh potential benefits. "FDA recommends that the physician advise the pregnant patient of the potential hazard if she intentionally or inadvertently used the drug."

The wording of this classification is an improvement over the previous blanket disclaimer for new drugs, but it still has serious failings. Its attitude toward animal studies is too simplistic. Although it is important to know about embryotoxic effects, it is more important to know whether these occur within the therapeutic range and what types of embryopathology are produced. Who is to make the determination that "the potential risk of a drug clearly outweighs potential benefits?" Vitamins A and D and acetylsalicylic acid could meet the criteria for being labeled in category X. The difficulty with this system is that 1) It will not prevent the introduction of a teratogen (Brent, '64; Fraser, '64; Ingalls and Klingberg, '65). 2) It creates a population of women who are therapeutic orphans (Shirkey, '68; Brent, '82). 3) It treats drugs marketed before 1966 much differently than new drugs (Brent, '82). 4) It miseducates physicians and lay individuals. 5) It causes unnecessary abortions (Brent, '82).

The classification and package inserts are inconsistent with what is known about teratological effects (Brent, '82). 1) They ignore the importance of dose. 2) They ignore the existence of a threshold effect for most teratogens. 3) They emphasize points in the package insert which are either misinterpreted or are confusing (Brent, '82). a) "This drug crosses the placental barrier." b) "This drug has not been proven safe for pregnant women and children." c) "This drug produces cleft palate in the mouse."

ANIMAL TESTING

It is well known that human teratogens have not been discovered from animal testing (Brent, '64, '72, '81; Fraser, '64, '77). Furthermore, animal testing which indicates that a drug or chemical is not teratogenic does not prove it safe for the human embryo (Lorke, 63; Fraser, '64, '77; Brent, '64, '69, '81; Loosli and Theiss, '64; Cahan, '64; Ingalls and Klingberg, '65; Gottscheski, '65; Frohberg and Oettl, '66; Tuchmann-Duplessis, '72, '73; Bertrand et al, '72; Grice et al, '75). Animal testing gives the investigator an inaccurate but necessary assessment of potential toxicity.

Animal testing has two other important functions: 1) studying the mechanism of action of known teratogens; 2) studying the pharmacodynamics of known or suspected embryotoxic or teratogenic agents.

METHODS OF EVALUATION

How should one approach the problem of evaluating the potential teratogenicity of a drug or chemical based on information that is available? In a recent exchange of letters in a scientific journal, two scientists disagreed on whether an epidemiological study indicated that a drug was teratogenic (Nora and Nora, '77; Yasuda and Miller, '77). Basic textbooks in epidemiology indicate that an initial epidemiological study that demonstrates an association of a toxic effect with a drug or chemical exposure does not prove and sometimes even suggests causality (Lilienfeld and Lilienfeld, '80). To prove causality 1) The epidemiological study should be repeated several times; 2) When appropriate, the frequency and severity of the pathology should be related to the dose; 3) An animal model should be developed; 4) The results should make biologic sense.

Several investigators have attempted to apply classical epidemiological dogma to the field of teratology (Shepard, '73; Brent, '78; Wilson and Brent, '81; Brent, '82).

The following method of evaluating alleged teratogenicity has been modified by applying the method to various drugs and chemicals that have been alleged to be teratogens and comparing the results with known teratogens.

1) Epidemiological studies consistently or repeatedly demonstrate a statistical association between exposure to the agent and an increase in congenital malformations, either a unique syndrome or a group of malformations.

a) The exposure to the agent occurred at a stage of pregnancy when the reported malformations could be produced.

b) The exposed population did not have some characteristic which by itself would be associated with an increase in congenital malformations.

c) The control population did not have an exceptionally low incidence of malformations or low ascertainment of exposure.

d) The exposed and control groups were not discrepant for the incidence of malformation from known causes (genetic), or for factors which are associated with malformations (twinning, diabetes, threatened abortion, etc).

2. A mammalian animal model for the teratogenesis was developed, utilizing exposures comparable to the therapeutic range in humans.

a) The chick is unacceptable for developing an animal model.

b) The animal model should not occur with exposures which make the maternal organism ill, decreases her food and water intake, or results in characteristic malformations for that species without other malformations (cleft palate in the mouse, anophthalmia in the rat, vertebral and rib malformations in the rabbit, omphalocele in the ferret (Szabo and Brent, '74, '75).

3. There should be a dose-response curve for teratogenicity in the animal model.

4. A plausible mechanism of teratogenesis can be established, and/or the teratogenic result makes biologic sense.

Known teratogens comply with most of these criteria. Alleged teratogens, such as Bendectin or Progestagens (Brent, '81; Wilson et al., '81), do not fit these criteria. Thus, although one cannot prove the negative, it is helpful to be able to utilize a formal process to evaluate an allegation.

CONCLUSIONS

In summary, the criteria utilized to 1) restrict the use of a drug or chemical, 2) implicate an agent as a human teratogen in the general thesis, or 3) implicate an agent as a human teratogen in an individual are very different. Confusion occurs when the same criteria utilized for restricting drug or chemical exposure are utilized to implicate that agent as a human teratogen. The present drug-labeling procedures add to this confusion and merit the attention of all those interested in applying the most modern concepts in teratology to the problems of protecting the public, educating physicians and the lay public, preventing unnecessary abortions, properly labeling drugs, and scientifically evaluating the allegation of teratogenicity in both the general thesis and in individual patients.

ACKNOWLEDGMENTS

The Stein Research Center Developmental Biology Laboratories are supported by NIH HD 7075, HD 19165, HD 18396, HD 18167, HL 7497; the Foeder Foundation, and the Harry Bock Charities.

LITERATURE CITED

Baker, J.B.E. et al. (1967) Principles for testing of drugs for teratogenicity. Die Pharmazeutische Industrie, *29:*759–763.

Berry, C.L., and S. Barlow (1976) Some remaining problems in the reproductive toxicity testing of drugs. Br. Med. Bull., *32:*34–38.

Betrand, M., E. Levet, J. Girod, M.F. Leperco (1972) L'Embryotoxicite des medicaments. Cah Med Vet, *2:*1–26.

Brent, R.L. (1964) Drug testing in animals for teratogenic effects: Thalidomide in the pregnant rat. J. Pediatr., *64:*762–770.

Brent, R.L. (1969) Implications of experimental teratology. Excerpta Med. Int. Cong. Ser., *204:*187–195.

Brent, R.L. (1978) Editorial: Methods of evaluating alleged human teratogens. Teratology, *17:*83.

Brent, R.L. (1981) The prediction of human diseases from laboratory and animal tests for teratogenicity, carcinogenicity and mutagenicity. In: Controversies in Therapeutics. L. Lasagna, ed. W.B. Saunders, Philadelphia, pp 134–150.

Brent, R.L. (1981) Drugs as teratogens: The Bendectin saga, another American tragedy. Teratology, *23:*28A.

Brent, R.L. (1982) Drugs and pregnancy: Are the insert warnings too dire? Contemp. Obstet. Gynecol. *20:*42–49.

Cahen, R.L. (1968) Evaluation of the teratogenicity of drugs. Clin. Pharmcol. Ther., *5:*480–514.

Fraser, F.C. (1964) Experimental teratogenesis in relationship to congenital malformations in man. In: Proceedings of the 2nd International Conference on Congenital Malformations. M. Fishbein, ed. Int. Med. Cong. Ltd., New York, pp 277–287.

Fraser, F.C. (1977) Relation of animal studies to the problem in man. In: Handbook of Teratology, Vol. 1., J.C. Wilson and F.C. Fraser, eds. Plenum Press, New York.

Frohberg, H. and H. Oettl (1966) Method for testing for teratogenicity in mice. Indus. Med. Surg., *35:*113–120.

Gottschewski, G.H.M. (1965) Konnen tierversuche zur losung der frage nach der teratogenen wirkung von medikamenton auf den menschlichen embryo beitragen? Arzneim Forsch, *15:*97–104.

Grice, H.C. et al. (1975) The Testing of Chemicals for Carcinogenicity, Mutagenicity, Teratogenicity. Marc Lalonde, Minister of Health and Welfare, Canada.

Ingalls, T.H., M.A. Klingberg (1965) Implications of epidemic embryopathy for public health. Am. J. Public Health, *55:*200–208.

Lilienfeld, A., R. Lilienfeld (1980) Foundations of Epidemiology. Oxford University Press.

Loosli, R. Von, E. Theiss (1964) Methodik und problematik der medikamentos-experimentellen teratogenese. Bull. Schweiz. Akad. Med. Wiss. *20:*398–416.

Lorke, D. (1963) Method for the investigation of embryotoxic and teratogenic effects on rat. Naunyn-Schmeidebergs Arch. Pharmacol., *246:*174–151.

Nora, J.J., A.H. Nora (1977) Letter to the editor concerning the paper of Yasuda and Miller. Teratology, *15:*332.

Shepard, T. (1973) Catalogue of Teratogenic Agents. Johns Hopkins University Press, p XV.

Shirkey, H. (1968) Editorial comment. Therapeutic orphans. J. Pediatr., *72:*119.

Szabo, K.T., R.L. Brent (1974) Species differences in experimental teratogenicity by tranquillising agents. Lancet, *1:*565.

Szabo, K.T., R.L. Brent (1975) Reduction of drug-induced cleft palate in mice. Lancet, *1:*1296–1297.

Tuchmann-Duplessis, H. (1972) Teratogenic drug screening. Present procedures and requirements. Teratology, *5:*271–286.

Tuchmann-Duplessis, H. (1973) Teratogenic screening methods and their application in contraceptive products. Meeting on pharmacologic models to assess toxicity and side effects of fertility regulating agents. Geneva, September 17–20.

Wilson, J.C. (1965) Embryological considerations in teratology. IV. Drugs and the mammalian embryo. Ann. NY Acad. Sci., *133:*129–227.

Yasuda, M., J.R. Miller (1977) Response to letter to the editor of Dr. Nora. Teratology, *15:*332.

TERATOGEN UPDATE: ENVIRONMENTALLY INDUCED BIRTH DEFECT RISKS, PAGES 203–214 (1986)

Medicolegal Aspects of Teratology

ROBERT L. BRENT
Department of Pediatrics, Thomas Jefferson University, Philadelphia, Pennsylvania 19107

The publicity accorded the thalidomide episode has increased the awareness of the public and the legal profession of the possibility that some human malformations are caused by non-genetic environmental influences. It is perfectly obvious that there has been an increase in the incidence of medicolegal cases involving malformed infants. Furthermore, these cases are receiving more attention in the lay press (1–5). The philosophy of some members of the legal profession and of the public is reflected in the concept that some one must be responsible for personal damages that have been incurred. Historically, the father or mother of a malformed infant was open to ridicule, criticism, or even prosecution (6,7). Folklore and superstition dominated the field, and the causes of malformations were attributed to evil spirits, fornication with animals, lewd thoughts or other immoral acts. Certainly, in the 1600's no one would have thought of receiving compensation for the birth of a malformed child. The following case presentation highlights the ignorance and superstition that surrounded the birth of a malformed offspring in the seventeenth century:

> "At a General court held at New Haven on 2 March 1641 (Hoadley, 1857) it transpired that on the preceding 14 February 'John Wakeman a planter and member of this church acquainted the magistrates thatt a sow of his which he had lately bought of Henry Browing, then with pigge, had now brought among divers liveing and rightly shaped pigs, one prodigious monster, which he then brought with him to be viewed and considered. The monster was come to the full growth as the other piggs for ought could be discerned, butt brought forth dead. Itt had no haire on the whole body, the skin was very tender and a redish white collour like a childs; the head most straing, itt had butt one eye in the middle of the face, and thatt large and open, like some blemished eye of a man; over the eye, the bottome of the foreheade which was like a childes, a thing of flesh grew forth and hung downe, itt was hollow, and like a mans instrument of generation. A nose, mouth and chinne deformed, butt nott much unlike a childs, the neck and eares had allso such resemblance.' This description is that of a typical cyclopean monster. The record continues '—a strange impression was allso upon many that saw the monster, (therein guided by the neare resemblance of the eye) that one George Spencer, late servant to the said Henry Browning, had beene actor in unnatureall and abominable filthynes with the sow--. (It came out during the proceedings that Spencer actually had not been in the service of Browning at the critical time!) The aforementioned George Spencer so suspected hath butt one eye for use, the other hath (as itt is called) a pearle in itt, is whitish Y deformed, and his deformed eye being beheld and compared together with the eye of the monster, seamed to be as like as the eye in the glass to the eye in the face.' There is little doubt that George Spencer had a cataract in one eye. That he 'had beene formerly notorious in the plantation for a prophane, lying, scoffing and lewd speritt' surely did not help his situation. Although professing innocence, he was committed to prison on 24 February. In jail he was visited by some of the magistrates and other fellow-puritans and under their strong moral suasion admitted to be guilty of the suspected crime, but almost immediately revoked his confession. There followed, up to the final day of the drama, a succession of admissions and revocations; but although he 'impudently and with desperate imprecations against himselfe denyed all thatt he had formerly confessed,' witnesses testified in court to his former admissions and their word was accepted as evidence. The court then 'judged the

Originally presented at the Mead-Johnson Symposium on Perinatal and Developmental Medicine (#7), Vail, Colorado, June 8–12, 1975.

> crime cappitall, and thatt the prisoner and the sow, according to Levit, 20 and 15, should be put to death—.' And so, on 8 April 1642, 'The sow being first slaine in his sight, he ended his course here. God opening his mouth before his death, to give him the glory of his rightousness, to the full satisfaction of all them present, butt in other respects leaving him a terrible example of divine justice and wrath" (7,8).

This is a cruel example of injustice. Injustices continue to occur, although they may not be as extreme as the case of George Spencer. In a recent time, however, when injustice occurs, it tends to favor the afflicted or the malformed. The following case, which was decided in the 1960's, is a good example of up-to-date injustice:

> In Sinkler vs. Kneal the "Plaintiffs filed a complaint containing four counts. In the first count plaintiff Nancy D. Sinkler claimed in her own right $100,000 damages for lacerations and contusions and *shock to her nervous system which resulted in the birth of a mongoloid child,* Rebecca, as well as for repairs to her 1952 Chevrolet coupe. In the second count, Emilie, daughter of plaintiffs Charles Sinkler and Nancy D. Sinkler, who was a passenger in her mother's automobile, claimed damages for lacerations and contusions, as well as shock to her nervous system. In the third count, Rebecca, a Mongoloid daughter, born November 11, 1958, sued defendant, alleging (a) he negligently ran into the rear of her mother's automobile and (b) *that at the same time of the accident and (c) 'as a result of the accident plaintiff was born a Mongoloid child'* Plaintiff claimed $100,000 for the pain, suffering and humiliation, as well as for medical expenses as loss of earnings and earning power. In the fourth count, the father of the minors claimed damages in the sum of $100,000 for money which he spent, or may be obliged to spend in the future, for medicine, X-ray, nursing and hospital care (9). The majority opinion of the court pertaining to the third count was reported September 26, 1960, several years after the genetic aspects of mongolism had been clarified (10). Yet, the majority opinion clearly devoted its entire discussion to the question of whether an injured unborn had the right to recover damages in a negligence suit (9,11).

The important question as to whether the malformation and the auto accident were related was not considered in the majority decision. There is no question that the majority decision was accurate and sound with regard to the biologic concept that the fetus is a separate organism. But, the court was grossly negligent in taking for granted an etiological relationship between a pregnant woman's automobile accident and the subsequent birth of a mongoloid child. It is obvious that a turnabout has occurred. The "malformed" offspring and his parents are no longer the accused. On the contrary they have become the plaintiff, seeking recompense and justice for the malformation and the "injured" family, when, in the eyes of a counselor and his medical consultants, the mother or infant had been treated negligently during the pregnancy. There is a great deal of confusion concerning the legal and medical aspects of the human malformation problem. Therefore, it is the purpose of this paper to:

1. Justify certain instances of plaintiff action on behalf of a malformed infant and family
2. Indicate the proper preparation of the case in behalf of the malformed infant
3. Indicate important concepts in the proper defense of the defendant; be it the physician, a lay individual, a business or corporation
4. Suggest preventive measure to reduce the circumstances that might result in a justifiable suit

LEGAL PROBLEMS PECULIAR TO THE FIELD OF TERATOLOGY

There are a number of factors or problems that are peculiar to the medicolegal aspects of teratology that separate it from the rest of the medicolegal field. These peripheral legal complications frequently consume much of the court's time so that the important issue of negligence and proof of causality may be ignored. Let us consider some of the problems that the court has to face besides determining the cause of the malformation and the existence of negligence.

Who can be the plaintiff? (2,3,5,9,11,113,114)

If the malformed infant survives, then the parents, siblings and malformed infant may all file suit for pain and suffering of the family; for loss of earning power and medical expenses for the malformed infant. If the malformed infant does not survive, it is still possible to bring suit in behalf of the estate of the dead malformed infant providing there is legal evidence that the fetus was once alive. It then becomes mandatory for the court to decide on the criteria that should be the basis for determining viability. The criteria vary and may include gestational age; evidence of a heart beat and/or respiration after severing the umbilical cord; or both. It has been decided that an abortus cannot bring suit, although the parents of the abortus have this right (11).

Who is the defendant?

It is possible that a physician, industrial firm, pharmaceutical firm, parent or lay person might be held responsible for a child's malformation. It is conceivable that parents may be held responsible for their hereditary defects or even for the occurrence of congenital syphilis (5). One important factor that must be considered in evaluating liability cases is the level of sophistication that is expected from a particular potential defendant. This can only be decided by the court. Should a lay individual be cognizant of the teratogenic consequences of rubella? Should an adult be held responsible for knowingly exposing a pregnant woman to rubella infection? Can a government which legally prevents therapeutic abortions be sued by a malformed infant whose mother was denied the right of having an abortion (3)? Is it possible that a parent or government might be sued by an illegitimate child for failing to request a therapeutic abortion? In the future any individual or group may be a potential defendant.

Who is the expert?

A third problem that the court faces is to decide "who is the expert." Who can provide expert testimony regarding the cause of a congenital malformation? This is made particularly difficult because no one medical specialty prepares a physician for testifying in this type of litigation. Thus, the quality of expert testimony will vary, since the expert testimony may include anyone from the family physician to an embryologist, and including almost every medical specialty. In essence there is no one group of physicians or specialists whom the lawyer can confidently consider as an authority in the field of medical teratology.

Most briefs dealing with malformed infants will include initial consultations with the family obstetrician and pediatrician. These opinions are often definite, concise, and undocumented. As an example, a pediatrician sent in the following reply to a legal consultation involving a mentally retarded infant whose mother was involved in an automobile accident during her pregnancy. The mother was hospitalized because of uterine hemorrhage. "In my opinion, this child's mental retardation could not be related in any way to the mother's automobile accident." The obstetrician of the mother contributed the following statement to the plaintiff's lawyer: "In my opinion, the psychologic trauma of the accident during the mother's pregnancy resulted in the congenital malformation of this offspring." Both consultations gave no other supporting documentation or information. The lawyer frequently utilizes the family physician as a consultant because he knows that the jury intuitively believes that the family pediatrician and obstetrician are the most informed about the circumstances of the case. In defense of the attorney, it must be stated that there is no one group of physicians or specialists with whom the lawyer can feel confident.

The etiology of congenital malformations

There is ample evidence to indicate that many environmental and genetic factors account for only a small portion of all human malformations (12–15,115,120). Pitt (15) estimated that 60 per cent of all malformations had no known cause. In 80.8 per cent the family history was not helpful. Even during epidemic years, rubella accounted for only .59 per cent of all malformations.

This means that the majority of malformations have no definite etiology resulting rather from a combination of unknown environmental or genetic influences (12–15). It is also possible that many malformations result from errors of growth and differentiation in the embryo which are unrelated to exogenous or hereditary factors. There is a statistical probability that a small percentage of embryos will fail to accomplish the intricate processes that are necessary for normal differentiation. Thus, it is possible that malformations may result from predictable but rare biological errors of embryonic growth and differentiation, comparable to predictable spontaneous mutation rates occurring at specific gene loci (14). If the majority of malformations fall into the etiological category, then environmental factors that can be considered potentially medicolegal in nature would be in the minority (Table 1).

The problem of multiple etiologies is further compounded by the fact that malformations are relatively common, in the order of 25–40 malformed infants per 1000 births. Furthermore, a similarly appearing malformation may be genetically determined, environmentally produced or have no known etiology. The problem of determining the etiology of a malformed infant is exasperatingly more complex than determining the causative factors in most other medicolegal cases.

Thus, the high incidence of malformations, the multiplicity of etiologies and the variety of malformations all complicate the evaluation process.

Oversimplification of the concept of a sensitive period

Although congenital malformations are most readily induced in the first trimester, one must remember that malformations can be induced in all three trimesters (12,16–20). Warkany and Kalter discuss the sensitive period in an excellent monograph dealing with congenital malformations (20). They emphasize the difference between the "determination" period and the "termination" period for congenital malformations. It is frequently stated that the younger the embryo the greater its sensitivity to teratogenic agents. Actually, there is ample evidence to indicate the mammalian zygote is quite resistant to teratogenic agents during the first weeks of gestation (21). Furthermore, syphilis and toxoplasmosis are more likely to inflict permanent damage to the embryo late in gestation. Growth failures in the latter part of pregnancy can result in certain types of digital abnormalities even though the original hand formation was normal. Central nervous system malformations can be produced in the latter part of pregnancy. Furthermore, one must consider that inflammatory or degenerative processes can occur in the fetus, resulting in destructive lesions which can mimic first trimester-induced malformations. Therefore, each individual case should be evaluated separately and should not be based on broad generalizations that have become embryological dogma.

The illogical extension of responsibility in negligence cases

The legal quest for compensation to a malformed infant is an emotionally charged situation. If the defendant's treatment of the pregnant mother is negligent, this in itself can be construed as satisfactory evidence that the malformation is the result of the negligent event or treatment. The following situations involving pregnant women are examples of malpractice or negligence, but in no way define the relationship between

TABLE 1. Relative contribution of various cases to the frequency of human malformations

Etiology	Malformed live births (%)
Cytogenic	5
Mendelian inheritance Spontaneous mutations }	15–20
Unknown	65–70
Polygenic	
Multifactorial	
Synergism	
Spontaneous errors of development	
Environmental (exposure of the embryo)	
Maternal infections (rubella, toxoplasmois, herpes simplex, C.I.D., syphilis, etc.)	3
Maternal disease states (diabetes, phenylketonuria, endocrinopathies and endocrine tumors, alcoholism, smoking, nutritional problems)	4
Problems of constraint	2
Drugs, chemicals, irradiation, hyperthermia	1

the malformation and the event under question:

1. A pregnant woman's physician made a diagnosis of abdominal tumor and performed a laparotomy.
2. A man passed through a red light and struck the car of the pregnant woman.
3. A pharmacist erred in filling a prescription and the pregnant woman received an overdose of medication.
4. A pregnant woman slipped and fell in an exclusive restaurant because the entranceway was icy.

In many instances the temporal association between obvious negligence and the birth of a malformed infant is considered proof of an etiological relationship. It is imperative that the court prove the existence of two separate events. First, that the environmental occurrence was the result of negligence on the part of the defendant; second, that a malformation resulted from the environmental occurrence. Both conditions must be proven in order to establish the defendant's responsibility.

CLASSIFICATION OF CONGENITAL MALFORMATIONS FROM A MEDICOLEGAL VIEWPOINT

In an effort to discourage litigation which is scientifically unsound and support just complaints, the following medicolegal classification of malformations is presented:

Malformations, syndromes and causes of human malformations have been divided into five categories based on the probability of the relationship between a particular cause and the resultant malformation (Table 2). The categories are:

1. Definite relationship
2. Probable relationship
3. Questionable relationship
4. Improbable relationship
5. No relationship

One must keep in mind that this Table has been prepared from the medicolegal viewpoint, which dictates that a stand has to be taken with the available facts. Although the information in Table 2 needs to be qualified and expanded, it is a starting point for the courts.

The items in the "definite relationship" category account for an extremely small segment of human malformations. The "probable relationship" category does include a few more common events. Both these categories, however, include problems that are infrequently brought to court in spite of the fact that a reasonable case could be prepared. One must keep in mind that proof of negligence is inherent in a decision in favor of the plaintiff. As an example, if an infant with congenital goiter resulted from the administration of an antithyroid drug to a pregnant mother, a suit might be brought in behalf of the malformed infant. The physician defendant should be prepared and be able to prove that 1) the antithyroid medication was necessary for the mother's health, 2) the mother was informed of the complications of antithyroid drugs during pregnancy, 3) the physician and family were aware of the complications and this was made part of the medical record. In a case such as this, there would be no aspect of negligence and the plaintiff would not have just cause for litigation. There are a number of drugs that have been reported to be teratogenic in one epidemiological series and have been reported to be harmless by others. These drugs have been placed in the "Questionable" category. It is possible that variations in dosage and genotype may account for the conflicting reports as well as the introduction of extraneous factors that make insignificant environmental factors appear to affect the population. The category labeled "Improbable relationship" contains those relationships that are most commonly involved in litigation. The three common problems are concerned with 1) diagnostic radiation exposure to the pregnant mother, 2) drug exposure to the pregnant mother, or 3) psychological or physical trauma to the pregnant mother. It is obvious that a large number of these cases will have no scientific basis and yet, in some instances, the plaintiff's view will preside. This does not mean that no human malformations have resulted from any of these causes. There is no doubt that on very rare occasions trauma to the pregnant mother has resulted in a congenital defect or fetal death. Therefore, this category is labeled improbable because past experience has told us that these environmental factors are unlikely causes of human malformations. In order to prevent injustice, however, each case must be evaluated individually.

There are certain syndromes or malformations that are listed in the category labeled "No relationship." This particular category is the most important item in Table 2. It offers the defendant a group of malformations or syndromes in which the causes can be demonstrated at any point in time, even

*TABLE 2. The relationship between teratogenesis or pathologic alterations of a fetus and the occurrence of an event or the administration of an agent during the gestational period from 12 days to term when the agent is utilized in its usual dosage form (for drugs)**

Definite relationship
1. Thalidomide embryopathy[25,26]
2. Androgenic masculinization[27–30]
3. Diethylstilbestrol adenosis and adenocarcinoma of the vagina[120]
4. Fluorescent tooth staining from tetracyclines[31–36]
5. Goiter resulting from antithyroid medications and iodine deficiency[16,17]
6. Syndromes resulting from infection with rubella virus, toxoplasmosis, cytomegalovirus infection, treponema palidum, herpes simplex, venezuelan equine encephalitis, varicella; with isolation or identification of the organism[12,18,37,38,39]
7. Documented drug induced hemolytic anemia in the fetus[16]
8. Cerebral palsy associated with maternal methylmercury exposure (Minamata disease)[121]
9. Nasal hypoplasia following warfarin exposure[122]
10. Virus infection of fetus with live virus vaccine
11. Retinoic acid and high doses of vitamin A

Probable relationship
1. Greater than 50 rad exposure[123]
2. Altered sex development following exposure to high dose of certain sex steroids[44,45]
3. Growth retardation, embryolethality and malformations following exposure to folic acid antagonists and certain other cancer chemotherapeutic drugs[46–49]
4. Maternal disease states[115]
   a. Diabetes
   b. Phenylketonuria
   c. Chronic alcoholism[124]
   d. Epilepsy associated with anticonvulsant therapy[125]
   e. Smoking addiction (tobacco)
   f. Mechanical or constant problems causing limb malformations, cleft lip and palate, open neural tube, omphalocele related to uterine malformations, oligohydramnios, amniotic rupture, bleeding, velamentous cord insertion and multiple pregnancies
5. Deafness following the administration of streptomycin to a pregnant women[41–43]
6. Documented hypoglycemia—insulin induced or idiopathic[55–57]
7. Fetal hydantoin syndrome (chronic drug administration)
8. Trimethadione syndrome (chronic drug administration)
9. PCB cola babies
10. Penicillamine
11. Valproic acid (chronic drug administration)
12. IUD (pregnancy loss)
13. Lithium

Questionable relationship[114,118,119]
1. Quinine
2. INH, PAS, ethionamide
3. Aspirin in toxic doses
4. Dexamphetamine, phenmetrazine
5. Tolbutamide, sulfonylurea
6. Hyperthermia

Improbable relationship
1. Most drugs including LSD, sulfonamides, meclizine, cortizone, antihistamines, bendectin and antiemetics[16,24,30,58–81,118,119]
2. Maternal physical trauma[83–89]
3. Maternal psychologic trauma[90–100]
4. Diagnostic radiation[21,101–103,123]
5. Active immunization with dead vaccines[16–20]
6. Hypoxic episode[82]
7. Imipramine
8. Anesthetic agents
9. Nongenital malformations and sex steroids exposure
10. Spermicides

No relationship
1. Dominant genetic disease present in complete or incomplete form in one parent
2. Dominant genetic disease due to a spontaneous mutation
3. Recessive metabolic defects and malformations
4. Cytogenetic abnormalities: trisomy, delections, translocations[10,104–107]

*12,15,16–24,117–119. Gestational age, dose, and the type of embryopathology are other relevant factors in establishing a relationship.

during the litigation. Furthermore, it can readily be demonstrated that no drug or environmental factor could have produced this group of diseases during the gestational period of from one week to parturition.

Each of the items in Table 2 could be discussed separately, listing all the pros and cons, the exceptions and the qualifications. It is not the purpose of this paper to defend the classification. As mentioned in the beginning of this section it is an attempt to discourage the initiation of unjust litigation and to support just claims.

MEDICOLEGAL WORKUP

In the trial of a malformation case, there is a minimal amount of essential information that both the plaintiff and the defendant should make available to the court. In many instances, judicial decisions are rendered without sufficient data to arrive at a just conclusion.

It has already been stated that there are certain malformations or groups of malformations which are related to environmental factors that occur between the end of the first week of gestation and the time of delivery (Table 2). Therefore, if the plaintiff is attempting to prove that an environmental event (resulting from the defendant's negligence) resulted in a congenital malformation, he must prove that the malformed infant is not an infant with a cytogenetic or genetic defect. On the other hand, the defendant's case would be irrefutable if a genetic defect could be demonstrated.

Therefore, the court should request that the malformed infant have a *cytogenetic evaluation* and a thorough, well-documented *genetic family history*. Certain screening procedures may be in order, such as *amino acid analyses* of the patient's and parents' serum and urine, especially if mental retardation is part of the patient's syndrome. Finally, the child's defects should be documented with regard to severity and prognosis. This is especially true with regard to mental retardation. It is not enough to state that a child is retarded. The severity of the retardation and the prognosis are essential pieces of information that should be available to the court.

The procedures that are necessary to prepare a case adequately will not remain the same over the years. As new and better diagnostic and prognostic tests are discovered, they should be added to the medicolegal workup.

THE PREVENTION OF MEDICOLEGAL PROBLEMS

Proper communication (116)

Failure of communication is one of the prime errors committed in many medicolegal cases. In fact, in many instances the negligence factor is decided on the basis of the adequacy of communication between patient and doctor. In the area of teratology, the communication problem is more complex, since it can involve relationships between doctor-patient, doctor-doctor, doctor-pharmaceutical firm, patient-lay individual, etc. In order that proper communication occur between the potential plaintiff and defendant, information that pertains to environmental teratology has to be disseminated adequately to the doctor by medical educators, by the Food and Drug Administration and by pharmaceutical firms. If a drug is known to have some detrimental effect on the fetus it should be clearly stated in the drug brochure in a special section in that brochure. In fact, *every* drug brochure should have a clear statement regarding its use in pregnancy. If there is a hazard to the fetus, then the hazards of the drug or the procedure, as well as its benefits, can be discussed with the family. A note should be made in the office or hospital record regarding this discussion and its outcome. Awareness and the communication of this awareness should reduce the initiation of a number of groundless suits.

There are other aspects of communication to be considered. It is possible to communicate erroneously, although unintentionally. Every physician knows that he cannot guarantee the outcome of a pregnancy and yet he can inadvertently be trapped into making such a guarantee. For example, a 22-year-old woman, six weeks pregnant with her second child, attended a birthday party with her first child. The next day the mother learned that one of the children at the party was ill and was diagnosed as having rubella. The mother made an appointment with her physician to receive an injection of gamma globulin. The next day the mother learned that the original diagnosis was in error, the other child's illness was not rubella. Her obstetrician did not give her the gamma globulin and informed the pregnant mother, "You no longer have to worry." The physician meant that she no longer had to worry about the rubella embryopathy, not congenital malformations in general. When the infant was born malformed, suit was brought against the physician, primarily because the mother was angry and guilty, but most of all surprised. The statistics dealing with the incidence of malformations should be discussed with any pregnant woman who asks for reassurance after some unusual event has occurred during her pregnancy. This discussion will eliminate the possibility of making inadvertent guarantees to the patient.

Establishment of authoritative sources of information to assist the court

Once a suit has been initiated, it is the purpose of the court to arrive at a just decision. It is obvious from reviewing previous court records that unjust decisions have been handed down because of the submission of erroneous scientific information or the failure to submit available medical data. This means that the proper expert testimony was not available to the court. In order to prevent unjust decisions against either plaintiff or defendant, it would seem appropriate to establish a national committee that could participate in medicolegal teratology cases as a friend of the court. The committee members could be apointed from National Scientific Societies representing Obstetrics, Pediatrics, Radiology, Human Genetics and Pharmacology. It would be the purpose of this committee to review court records and keep an up-to-date file of court decisions and scientific literature that pertains to the medicolegal aspects of teratology. The existence of such a national committee would be a deterrent to nuisance suits and an aid to both the plaintiff and the defendant. It would be essential that this committee confine itself to the determination of the etiology of the malformations and not get involved in the negligence aspects of the case; that is, the decision as to whether the potentially teratogenic situation resulted from negligence.

Changing the laws (114,117)

New legislation may be necessary in order to protect all who may be involved in cases involving malformed infants. Before legislation is considered, one has to decide whether parents should be protected or made liable for malformations in their offspring. For example, should parents with a dominantly inherited malformation be protected or made vulnerable by the new laws? Should a child with syndactyly or retinoblastoma be prevented from suing or encouraged to seek damages from his parents? Should a child with kernicterus or congenital syphilis be allowed to seek damages for his stigmata?

Inherent in these situations is the question of how much should a parent know before becoming a parent. Is ignorance an acceptable defense in such a case? Should there be an altered statute of limitations to protect the child or the parent? This paper does not intend to answer these questions, but only to pose them, since they are unusual questions and pertain to moral and religious concepts beyond the field of teratology. They are also directly related to other problems, such as eugenics, legal abortion and contraception.

Legislation

The legal heritage of this nation is almost by definition intimately related to ethical and moral standards of our culture. The legislative process is a very slow reflection of changes in ethical and moral standards and marked social changes. Because of the varied religious and ethnic backgrounds of our population, it is difficult to obtain a consensus about many of the ethical questions that directly relate to the problems of reproduction, abortion and fetal research. In fact, recent rulings of the Supreme Court which liberalized abortion have further polarized various factions, so that the disagreements about abortion policy have activated controversies dealing with fetal research, genetic counseling, family planning, etc. If one views these issues from a historical perspective, one should be optimistic since, eventually, the ethical and moral standards of the people of our democracy will be reflected in the laws of the land. Ethical and moral positions of responsible groups are frequently viewed by protagonists as being right or wrong. Like feelings they are neither right nor wrong but only reflect the inner rules of a culture. Each of us tends to be quite "noncritical" of the rules of our personal culture and very "objective" about the morals and ethics of other cultures or religions. This concept is exemplified superbly by the response of the leader of a tribe of cannibals when asked by an inquisitive missionary, *if it was true that in his tribe they killed people and ate them?* The leader of the tribe answered the civilized missionary with a question. "Is it true in your world that you kill people and don't eat them?"

There are many controversial issues that have developed that will directly affect the incidence of congenital malformations, the incidence of morbidity and mortality in newborn infants, the extent of future developments in biomedical research and the quality of health care. The resolution of these issues can occur by decisions of the courts, by state and national legislative changes, or both. Since we previously indicated that these issues reflect emotionally charged ethical opinions, in many instances they are neither right nor wrong. Therefore, the legislative alternatives will be provided and the impact of these alternatives discussed.

The congress and state legislatures will have to become cognizant of the rising level of sophistication of the public. Frequently, laws are altered by important court decisions. It would seem much wiser to face the problems squarely and ask ourselves whether drastic legislative measures are indicated. The important areas for legislative consideration are:

1. Resolution of the abortion problem (4,108,111,114)
2. Indications for voluntary or mandatory family planning for eugenic purposes.
3. Laws dictating the types of information with which the court should be provided before permitting the initiation of a trial involving a malformed child.
4. Establishment of the criteria upon which the fetus can be considered to have the rights of a plaintiff.
5. Parental responsibility toward the health of their unborn offspring.
6. Limits and extent of responsibility of pharmaceutical firms for the safety of drugs.
7. Legislation that would provide the mechanism for rapid computer recording of agents or environmental factors that are harmful to the fetus (112).
8. Resolution of the problem of consent.
9. Adoption of a new system of a malpractice awards.
10. Guidelines for fetal research, fetal clinical care, fetal therapy and fetal diagnosis.

It is obvious that the problem of medicolegal litigation involving the unborn fetus will not be resolved without the active participation of the legal and medical profession and the national and state legislatures. The crisis in malpractice insurance is the result of permitting a problem to get out of hand. The present flurry of legislative attempts to resolve the problem has occurred because the situation has become untenable. Hopefully, we should initiate some of the legislative reforms mentioned before other crises in the area of litigation arise. The purpose of the recommended legislation would be to prevent situations from arising that might lead to litigation and to aid in arriving at a fair decision when litigation is necessary.

SUMMARY

The medicolegal aspects of teratology have some unique problems which separate this field from other medicolegal problems. These problems include:

1. Who can be the plaintiff?
2. Multiplicity of defendants.
3. The legal rights of the unborn fetus.
4. Multitude of etiologies of congenital malformations. (Table 1)
5. The problem of available expert testimony.
6. The necessity of dual proof: negligence and causality (the illogical extension of defendant responsibility in negligent cases).
7. Dogmatic application of the so-called sensitive period.

In an effort to discourage litigation which is scientifically unsound and support just complaints, the following medicolegal classification of malformations is presented. Malformations, syndromes and causes of human malformations have been divided into five categories based on the probability of the relationship between a particular cause and the resultant malformation. (Table II). The categories are:

1. Definite relationship.
2. Probable relationship.
3. Questionable relationship.
4. Improbable relationship.
4. Improbable relationship.
5. No relationship.

One must keep in mind that this table has been prepared from the *medicolegal viewpoint,* which dictates that a stand has to be taken with the available facts.

The concept of a *medicolegal workup* is introduced: No case should be permitted into court without adequate preparation and documentation.

There are several phases to the prevention of medicolegal litigation involving the malformed child. *Proper communication*-i.e., between the doctor and patient; the doctor and pharmaceutical firm; the pharmaceutical firm and the government; the patient and a lay individual, etc.-is an excellent preventive measure for the misunderstandings that lead to litigation. If one can eliminate the element of surprise, you have eliminated one major factor present in many malpractice or negligence suits. Proper communication and excellent record keeping is the best deterrent to the initiation of negligence suits.

National committees should be set up as a friend of the court to determine the etiological relationship between the proposed cause of the malformation and the malformation.

Of course, the committee would have nothing to do with the negligence aspect of any suit.

The passage of new legislation at the national or state level could clarify the controversial aspects of the rights of the unborn plaintiff and also define the responsibility of parents, lay individuals, doctors and industrial firms in this regard. The legislation should contend with present and future problems in the area of congenital malformations, abortion and eugenics.

It is obvious that the problem of medicolegal litigation involving the unborn fetus will not be resolved without the active participation of the legal and medical profession and the national and state legislative bodies. It is, therefore, proposed that the above be considered in order to eliminate unnecessary litigation and aid in obtaining just decisions when litigation is initiated.

ACKNOWLEDGMENTS

This paper was supported by research grants NIH HD 18396, 19165, 7075, the Foederer Foundation, and Harry Bock Charities.

LITERATURE CITED

1. Symposium on congenital anomalies as a social problem. (1961) Founding meeting of Japan Association foor Study of Congenital Anomalies, Kyoto University, Kyoto, Japan, Feb. 22.
2. New York State Court of Claims granted an illegitimate child the right to sue for having been born, Philadelphia Evening Bull., June 26, 1964.
3. Litigation, the unborn plaintiff. Time, p. 58, April 30, 1965.
4. Niswander, K.R., M. Klein, C.L. Randall (1966): Changing attitudes toward therapeutic abortion, JAMA *196:*1140.
5. Gordon, D. (1965) The unborn plaintiff. Michigan Law Rev., *63:*579.
6. Warkany, J, and H. Kalter (1962) Maternal impressions and congenital malformations. Plast Reconstruct. Surg., *30:*628.
7. Landauer, W. (1961) Hybridization between animals and man as a cause of congenital malformations, Extra Arch. Anat. Histol. Embryol. Normales. et Exper. *14(Suppl.):*155.
8. Headley, C.J. (1857) Records of the Colony and Plantation of New Haven from 1638 to 1649. Case, Tiffany & Co., Hartford.
9. Sinkler, appellant, v. Kneale, 401 Pa., Appeal No. 124, January 1960, from order of the Court of Common Pleas of Chester County, March 1, 1959. No. 49, of Sinkler v. Kneale, 267–278, 1960.
10. Lejeune, J., R. Turpin and M. Gautier (1959) Le mongolisme, maladie chromosomique (trisomie). Bull. Acad. Nat. Med. (Paris) *143:*256.
11. Caroll v. Skloff 159: In the Supreme Court of Pennsylvania, Eastern District No. 131, January 1, 1964. Appeal from the Judgement of the Court of Common Pleas No. 1 of Philadelphia County, March Term, 1963, No. 5407, sustaining appellees' preliminary objections and dismissing appellants' complaint, Entered October 25, 1963.
12. Fraser, F.C. (1959) Causes of congenital malformations in humans. J. Chron. Dis. *10:*97.
13. Landauer, W. (1961) The interplay of intrinsic and extrinsic factors in the origin of congenital malformations. In: Papers and Discussions Presented at the First International Conference on Congenital Malformations. London, England, July 12–22, 1960. JB Lippincott Co., Philadelphia and Montreal.
14. Brent, R.L. (1965) Effect of proteins, antibodies, and autoimmune phenomena upon conception and embryogenesis, In: J. Wilson and J. Warkany, ed. Teratology, Principles and Techniques. University of Chicago Press, Chicago.
15. Pitt, D.B. A study of congenital malformations, Part II. Aust. NZ J. Obst. Gynecol., *2:*82.
16. Cohlan, S.Q. (1964): Fetal and neonatal hazards from drugs administered during pregnancy, NY J. Med., *64:*493.
17. Connelly, J.P. S. Reynolds, J.D. Crawford and N.B. Talbot (1964) Viral and drug hazards in pregnancy. Clin. Pediatr., *3:*597.
18. Fraser, F.C. (1961) Congenital defects—intrinsic and extrinsic factors. Acad. Med. Bull., *7:*763.
19. Wilson, J.G. (1960) Factors involved in causing congenital malformations. Bull. NY Acad. Med., *16:*145.
20. Warkany, J., and H. Kalter (1961) Congenital malformations. N. Eng. J. Med., *265:*993, 1046.
21. Apgar, V. (1961): Human congenital anomalies, Am. J. Dis. Child. *101:*249.
22. Haring, O.M. and F.J. Lewis. (1961) The etiology of congenital developmental anomalies. Surgery, *113:*1.
23. Karnofsky, D.A. (1965) Drugs as teratogens in animals and man, Ann Rev. Phamacol., *5:*447.
24. Schull, W.J. (1961) Congenital malformations: Current knowledge of etiology. Clin. Obst. Gynecol. *4:*365.
25. Lenz, W. and Knapp K. (1962) Die thalidomidembryopathie. Deutsch med Wchnschr., *87:*1232.
26. Speirs, A.L. (1962) Thalidomide and congenital abnormalities. Lancet, *1:*303.
27. Grundwaldt, E. and T. Bates (1957) Nonadrenal femal pseudohermaphroditism after administration of testosterone to mother during pregnancy. Pediatrics *20:*503.
28. Grumbach, M.M. and Ducharme J.R. (1960) The effects of androgen on fetal sexual development, Fertil. Steril. *2:*157.
29. Jost, A. (1963) Hormones et teratogenese. In: Proceedings of the European Society for the Study of Drug Toxicity, Effects of Drugs on the Foetus *1:*35. Excerpta Medica Internat. Cong. Ser. No. 64.
30. Bongiovanni, A.M. and A.J. McPadden (1960) Steroids during pregnancy and possible fetal consequences, Fertil. Steril *2:*181.
31. Bevelander, G. G.K. Rolle and S.Q. Cohlan (1961) Effect of the administration of tetracycline on the development of teeth. J. Dent. Res. *40:*1020.
32. Frankel, M.A. and R.R. Hawkes (1964) Tetracycline antibiotics and tooth discoloration. J. Oral Ther. Pharmacol., *1:*147.
33. Johnson, R.H. and D.F. Mitchell (1966) The effects of tetracyclines on teeth and bones. J. Dent. Res., *45:*86.
34. Swallow, J.N. (1964) Discoloration of primary dentition after maternal tetracycline ingestion in pregnancy. Lancet, *i:*611.
35. Wallman, I.F. and H.B. Hilton (1962) Tooth pigmentation by tetracycline. Lancet, *1:*827.
36. Witkop, C.J. and R.O. Wolfe (1963) Hypoplasia and intrinsic staining of enamel following tetracycline therapy. JAMA, *185:*1008.

37. Feldman, H.A. (1958) Toxoplasmosis. Pediatrics, *22:*559.
38. Weller, T.H., J.B. Hanshaw, and D.E Scott (1960) Virologic and clinical investigatins on cytomegalic inclusion disease. Proc. Soc. Pediatr. Res. *8*.
39. Giles, J.P., L.Z. Cooper, and S. Krugman (1964) The rubella syndrome. J. Pediatr. *66*:434.
40. Gregg, N. (1941) Congenital cataract following German measles in the mother. Tr. Ophthalmol. Soc. Aust. *3:*35.
41. Bolletti, M. and L. Croatt (1958) Deafness in a five-year-old girl resulting from streptomycin therapy during pregnancy. Acta Paediat. Lat. *11:*1.
42. Robinson, G.E. and K.G. Cambon (1964) Hearing loss in infants of tuberculous mothers treated with streptomycin during pregnancy. N. Eng. J. Med., *271:*949.
43. Varpela, E. (1964) On the effect exerted by first-line tuberculosis medicines on the foetus. Acta Tuberc. Scand., *35:*53.
44. Bongiovanni, A.M. A.M. DiGeorge and M.M. Grumbach (1959) Masculinization of the female infant associated with estrogenic therapy alone during gestation. J. Clin. Endocrinol., *19:*1004.
45. Wilkins, L, H.W. Jones, G.H. Holmar and R.S. Stempfel (1958) Masculinization of the female fetus associated with administration of oral and intromuscular progestins during gestation: non adrenal female pseudohermaphroditism. J. Clin. Endocrinol., *18:*559.
46. Meltzer, H.J. (1956) Congenital anomalies due to attempted abortion with 4-aminopteroylglutamic acid. JAMA, *161:*1253.
47. Sokal, J.E. and E.M. Lessmann (1960) Effects of cancer chemotherapeutic agents of the human fetus. JAMA, *172:*1765.
48. Thiersch, J.B. (1952) Therapeutic abortions with folic acid antagonist. 4-aminopteroylglutamic acid(4-ami-
no P.G.A.) administered by the oral route. Am. J. Obst. Gynecol., *63:*1298.
49. Warkany, J. P.H. Beaudry and S. Hornstein (1959) Attempted abortion with aminopterin (4-aminopteroylglutamic acid). J. Dis. Chil., *97:*274.
50. Brent, R.I. (1960) The effect of irradiation on the mammalian fetus. Clin Obst Gynecol 3s:928.
51. Murphy, D.P., M.E. Shirlock, and E.A. Doil (1942) Microcephaly fo llowing maternal pelvic irradiation for the interruption of pregnancy. Am. J. Roontgonol. *18:*356.
52. Yamazaki, J.N, S.W. Wright and P.M. Wright (1954) Outcome of pregnancy in women exposed to the atomic bomb in Nagasaki. J. Dis. Child. *87.*448.
53. Murphy, D.P. (1929) The outcome of 625 pregnancies in women subjected to pelvic radium or roentgen irradiation. Am. J. Obst. Gynecol., *18:*179.
54. Hicks, S.P., and C.J. D'Amato (1966) Effects of ionizing radiation on mammalian development. In: Advances in Teratology. D.H.M. Woolam, Logos Press, vol I, London, p. 196.
55. Boyd, B.A., and D.W. Brown (1948): Electric convulsive therapy in mental disorders associated with child bearing. J. Miss. State Med. Assoc., *45:*573.
56. Sobel, D.F. (1960) Fetal damage to ECT, insulin coma, chlorpromazine or reserpine. Arch. Gen. Psychiatr., *2:*606.
57. Wicks, I.G. (1954) Fetal defects following insulin coma therapy in early pregnancy. Br. Med. J., *2:*1029.
58. Beyer, K.H. (1964) Proportionate costs of drug testing in animals, Lab Anim. Care *14:*404.
59. Bonfield, C.T. (1964) Proportionate costs of drug testing in animals, Lab Anim. Care, *14:*404.
60. Brent, R.L. (1964) Drug testing in animals for teratogenic effects: Thalidomide in the pregnant rat. J. Pediatr., *64:*762.
61. Cahen, R.L. (1964) Evaluation of the teratogenicity of drugs. Clin. Pharmacol. Ther., *5:*480.
62. Cobrink, R.W., J. Hood, and E. Chusid (1959) The effect of maternal narcotic addition on the newborn infant. Pediatrics. *24:*288.
63. DeCosta, E.J., and M.A. Abelman (1952) Cortisone and pregnancy: Experimental and clinical study of effects of cortisone on gestation. Am. J. Obst. Gynecol. *64:*746.
64. Dunlop, D. (1965) The problem of drug toxicity. *In:* Symposium on Drug Toxicity. Practitioner, *194:*5.
65. Harley, J.D. (1964) Gross congenital malformations in siblings of children with glucose-6-phosphate dehydrogenase-deficient erythrocytes. Aust. Ann. Med. *13:*204.
66. Kelsey, F.O. (1964) Control of investigational drugs. Presented at the Annual Pharmacy Congress of the College of Pharmacy, St. John's University, March 17.
67. King, C.T.G., S.A. Weaver, and S.A. Narrod (1965) Antihistamines and teratogenicity in the rat. J Pharmacol. Exp. Ther., *147:*391.
68. Kretchmer, N. (1962) Primun non nocere. Pediatrics, *30:*513.
69. Krop, S. (1964) Pharmacological aspects of teratogenicity of laboratory animals. Am. J. Pharmaceut. Ed., *28:*719.
70. Leck, I. (1964) Examination of the incidence of malformations for evidence of drug teratogenesis. Br. J. Prev. Soc. Med., *18:*196.
71. Lorke, D. (1963) Method for the investigation of embryonic and teratogenic effects on rat, Naunyn-Schmiedebergs. Arch. Exp. Path. Pharmak., *246:*147.
72. Lucey, J.F.: (1963) Primates, drugs and fetal safety. Pediatrics, *32:*953.
73. Mellin, G.W. (1964) Drugs in the first trimester of pregnancy and fetal life of Homo sapiens. Am. J. Obst. Gynecol., *90:*1169.
74. Modell, W. (1963) Hazards of new drugs. Science, *139:*1180.
75. Parker, R.P. (1964) Self-regulation in the drug industry. Food, Drug & Cosmetic Law J. *661*.
76. Peck, H.M. (1963) Preclinical evaluation of drugs for evidence of teratogenic activity. J. Pharmaceut. Soc. *52:*1115.
77. Rising, J.D. (1964) The practicing physician's approach to the evaluation of new drugs. Can. Med. Assoc. J., *19:*1046.
78. Robson, J.M. (1963) The problem of teratogenicity. *In:* Symposium on Congenital Abnormalities. Practioner, *191:*136.
79. Sandberg, D.H. (1961) Drugs in pregnancy. California Med., *94:*287.
80. Smith, A. (1963) Legal considerations in drug research. Clin Pharmacol. Ther., *4:*704.
81. Zbinden, G. (1964) The problem of the toxicologic examination of drugs in animals and their safety in man. Clin. Pharmacol. Ther. *5:*537.
82. Ingalls, T.H., F.J. Curley, and R.A. Prindle (1950) Anoxia as a cause of fetal death and congenital defects in the mouse. Am. J. Dis. Child *80:*34.
83. Hinden, E. (1965) External injury causing foetal deformity. Arch. Dis. Child., *40:*80.
84. Ozan, H.A., and A.A. Gonzalez (1963) Post traumatic fetal epilepsy. Neurology (Minneapolis), *13:*541.
85. Torpin, R., G.T. Miller, and B.W. Culpepper (1964)

Amniogenic fetal digital amputations associated with clubfoot. Obst. Gynecol. *24:*379.
86. Turner, E.J. (1960) Intrauterine constriction band. J. Pediatr., *57:*890.
87. Streeter, G.L. (1930) Focal deficiencies in fetal tissues and their relation to intra-uterine amputation. Contrib. Embryol. Carnegie Inst. *22:*1.
88. Whitehouse, D.B., and T. McKeown (1956) A note on the significance of attempted abortion in the aetiology of congenital abnormalities. J. Obst. Gynecol. Br. Emp., *63:*224.
89. Wiedemann, H.R. (1955) Schadigungen der Frucht in der Schwangerschaft. Med. Monatschr., *9:*141.
90. Abramson, J.H., R.S. Ansuyah, and V. Mbambo (1961) Antenatel stress and the baby's development. Arch. Dis. Child., *36:*42.
91. Davids, A., S. DeVault, and M. Talmadge (1961) Anxiety, pregnancy and childbirth abnormalities. J. Consult. Physchol., *25:*74.
92. Davids, A., and S. DeVault (1962) Maternal anxiety during pregnancy and childbirth abnormalities. Psychosomat. Med., *24:*464.
93. Ferreira, A.J. (1965) Emotional factors in prenatal environment. J. Nerv. Ment. Dis *141:*108.
94. Hartel, A., and G. Hartel (1960) Experimental study of teratogenic effect of emotional stress in rats. Science, *132:*1483.
95. Lieberman, M.W. (1963) Early developmental stress and later behavior. Science, *141:*824.
96. Sobel, D.E. (1961)Infant mortality and malformations in children of schizophrenic women. Psychiatr. Q., *35:*60.
97. Scott, D.H. (1961) Mongolism related to emotional shock in early pregnancy. Vita Hum., *4:*57.
98. Thompson, W.R., and S. Quinby (1964) Prenatal maternal anxiety and offspring behavior: Parental activity and level of anxiety. J. Genet Psychol., *106:*359.
99. Turner, E.K. (1960) Teratogenic effects of the human foetus through maternal emotional stress: Report of a case. Med. J. Aust., *2:*502.
100. Warkany, J. (1959) Congenital malformations in the past. J. Chron. Dis., *10:*84.
101. Spiers, F.W., P.R.J. Burch, and G.W. Reed (1960) Background radiation as a cause of fetal congenital malformations. Int. J. Rad Biol., *2:*235.
102. Russell, L..B., and W.L. Russell (1952) Radiation hazards to the embryo and fetus. Radiology, *58:*369.
103. Russell, L.B. (1954) The effects of radiation on mammalian prenatal development. *In:* A. Hollaender, ed. Radiation Biology, Vol 1, McGraw-Hill Book Company, Inc, New York, p. 861.
104. Makino, S (1964) Chromosomal studies in normal human subjects in 300 cases of congenital disorders. Int. J. Cytol., *20:*12.
105. Polani, P.T. (1964) Chromosome anomalies. Ann. Rev. Med., *15:*93.
106. Patau, K., D.W. Smith, E. Therman, S.L. Inhorn, and H.P. Wagner (1960) Multiple congenital anomaly caused by an extra autosome. Lancet, *9:*790.
107. Lewis, A.J. (1964) The pathology of 18 trisomy. J. Pediatr., *65:*92.
108. Brown, K.L. (1965) You do have medical-legal responsibility, doctor. JAMA, *191:*746.
109. Gold, E.M., C.L. Erhardt, H. Jacobziner, and F.G. Nelson (1965) Therapeutic abortions in New York City, A 20-year review. Am. J. Pub. Health., *55:*964.
110. Lader, L. (1965) The scandal of abortion laws. New York Times Magazine, p 32, April 25.
111. Uhrus, K. (1964) Some aspects of the Swedish law governing termination of pregnancy. Lancet, *2:*1292.
112. Ingalls, T.H., and M.A. Klingberg (1965) Implications of epidermic embryopathy for public health. Am. J. Pub. Health., *55:*200.
113. Churchill, J. (1973) Rights of the fetus to sue. Br. Med. J., January 27, p. 224.
114. Ladimer, I. (1976) The law, *in:* The prevention of embryonic fetal and perinatal disease. R.L. Brent and M. Harris, eds. US Govt Publication; DHEW NH 76–853; Bethesda, p 411.
115. Brent, R.L., and M. Harris (1975) The prevention of embryonic fetal and perinatal disease. US Govt Publication; DHEW Publ. NIH 76–853, Bethesda, p. 411.
116. Temple, R. (1974) Legal implications of the package insert. Med. Clin. N. Am., *58:*1151–1159.
117. Brent, R.L. (1967) Medicolegal aspects of teratology. J. Pediatr., *71:*288–298.
118. Shepard, T.H. (1973) Catalog of teratogenic agents. Johns Hopkins University Press, Baltimore.
119. Wilson J.G. (1973) Environment and birth defects. Academic Press, New York.
120. Herbst, A.L., H. Ulfelder, and D.C. Poskanzer (1971) Andenocarcinoma of the vagina: Asociation of maternal stilbestrol therapy with tumor appearance in young women. N. Engl. J. Med., *284:*878–881.
121. Matsumoto, H., G. Koya, and T. Takeuchi: Fetal Minimata disease: A neuropathological study of two cases of intramuterine intoxication by methyl mercury compound. J. Neuropathol. Exp. Neurol., *24:* 563–574.
122. Kerber, I.J., O.S. Warr, and C. Richardson (1968) Pregnancy in a patient with prosthetic mitral valve. JAMA, *302:*223–225.
123. Brent, R.L., and R.O. Gorson (1972) Radiation exposure in pregnancy. *In:* Current Problems in Radiology. R.D. Mosley, Jr., *et al*, eds. *2:*1–48. Yearbook Med. Publishers Inc, Chicago.
124. Lemoine, P. H. Harrousseau, J.P. Borteyru, and J.C. Menuet (1968) Les enfants de parents alcooliques. Anomalies observees. A propos de 127 cas. Cuest Medical, *25:*477.
125. Hanson, J.W., and D.W. Smith (1975) The fetal hydantoin syndrome. Teratology, *11(2):*20A.

TERATOGEN UPDATE: ENVIRONMENTALLY INDUCED BIRTH DEFECT RISKS, PAGES 215–227 (1986)

Litigation-Produced Pain, Disease and Suffering: An Experience With Congenital Malformation Lawsuits

ROBERT L. BRENT
Departments of Pediatrics, Radiology and Anatomy, Thomas Jefferson Medical College, Philadelphia, Pennsylvania 19107

ABSTRACT The exponential rise in malpractice litagation is due to attitudes and happening in the medical, legal and lay sectors of our society. Evaluation of congenital malformation lawsuits provides a unique opportunity to evaluate the process of litigation. Because the cases are rarely meritorious, the litigation process is detrimental to the plaintiff, society and frequently unfair to the defendant. There is no area of our legal system with such a high percentage of innocent defendants. When the family of a malformed infant becomes orchestrated by an attorney into a position of devoting their energy to winning a lawsuit, many high priority family responsibilities may be ignored and important ethical standards are distorted. To win at all costs may be appropriate for a football team but it can be detrimental to a family. The family enters the litigation arena unaware of the lengthiness of the litigation process and ignorant of the fact that only a small portion of the malpractice premium dollar ever reaches the patient. The plaintiffs are not the only participants who lose their objectivity and lower their ethical standards. The quality and veracity of the testimony of expert witnesses has deteriorated to the point that drastic corrective measures have to be instituted. It is believed that recommendations for solving the malpractice crisis, which are based on the experience with congenital malformation lawsuits, should have applicability to the overall malpractice problem and must involve changes in the medical, legal and lay sectors of our society. These recommendations are discussed in detail. It must be recognized that it is difficult to alter the laws and procedures that are not of benefit to the legal profession because so many legislatures are dominated by elected officials who happen to be attorneys. But it is emphasized that of all the recommendations put forth, the one having the greatest beneficial effect on the present malpractice crisis would be the elimination of the contingency fee system and replacing it with no-fault compensation or legal-fee insurance. The contingency fee system provokes and promotes negligence litigation. The process of litigation in congenital malformation lawsuits rarely solves the patient's problems and frequently develops into a disease all its own.

"Woe unto you also, ye lawyers! for ye lade men with burdens grievous to be born, and ye yourselves touch not the burdens with one of your fingers." (Luke: 11:46)

The comments which follow are based on familiarity acquired over the past 22 years with over 100 lawsuits and potential suits concerning malformed infants and children. While this is a narrow area of medical negligence litigation, I believe that the lessons learned are generally applicable to the problem of alleged malpractice. Many suits were withdrawn and some were settled. Approximately 25 went to trial. The increase in malformation suits, which has occurred in recent years, is simply a reflection of the exponential increase in the incidence of general malpractice litigation. In 1967, the paper, "Medicolegal Aspects of Teratology," foretold that increase and made certain recommendations to reduce or eliminate unwarranted litigation in the area of congenital malformations (Brent, '67). These recommendations, the adoption of which is now urgent, will be repeated at the end of this paper. On the basis of new experience since the 1967 publication, it is now my thesis that the process of medical malpractice negligence litigation is, itself, often so deleterious to the plaintiff that even a "successful" outcome rarely benefits him or the injured child in whose name the suit is brought. The litigation process is enervating for the family. Case histories show that when a family becomes orchestrated by a lawyer into devoting much of their energies into the litigation process, many high priority family responsibilities are ignored and important cultural standards are distorted. To win at all costs may never be good; it is surely bad for a family.

The following case histories illustrated this thesis:

Case History 1

A woman in her mid-thirties had been visiting a fertility expert in order to conceive. She had several previous children and one abortion at three months gestation. She had not been able to conceive for the past several years, was receiving triiodothyronine daily, and was recording her temperature daily. On the 25th of the month, she noted a temperature rise and had intercourse on the 25th and 26th, which were the only times she had intercourse that month. Two days later she sustained a serious fall. In the process of evaluating the injuries, a series of roentgenograms were obtained on the fourth and fifth day of pregnancy. The total maximum dose to the embryo was 1.8 R. During the remainder of the pregnancy, the patient was treated for her back injuries and for other problems. The medications included Darvon®, Codeine, Cytomel®, Chlorpheniramine Maleate, Stilbesterol, vitamin K, P and C and various sedatives. Near term a baby with Beckwith's syndrome was delivered by Cesarian section. I was called as a consultant to determine whether the X-irradiation could have produced these anomalies. This consultation report was submitted to the plaintiff's attorney. My report indicated that the dose of radiation was too low to produce malformations at any stage of pregnancy and, furthermore, the embryonic age at the time of the accident and at the time of radiation exposure occurred during the period when the mammalian embryo is insensitive to the teratogenic effects of radiation. The plaintiff's attorney called me and requested that the report be altered. I refused and had no further communications from that attorney. The mother of the malformed child was a bright, well-bred individual from the upper-middle socio-economic strata who became very interested in the causes of malformations. She visited my office and I discussed this subject with her.

Approximately six years after the birth of this baby, I received a subpoena a 5 o'clock one afternoon ordering me to appear in court the next morning. The defense attorney had obtained from the hospital chart my original consultation in this case and was puzzled by the fact that I had not been called as the plaintiff's witness. In this rare instance, both the plaintiff and defense attorneys considered me a hostile or non-supportive witness. When I entered the courtroom the plaintiff's mother turned pale as did the plaintiff's attorney. I sensed a tremendous amount of anger and resentment as the plaintiff's attorney initiated his questions. Issues and facts were ignored and the main approach of the plaintiff's attorney was to indicate that I was a "professional" witness (although this was my first appearance in Court) and that I was in collusion with the defense attorney (an individual whom I had never seen or heard of before that morning). The countenance of the mother and the demeanor of the plaintiff's attorney became understandable when it was revealed that the mother of the plaintiff had altered her story by changing the dates so that the embryo would have been three weeks old at the time of radiation exposure, a stage that would be susceptible to teratogenesis. Alteration of data and suppression of the original expert testimony undoubtedly played a significant part in the loss of the suit by the plaintiff.

Comment. Preparation for the litigation and the trial itself occupied seven years of this family's time and energy. It is not uncommon for the enthusiasm of the attorney to be interpreted by the plaintiff to mean that the case is so meritorious that he or she deserves to win by any means. It is likely that the attorney and the mother knew that they were changing important data in order to make a better case. They were able to support each other's behavior because the child's malformations were real and they believed that someone in this society must be responsible for the occurrence of the malformations. Because of the lack of medical, psychological and social supports in our society, it is easier for a family to project their anger and frustration on someone rather than bear their burdens with equanimity. The lawyer may aid and abet this process. The story does not end here, because this mother was firmly convinced that her infant was malformed by something related directly or indirectly to her original accident. Although the court, the attorneys and the other witnesses could forget the litigation and go about their business, the plaintiff's mother was convinced that an injustice had been done and her anger and anguish remained unresolved. On several occasions many months later, she verbally accosted me in public places at which time she displayed quite bizzare behavior.

Case History 2

During the eleventh week of pregnancy, an expectant mother was sitting in the rear seat of an automobile which was hit broadside by another. Her car overturned and she sustained a comminuted fracture of the right femur. There was no obvious injury to the abdomen, no abdominal pain or tenderness and no vaginal bleeding. Examination by her obstetrician over the next ten days revealed all aspects of the pregnancy to be normal. She was eating well in the hospital. Members of the family suggested that she obtain an attorney following her discharge from the first hospital 11 weeks after the accident. A well-known negligence attorney was retained who discharged the expectant mother's physicians and selected another physician. This physician, an obstetrician, examined the patient for the first time in the twenty-ninth week of pregnancy and admitted her to another hospital for the remainder of the pregnancy because "she appeared markedly undernourished" and the patient complained of a 10-pound weight loss. During the first and second hospitalization all the records indicated that the fetal heart rate and movements were normal. During the thirty-eighth week of pregnancy she delivered the plaintiff. During the course of her labor, her blood pressure dropped precipitously and the fetal heart rate dropped simultaneously. With the infant in an arrested transverse position, vasopressors and pitocin were administered to the mother while a midforces delivery was attempted. The transverse position was converted by fundal pressure and the infant was delivered 35 minutes after the maternal blood pressure dropped. The umbilical cord was within the birth canal during the second stage of labor and was compressed by the infant's neck and shoulder. At birth the infant was deeply cyanotic, did not breathe for two minutes nor cry for 45 minutes. There was absence of muscle tone, failure to respond to painful stimuli and convulsions occurred on the second day of life. At the time of the trial the child was a little girl approximately nine years old with severe spastic quadriplegia.

The plaintiff's attorney's obstetrician testified that in his opinion the cerebral palsy was due to the automobile accident in the eleventh week of pregnancy which resulted in damage of the placenta. He also testified that the placenta was 70–80% infarcted at birth and that these infarctions were due to the trauma of the automobile accident. An authority in cerebral palsy and an embryologist and pediatric rehabilitationist both testified that in their opinion the automobile accident produced the placental infarctions and the resulting cerebral palsy.

My testimony was as follows: The work of Windle and Meyers clearly indicates that the lesions of cerebral palsy are produced in the perinatal period and not during the first trimester. There were at least four obstetrical mishaps in this case which are etiologically correlated with perinatal fetal brain injury. If the placenta was infarcted 70–80% by the accident in the eleventh week, it would be impossible for the fetus to reach almost seven pounds at the thirty-eighth week. One would expect severe growth retardation if the placenta actually was 70–80% infarcted and, in fact, the embryo probably would not survive. There is no clinical or experimental data to indicate that environmental insults in the first trimester result in brain lesions that are observed in cerebral palsy. Although the plaintiff's mother had been awarded damages to herself for her personal injuries, the jury did not conclude that the automobile accident contributed to the plaintiff's cerebral palsy.

Comment. Once this mother retained an attorney, her entire approach to this pregnancy changed. While the original obstetrician could find nothing objectively wrong with this pregnancy, she retrospectively complained of abdominal cramps and vaginal spotting. Her recorded weight gain was better than her previous pregnancies but she complained of weight loss. Her visit with the attorney-appointed obstetrician resulted in readmission to another hospital for the remaining two months of her pregnancy. This admission was only to make the plaintiff's case more impressive. The mother did not consciously change her priorities, but this pregnancy and her family responsibilities, in fact, became secondary to the goal of winning a legal battle. What prompts an individual to discharge her family obstetrician and allow herself to be readmitted to a hospital many miles from her home and family, in spite of the fact that she is well? What prompts physicians and scientists to testify for the plaintiff or defense when the data they are presenting are unsound and sometimes untrue? Why does a patient permit an attorney to direct his medical care in medicolegal cases? There is the driving interest in the monetary reward for those participating in the process, be they plaintiff, attorney or expert witness. For the patient, it may be misdirected anger and revenge. For the expert witness, it may be the ego gratification of being called an expert. For the attorney, it is the error in thinking that winning the case will solve the patient's or plaintiff's problems. It may make the problem worse. If anyone contributed to the occurrence of cerebral palsy in the plaintiff, it was the plaintiff's attorney, the second obstetrician and the medical profession and state licensing laws that permitted the second obstetrician to practice medicine.

Case History 3

A mother who recently immigrated to the United States and spoke no English delivered a child with phocomelia. She had been given an antibiotic for an upper respiratory infection by her obstetrician in the latter part of the third trimester. The family on behalf of the plaintiff sued a large pharmaceutical firm indicating that the antibiotic had produced the malformations. Pre-trial briefs were presented to the court. The defense presented experimental and epidemiological data that indicated the antibiotic did not cause this child's malformations. The plaintiffs could not find an expert witness to support their claim. They did, however, present data which indicated that high doses of this antibiotic could interfere with mouse embryonic development and there were several isolated case reports of malformations in infants whose mothers took the antibiotic plus other drugs. The court ruled that there was not enough evidence to warrant a trial and the case was dismissed. The mother of the malformed infant was distraught, displaying hysterical antics following the court's ruling. The plaintiff's attorney did not abandon the case, however. After two years of searching, the attorney found a general practitioner in a small town who was willing to testify on behalf of the plaintiff as an expert witness. The brief to reopen the case was identical to the original complaint, but now it had the authenticity of an "expert" witness. The case was reopended and went to trial.

Comment. None is needed.

DISCUSSION

The incidence of medical malpractice litigation has passed epidemic proportions (Ragan, '73; Brierly et al., '75; Geekie, '75; Schwartz, '75; Welch, '75; Wiseman, '75), with a possible future malpractice rate per physician of greater than 10% per year and premiums running into billions of dollars (Brierly et al., '75). Numerous changes in the present system have been suggested, including the possibility of "no fault" malpractice insurance (Ragan, '73; Brierly et al., '75; Welch, '75; Krugman, '75). Utilizing a judicial process to solve malpractice disputes has been called an "archaic social tool" unfit for present-day medicolegal problems (Wiseman, '75). This statement is supported by the fact that 85% of malpractice premiums are accounted for by defense and plaintiff lawyers' fees and insurance companies administrative costs.

The case histories presented in this paper emphasized that there is a dimension beyond the legal and financial aspects of malpractice litigation. The social and psychological aberrations demonstrated by lawyers, patients and physicians in these three cases were present to a greater or lesser degree in almost all the 100 cases with which I have been involved and in every single one that went to trial. In these cases, it was rare that a family benefitted from the litigation process. Most families would have suffered less and resolved their problems sooner had they not engaged in litigation.

CONTRIBUTING FACTORS AND POSSIBLE SOLUTIONS TO THE MALPRACTICE EPIDEMIC

Some of the following comments and recommendations related only to the problem of litigation involving malformed infants, but many apply to malpractice in general. A unique aspect of litigation involving malformed infants is that the alleged malforming agent, or drug, is rarely responsible for the infants' malformations or embryopathology (Brent, '76a,b,c; Wilson, '73; Holmes, '76). The fact that hundreds of lawsuits have been initiated in this area may provide some insight into the magnitude of the litigation epidemic. *The patient, the physician, the attorney* and *the legal and health care systems* all are contributing forces to the malpractice epidemic.

The patient as a plaintiff

Most families that become involved in litigation concerning the causation of malformations in their child do not realize how long the litigation will last. Nor are they aware of the energy and time that will be involved—for all parties. Yet, these are minor problems compared to what else happens to the patient or the family.

In few other circumstances would a patient solicit an attorney's advice in selecting a physician. The plaintiff is ready and willing to have his medical problem managed by his attorney. First, the patient abandons his regular physician. Then he will visit physicians, therapists, photographers and psychologists, in spite of the fact that it is perfectly obvious that the main goal of the attorney's medical consultants is to win a legal case and not to provide excellent medical care. The patient knows that the visits are more frequent than is necessary and that the interaction between the doctor and patient is a charade.

The family of a malformed child frequently interprets the malformations as a stigma. The associated shame and guilt is sometimes projected outside the family (Brent, '76; Drotar et al., '75). The physician, place of employment or pharmaceutical firm may become a convenient scapegoat. Thus, the litigation process may be one method of projecting blame for a congenital malformation outside the family unit.

Litigation may also be a mechanism for expressing anger. Drotar et al. ('75) studied the adaptation of parents to the birth of a child with congenital malformations. The authors found that these families had a predictable course of parental reactions which included *shock, denial, sadness, anger, adaptation* and *reorganization*. They advise early intervention with professional help to assist the family through the painful stages so that the family may become reorganized as soon as possible.

Litigation prolongs and amplifies the family's anger. Its initiation aborts the process of reorganization. Since the litigation process may last for years, we frequently observe an "anger fixation" that modifies the personality of the family beyond recognition. The attorney's role in this process is interesting and will be discussed later.

When families or individuals psychologically decompensate under the stress of prolonged litigation, it is difficult to determine whether the litigation process or the individual's basic personality was the more important factor. We do know that the pathological pursuit of the resolution of problems via litigation is clinical evidence of psychological decompensation (Polsky, '69). Although it is difficult to obtain objective data, it appears that the guilt feelings (Solnit and Stark, '61; Johns, '71), remorse and depression are also prolonged by the litigation process. Even more important, the resolution of the legal problem exacerbates many of the early reactions which should have been resolved long ago (Smithells, '65).

Lying and distortion of facts are common occurrences in medical negligence suits (Table 1). In Case 1, the mother changed the dates of her LMP so that the embryo was in a more susceptible period. In Case 2, the mother complained of cramps, bleeding and weight loss, although there was never any objective evidence of these findings and, furthermore, the symptoms and signs occurred only after the mother retained an attorney. In Case 3, the mother admitted to taking only the suspected drug during her pregnancy; no other medications. It is interesting that the average mother either takes or is administered 11 medications during preg-

TABLE 1. Distortions of the facts by participants in medical negligence litigation[1]

	Plaintiffs	Plaintiffs' lawyers	Plaintiffs' experts	Defendants	Defendants' attorneys	Defendants' experts
Number/total cases	17/17	19/23	19/31	6/24	1/21	2/27
Percent	100	82.6	61.2	25.0	4.7	7.4

[1]These figures were obtained by reviewing the depositions and trial minutes in each case. The occurrence of distortion of data was recorded only when it was very obvious.

nancy, unless she is involved in litigation. Mothers involved in litigation rarely remember taking anything during their pregnancy except the suspected drug.

Why are the facts so frequently distorted in malformations cases? First of all, the plaintiff's case is frequently very weak, yet the plaintiffs are usually convinced they are in the right. If they are right, then the defendant has wronged them. To win the case would confirm their position. Distortion of the data seems an appropriate method of guaranteeing that the defendant is punished. The plaintiff's attorney is an active, but silent partner in the process, since the attorney's primary goal is to win the case.

The consequences of the litigation process are rarely considered by the plaintiff or the attorney. If the family has altered its moral behavior in order to win a lawsuit, the family could be seriously affected long after the litigation is complete. During the litigation process, the home, the other children and one's profession or job may be neglected, since most individuals do not realize the length of the litigation process and, therefore, do not understand the extent of their original commitment. The psychological liability of being in a perpetual state of belligerency cannot be measured. The moral and social liabilities are rarely measured against the financial rewards of litigation and, when these intangibles are not considered by either the plaintiffs or their attorney, the scale tips heavily toward litigation.

The defendant

In these United States, it has always been psychologically easy, although difficult in practice, to sue "impersonal" corporate bodies and governmental agencies. The assumption by the public is that the malpractice award is "no one's" money and it "doesn't hurt anyone." Furthermore, the public in general has a continuing hostility toward large corporations and governmental agencies for both rational and irrational reasons. Unfortunately, it has become easier to sue the physician as his image has changed from that of a caring family doctor. Although the medical profession still has the respect of the lay community, it no longer has the patient's affection.

Caustic and sarcastic comments about physicians have been recorded for years.

> "With the exception of lawyers, there is no profession which considers itself above the law so widely as the medical profession." (Adams, '68)
>
> "Doctors are just the same as lawyers, the only difference is that lawyers merely rob you, whereas doctors rob and kill you." (Chekhov, '68)

The vindictiveness of the preceding quotations from the past differ from the present climate only in quantity, not quality. In a recent discourse Hardy ('75) elaborated on the materialistic image of the physician. She used such phrases as, "He has a cash register mind." "Are you planning to be a two-Cadillac ambitious doctor?" "He must have killed a great many people to get so rich." Those physicians who charge reasonable fees, live modestly and are dedicated to delivering quality care are obviously having little impact on the physician's public image. When I recently visited several retirement communities in southern Florida, I was overwhelmed by the animosity of the aged population to impersonal service and exorbitant fees.

In the past, physicians generally could become wealthy only by participating in financial matters outside the field of medicine. Today, the manipulation and, in some instances, the exploitation of third party payers has enabled some physicians to become rich directly from the practice of medicine. Furthermore, in the past, physicians provided a significant amount of free medical care. The third party payer system and the higher costs of running a medical practice have practically eliminated these charitable services. Thus, the doctor, once seen as considerate and generous, has, for many, metamorphosed into a materialistic business man.

Although most patients do not consider physicians to be malpractitioners or incompetent, there has been an increase in the notoriety given to the notion that physicians do commit a great deal more malpractice than is revealed. Furthermore, there are data to indicate that many physicians are aware of instances of malpractice, dyspractice or incompetence, but are unwilling to report them to the local medical society or the licensing agency of the state (Rensberger, '76). The widening knowledge of these instances, together with the doctor's new materialistic image, psychologically tips the scale toward litigation.

The physician expert witness

It is alleged that malpractice litigation was uncommon years ago because attorneys were unable to obtain expert medical witnesses to testify against other physicians (Robitscher, '69; Rubsamen, '75). The allegation is probably partially correct. Today, the expert medical witness for the plaintiff is no longer a rarity. Robitscher describes the plaintiff expert medical witness as follows: ". . . a small fraction of medicine that relishes the attention and sometimes also welcomes the remuneration that results from court testimony . . . who is ready to see causal connections—a blow by a taxi door and the resulting development of cancer. . . Lawyers use these witnesses frequently, but they do not always respect them." They are a "few of the best doctors and most of the worst doctors" (Robitscher, '69).

Since not all litigation involving malformed infants involves a physician defendant, it has been somewhat easier for the plaintiff's attorney to obtain an expert witness, especially if the defendant is a pharmaceutical firm, industrial firm or branch of government. My experience in malpractice litigation is limited to areas of radiation hazards and the etiology of malformations, but in these cases I have been amazed at the lack of veracity and objectivity of many plaintiff's expert witnesses (Table 1). As an example, a scientist who published a paper in which he listed a drug as non-teratogenic was willing to testify for the plaintiff when the same drug was implicated as a cause of a child's malformations. In Case 3 presented in this paper, an unfounded lawsuit which had been discontinued was reinitiated when the plaintiff's attorney was able to locate a general practitioner to testify as a medical expert witness in the field of teratology. The medical expert who testifies for the plaintiff usually demands and receives substantial fees resulting in a sycophantic alliance between the expert witness and the plaintiff's attorney.

The expert witness could measurably improve the malpractice situation by being more critical of his/her role as an expert witness. Some expert witnesses assume the role of partisan. It is an untenable position for an expert medical witness if he—

> "automatically sorts the facts newly brought to light. He retains those, even the modest ones that seem to prove him right and neglects the others, even the clearest and most precise and convincing ones if they appear to indict him. Blinded by his passion, that is, by his immoderate love for his theory, he has recourse to all means, honorable or not, in order to defend it, for to him all means have become legitimate. He has ceased to be a scientist and has become a partisan." (Arthus, '43)

In the past, expert witnesses did not testify on a contingency fee basis because it might distort the objectivity of the expert witness. At the present time there is a suggestion in some legal circles to allow expert witnesses to be paid on a contingency fee basis. If this came about, it would exponentially increase the incidence of partisan expert witnesses and destroy the credibility of all expert witnesses.

The plaintiff's attorney

The evils of malpractice litigation are related more to the litigation process than to any sinister qualities of the plaintiff's attorney. In most instances, the attorney is a bright, energetic individual who is utilizing the legal system to obtain compensation for his injured client. Although the plaintiff's attorney admits freely that the tort system has many disadvantages for the client, he believes that society has not provided a better means to solve the injured client's dilemma. Furthermore, the legal profession has no incentive and little inclination to provide a better method of compensating injured victims.

There are a number of abuses practiced by attorneys that contribute to the increasing incidence of malpractice and negligence litigation. *Attorneys are presently actively seeking malpractice cases.* Informants have been placed in hospital record rooms by law firms engaged in negligence law. Ambulance chasing appears to be on the increase. At a postgraduate seminar in Wellsboro, Pennsylvania, I was told by one of the family physicians that a patient of his received a telephone call from a large Philadelphia law firm.The patient had just returned from an eye hospital in Philadelphia following surgery for a retinal detachment. The law firm wanted to know whether "everything was all right." This is a sophisticated approach, because the attorney had enough medical knowledge to select a disease category in which it is unlikely that everything would be all right.

In the area of human malformations, the physician or pharmaceutical firm is extremely vulnerable to the plaintiff's attorney who actively solicits business. As an example, one percent of the three million annual pregnancies have some exposure to diagnostic radiation. Four percent or 120,000 of these pregnancies will result in some type of congenital abnormality which is unrelated to the radiation. Therefore, by chance alone there are 1,200 malformed infants born each year to mothers who received diagnostic X-ray exposure. The potential number of lawsuits involving malformed infants is staggering.

Attorneys are also willing to accept a malformation case that has no merit because of the possibility of obtaining a small out-of-court settlement. The cost of the legal process has become so expensive that insurance companies are sometimes inclined to settle non-meritorious lawsuits for several thousand dollars. In most instances, the defendant is not sympathetic to the insurance company's willingness to settle. These numerous small claims and settlements have been one of the causes for the increase in malpractice premiums and are of minimal benefits to the injured patient or to society as a whole, but do provide some income for the negligence attorney.

Even more ominous than the settlement or non-meritorious nuisance claims for small amounts of money is the settlement of non-meritorious suits by large corporations in an effort to avoid publicity. In the past three years, two very large suits were settled out of court because the manner in which the plaintiff was dealt with by a physician or supervisor was less than optimal. In one instance a physician did not realize a patient was pregnant and did an exploratory laparotomy. In the other instance, a pregnant woman working with a very "safe" piece of X-ray equipment was refused permission to be transferred during her pregnancy. Although the resulting malformations were unrelated to the plaintiff's accusations, the cases were settled to avoid bad publicity. The plaintiff's attorneys used the "double jeopardy" concept prevalent in congenital malformation lawsuits in order to blackmail the defendants into submission (Brent, '76a). This turn of events is very ominous and will measurably worsen the already serious epidemic of negligence and malpractice lawsuits.

The pursuit of non-meritorious lawsuits by attorneys may even continue after several expert witnesses have rendered an opinion contrary to the attorney's wishes. In several instances the attorneys have requested that I alter my expert opinion in order to strengthen their position enough to obtain an out-of-court settlement (Table 1). Let me quote from an attorney's letter.

> "I am struggling hard, hoping to recoup some of the out-of-pocket costs in this matter by some kind of settlement."

In another letter, the plaintiff's attorney states,

> "I would certainly appreciate a response to my letter and the strongest and most affirmative statements, conclusions and opinions that you can make and state, even though they may be strictly your own. I would appreciate this even though I certainly understand the probability that from a medical-legal standpoint, any such statements or opinions may not technically qualify as admissible evidence. As you know, the defendants and their carriers in settling a case need something to 'hang their hats on' and, for such purposes, the complete technical requirements of admissibility are not always controlling."

The plaintiff's attorney is frequently insensitive to the impact of the litigation process on the family. There is no evaluation of a family's stability or suitability to enter the litigation arena. Just as there are people who are psychologically unsuited to drink, gamble or play the stock market without damage to themselves, there are families who suffer immensely from the strain of the litigation process. *I have never seen a family counseled to avoid litigation because it may be hazardous to their health.* Since the true pursuit of justice often plays no part in initiating malpractice suits, and since most malformation lawsuits have no merit, the plaintiffs may be trapped into litigation only to provide fodder for the litigation process. How many would be spared if they heeded Edmund Burke's wise counsel—"It is not what a lawyer tells me I may do: but what humanity, reason and justice tells me I ought to do" (Burke, '68). This admonition from long ago remains largely unheeded by the public.

One must not be too critical of the lawyer since "lawyers are trained to win cases rather than solve problems" (Boulding, '75), while some recognize that society and the plaintiff would benefit from less costly ways of shifting burdens. It is unlikely that alternative methods for solving the plaintiff's problems will come from the legal profession, since they have a vested interest in preserving the tort system and control most of the legislative bodies in the country.

The medical care and legal systems

If all medical care, rehabilitation, custodial care and social-psychological services were freely available to everyone, the frequency of malpractice lawsuits would, of course, be drastically reduced. Since we are a long way from that extreme of socialized medicine, we must recognize that the fragmentation and the high cost of medical care is a contributing factor in malpractice litigation. Just as patients may become angry at the physicians, so have they become angry at many aspects of the health care system.

The most controversial aspect of this entire topic deals with the appropriateness of utilizing litigation for compensating injured patients. Some competent individuals are firmly convinced that the legal system is a satisfactory mechanism for compensating injured patients (Robitscher, '69).

> "It is in the legal arena, more than any other part of our society, where medicine can be made aware of its lack of certainty . . .
>
> "It seems to me that the adversary system is the honest way of exposing the truth . . .
>
> "Civilization has yet to produce a better system of adjudicating the differences between man and man and man and institution, than the Anglo-Saxon administration of law." (Robitscher, '69)

My experience in malpractice litigation leads me to disagree vehemently with the concept that litigation is a proper and suitable means of solving an injured patient's problem. Justice is an accidental by-product of the litigation process. What has been most disconcerting to me is that, in many cases that were deservedly lost, the plaintiff's attorney could have been provided with an approach that may have reversed the results of litigation, in spite of the fact that malpractice had not been committed. Should a plaintiff's future or a defendant's reputation depend on a game of skill between opposing attorneys and expert witnesses?

Rubsamen ('75) says, "the jury system is basically irrational." Wiseman ('75) sums up the frustration of the litigation process as follows:

> "The assertion that society must accept the tort system as the only available solution for the problem of medical malpractice is obviously not valid. It is the last desperate argument of legal chauvinism. Social engineering has advanced to a point where the public is no longer restricted to the crude choices of frontier days.
>
> "The tort system in medicine was designed, created, and administered by lawyers; it is not criticism of law as a profession but a general commentary on human nature to observe that it now benefits no one but lawyers. It hurts everyone else . . .
>
> "The tort system can no more be reformed to fit modern medical requirements than could a dinosaur be made into a creature suited to the present. The tort system belongs to the history books like covered wagons and knights in armor. The facts speak for themselves; res ipsa loquitur."

The worst aspect of the tort system is the contingency fee basis for funding litigation. Directly or indirectly, it has become a significant cost of medical care. The defenders of the contingency fee claim to be convinced that it permits the poor to recover damages, something which could be accomplished equally well with some kind of legal insurance. Actually, the contingency fee not only allows the poor to sue but it stimulates litigation from all economic classes. Countries without a contingency fee have few malpractice lawsuits (Geekie, '75; Rubsamen, '75).

> "Without a contingent fee system, malpractice litigation unquestionably would be dormant in the United States. The likelihood of recovery in many substantial meritorious cases is sufficiently equivocal to forestall litigation unless the plaintiff's attorney can look for a high return in the case of a win. So the plaintiff's bar seems to have the better part of the argument in retaining the contingent fee. But the fact remains, that the scale of recovery under our contingent fee system is almost totally irrational." (Rubsamen, '75).

The quotation by Rubsamen ('75) defends the contingency fee because it provides a mechanism for a meritorious client to recover damages. Rubsamen would modify the fee structure so that the awards were more appropriate and the attorney's remuneration was lower. Thus, Rubsamen defends the contingency fee in the name of justice. But the majority of congenital malformation malpractice suits prove to be without merit, and the contingent fee system stimulates these lawsuits. Is it not injustice to accuse and malign a very large number of non-negligent defendants? It is apparent that much "malpractice" is truly "dyspractice" (Krugman, '75). Reichman ('76), in discussing quality medical care, stated "A satisfactory outcome is never guaranteed for the patient, even when the process of care is excellent." Therefore, "the allegation that a physician is a malpractioner . . . is not necessarily an accusation that he is inept" (Willig, '69). This indicates that physicians and other potential defendants are expected to assume the burden of negative results that may not be associated with malpractice. It is this new concept of unrealistic expectations in malpractice and medical negligence litigation that has exponentially increased the number of lawsuits. In malpractice law, what may be "justice" to the plaintiff may be "injustice" to the defendant and vice versa.

EPILOGUE

Many recommendations for changing the litigation process have been presented in the Appendix. These recommendations have been made in the belief that it will literally be impossible to eliminate the litigation process as the method of settling malpractice claims. But, I wish to emphasize that in the long run I believe, the greatest benefit to all would come from elimination of the contigency fee and replacing it with either no-fault medical insurance or comprehensive law insurance. There would be an immediate reduction in the frequency of non-meritorious negligence litigation. Society would then be forced to utilize other means to solve problems which had been left in the inefficient and unjust hands of the litigation process.

The elimination of the litigation process is nothing other than "good medicine." When a physician observes that a drug harms more patients than it helps, he stops using the drug. It is easy to observe that the litigation process is very bad for the patient and for most others who are involved in the process.

I have learned from past experience that the analysis and criticism of a problem in a scientific journal does not solve problems (Brent, '67, '76). However, it is a useful first step in pointing out that the problem exists and solutions are available. The next step must follow. Those who believe that the contingency fee and malpractice litigation are archaic social tools will have to enter the political arena or convince those who are there that these matters should have a high priority.

SUMMARY

In 1967, I indicated that the number of lawsuits involving malformed infants seemed to be increasing, not realizing that the increase was foretelling an epidemic. The reasons for this epidemic are described in this paper and are due to attitudes and happenings in the medical, legal, and lay sectors of our society. Case histories have been utilized to demonstrate that the litigation process can produce pain and suffering and, in some instances, even disease. The case histories also indicate that, when a family becomes orchestrated by a lawyer into the position of devoting a great deal of their energy to litigation, many high priority family responsibilities are ignored and important ethical standards are distorted. To win at all costs may be good for a football team, but it is obviously bad for a family. We must take drastic changes in the method of supporting the victims of disease and injury so that litigation is no longer necessary to compensate and support patients and families whether negligence is or is not a factor.

Recommendations for diminishing the malpractice crises include: (1) education of the patient about the consequences of the litigation process—the fact that only a small portion of the malpractice premium dollar ever reaches the patient and the fact that most human malformations are not produced by medical negligence; (2) altering the deteriorating physician image, reversing the increase in irresponsible medical expert testimony and changing the laws pertaining to medical licensure and loss of medical licensure; (3) improving the health care system; (4) making the awards more realistic by taking into consideration community and insurance resources of the patient and by eliminating lump sum awards and "punitive" awards; (5) decreasing lawyer representation in legislative bodies so that legal reforms will become a possibility and, (6) eliminating the contingency fee system by replacing it either with legal insurance so that the attorney is working for the patient or by adopting no-fault malpractice insurance with binding arbitration so that the negligently injured patient is properly compensated. The process of litigation rarely solves the patient's problems and frequently develops into a disease all its own.

ACKNOWLEDGMENTS

The Stein Research Center Developmental Biology Laboratories are supported by NIH HD 7075, HD 18396, HD 19165, HD 18167, HL 7497; the Foederer Foundation, and the Harry Bock Charities.

LITERATURE CITED

Adams, S.H. (1968) The health master. In: Familiar Medical Quotations. Chap. I. Maurice B. Strauss, M.D. ed. Little, Brown & Co., p. 458.
Arthus, M. (1943) Philosophy of Scientific Investigation. Henry Sigerist (translator). The Johns Hopkins Press, Baltimore.
Boulding, K.E. (1975) Truth or power? Science, *190:*4213.
Brent, R.L. (1967) Medicolegal aspects of teratology. J. Pediat., *71:*288–298.
— (1976a) Medicolegal aspects of teratology. In: Biologic and Clinical Aspects of Malformations. R.S. Bloew, J.C. Sinclair and J.B. Warshaw, eds. Mead Johnson Symposium on Perinatal and Developmental Medicine No. 7, Vail, Colorado, June 8-12, 1975, pp. 65–76.
— (1976b) Contributions of experimental teratology to clinical medicine. In: Biologic and Clinical Aspects of Malformations. Mead Johnson Symposium on Perinatal and Developmental Medicine No. 7, Vail, Colorado, June 8-12, 1975, pp. 54–56.
— (1976c) Environmental factors, Miscellaneous. In: Prevention of Embryonic, Fetal and Perinatal Disease, Robert L. Brent and Maureen Harris, eds. DHEW Publication No. (NIH) 76–853, 1976, *3:*211–218.
Brierly, C., J. McDonald, J. Giacalone, L. Kempinski-York and M. Franks (1975) Malpractice in focus. A national problem the states must solve. AMA source document. Prism, Chicago, 32 pp.
Bucy, P.C. (1975) The medical expert witness in malpractice suits. J.A.M.A., *232:*1352–1353.
Burke, E. (1968) Second speech on conciliation with America. The Thirteen Resolutions (March 22, 1775). In: Bartlett's Familiar Quotations, Fourteenth ed. Little Brown & Co., Boston, pp. 452–453.
Chekhov, A.P. (1968) Ivanov, Act I, Scene 2. In: Familiar Medical Quotations. Chap. 1. Maurice B. Strauss, M.D., ed. Little, Brown & Co., p. 458.
Drotar, D., B.A. Baskiewiz, N. Irvin, J. Kennell and M. Klaus (1975) The adaptation of parents to the births of an infant with a congenital malformation: A hypothetical model. Pediat., *56:*710–711.
Geekie, D.A. (1975) The crisis in medical malpractice: Will it spread to Canada? Canad. Med. Assoc. J., *113:*327–334.
Hardy, H.L. (1975) Annual discourse—risk and responsibility. New Eng. J. Med., *293:*801–806.
Holmes, L.B. (1976) Congenital malformation incidence: Racial differences, recognized etiologies. In: Biologic and Clinical Aspects of Malformations. Mead Johnson Symposium on Perinatal and Developmental Medicine No. 7, Vail, Colorado, June 8-12, 1975, pp. 3–9.
Johns, N. (1971) Family reactions to the birth of a child with a congenital abnormality. Med. J. Aust., *7:*277, 1971.
Krugman, R.D. (1975) Immunization "dyspractice": The need for "no-fault" insurance. Pediat., *56:*159–160.
Polsky, S. (1969) Psycholegalities of everyday medical practice. Modern Medicine (June 30), pp. 82–85.
Ragan, C.A. (1973) Pros and cons of "no-fault" malpractice insurance. Resident and Staff Physician, *19:*31–32.
Reichman, S. (1976) Quality assessment and ambulatory care. Bull. N.Y. Acad. Med., *52:*75–80.
Rensberger, B. (1976) Doctor's incompetence. New York Times, January 29, pp. 1,24 (pd 1112).
Robitscher, J. (1969) The doctor as an occasional witness. Modern Medicine (June 30), pp. 78–81.
Rubsamen, D.S. (1975) The evolution of medical malpractice litigation in the United States. Canad. Med. Assoc., *113:*334–341.
Schwartz, H. (1975) Will malpractice socialize United States Medicine? Medical Economics, *52:*114.
Smithells, R.W. (1965) The thalidomide legacy. Proc. Royal Soc. Med., *58:*491–492.
Solnit, A.J., and M.H. Stark (1961) Mourning and the birth of a defective child. Psychol. Stud. Child., *16:*523.
Welch, C.E. (1975) Medical malpractice. New Eng. J. Med., *292:*1372–1376.
Willig, S.H. (1969) Balance of benefits to risk. Modern Med. (June 30), pp. 68–69.
Wilson, J.G. (1973) Environment and Birth Defects. Academic Press, N.Y.C., 305 pp.
Wiseman, L.W. (1975) Rep ipsa loquitur. West J. Med. *123:*71–75.

APPENDIX

Recommendations

Recommendations made in 1967 (Brent, '67, '76) in order to decrease the number of non-meritorious congenital malformation lawsuits: (1) Establishment of authoritative sources of information to assist the court, such as a national committee of authorities that could render an unbiased scientific opinion about the merits of a malformation case as a friend of the court; (2) Introduction of the concept of a mediocolegal workup. In many instances, a preliminary evaluation which includes a genetic history, amino acid analysis, cytogenetic study and documentation of the defect can indicate that the particular case does or does not have merits. If the courts required such a basic workup before litigation could be initiated, many cases would never come to trial; (3) Creation of new laws to define responsibility and the rights of fetus, parent, physician and pharmaceutical firm or other industries; (4) Teaching physicians and industrial corporations the arts and sciences of proper communication.

The public should be educated to the fact that few congenital malformations are caused by drugs and radiation. The plaintiff should also be made aware of the length of the litigation process; the disorganizing and enervating effect that litigation can have on a family; and the fact that in nuisance settlements the attorney's fees and expenses may consume most of the award. The patients should also be aware of the fact that the litigation process, which is supposedly for their benefit, delivers only 15% of the billions of dollars of malpractice premiums to the injured party. The lawyer's own medical team is more interested in assisting in litigation preparation than in treating the patient. Therefore, only under unusual circumstances should the patients abandon their usual physician.

The materialistic image of the physician has taken some time to develop. It is very likely that it will remain with us until national health insurance becomes a reality or there are drastic changes in the methods of reimbursing physicians and delivering health care.

It may be possible to drastically alter the contribution of unscrupulous expert medical witnesses to malpractice cases by making their testimony available to their hospital staff or their academic department chairman. Professional witnesses rarely announce their participation in lawsuits. When confronted with the knowledge that they had participated in a lawsuit as an expert witness, they will deny it or claim that they took a very peripheral role. Physicians would be amazed at the number and position of their colleagues who have become expert witnesses. I suggest that medical societies require their members to file reports or at least report their participation in litigation as part of the requirement to remain in the medical society. I believe that some mechanism shedding the light of day on expert testimony would go a long way in increasing the responsibility and accuracy of this testimony.

It is necessary to educate medical students and physicians about the proper role of an expert medical witness as well as to the fact that this role has been distorted by the lure of money and reputation (Bucy, '75).

If attorneys could honestly evaluate the burdens and benefits of the present malpractice crisis, they would support drastic changes in the methods of compensating the injured. The problem is, as the previous paragraphs have indicated, they have vested interest in maintaining the status quo. We, therefore, must recognize that we cannot expect major reforms to emanate from the legal profession.

Litigation would be reduced if the health care system provided acute, intermediate and chronic care for injured patients. A medical-social welfare system that provides total care would eliminate the necessity for the exorbitant awards and, in many instances, the necessity for litigation. At the present time, a total social-medical welfare program is not on the horizon.

The size and appropriateness of compensation awarded by the court would be more realistic if all the resources available to an injured party were known to the judge and jury. It seems ridiculous to ignore already paid-for-medical care programs provided by the government or insurance system. Furthermore, the lump-sum award is also fiscally irresponsible, since it frequently benefits the relatives and estate of the injured patient rather than the patient. The cost of total awards would diminish if an appropriate award could be paid monthly or quarterly for the duration of the patient's life. There are many instances wherein a patient received a large financial award and died within the year. This type of an award distorts the purpose of the litigation process and primarily serves the needs of the attorney whose fees are based on a contingency fee.

This brings us to the most controversial topic of all and that is the contingency fee. I believe that the patient would be better off in the long run if there were no contingency fee. It would decrease the incidence of negligence lawsuits drastically. It might force the health care system to provide total care for the injured patients. It might even decrease the incidence of malpractice occurrence by forcing the licensing agencies to modernize the process whereby medical licenses are granted and revoked. At the present time, the loss of a malpractice suit is the only form of formal punishment the physician or defendant receives. It is much too severe a punishment for the dyspractitioner and frequently too mild for the malpractitioner.

It is obvious that the legal profession will resist the elimination of the contingency fee with all the resources at its command. Furthermore, it is very likely that it will prevail, since attorneys maintain a majority in legislative bodies in these United States. Probably one of the greatest benefits that might result from the malpractice crisis is the recognition by the public that the legal profession is too highly represented in legislative bodies to permit any reforms that relate to the legal profession. We have been very concerned about the racial and sexual representation in jobs and schools. We might begin to look at professional monopolies. All aspects of the democratic process might benefit if no vested interest group (including lawyers) were in control of our legislative bodies. This will evolve only if more non-lawyers enter politics and the electorate recognizes the benefit of decreasing the number of lawyers in legislative bodies.

The contingency fee system increases the total cost of legal services and discourages people from utilizing needed legal services that must be paid. While a middle class or lower socioeconomic class individual might be willing to sue on a contingency basis, he is unlikely to utilize legal services for other important activities. Thus, the promotion of law insurance for all legal services, including malpractice, might be the best containment for litigation costs and place the client in a better position to utilize all legal services appropriately.

A second alternative to law insurance would be no-fault medical malpractice insurance. It would eliminate the necessity for a contingency fee, and the litigation process. Compulsory arbitration by a representative panel would guarantee that most of the malpractice insurance premiums would end up in the rightful hands of the injured patient rather in legal fees and litigation costs.

At the present time, the medical profession is accused of permitting malpractitioners to continue to practice (Rensberger, '76). If this is the case, then it is up to the legislative bodies to alter the laws pertaining to medical licensure so that malpractitioners can have their license revoked. In the present situation, a physician who is aware of an instance of malpractice is placed in a serious dilemma. As an informant, he enjoys no protection against civil libel suit by the accused physician. He could be consumed in a legal process which could be costly and enervating.

TERATOGEN UPDATE: ENVIRONMENTALLY INDUCED BIRTH DEFECT RISKS, PAGES 229–239 (1986)

The Irresponsible Expert Witness: A Failure of Biomedical Graduate Education and Professional Accountability

ROBERT L. BRENT
Departments of Pediatrics, Radiology, and Anatomy, Jefferson Medical College, Thomas Jefferson University, Philadelphia, Pennsylvania 19107

ABSTRACT Many forces have created the epidemic of negligence and malpractice litigation. One of the contributing factors to the rising rate of nonmeritorious litigation is the increasing number of unqualified and irresponsible expert witnesses. The high remuneration has attracted physician-scientists who are unaware of the proper role of an expert witness. They are frequently manipulated by the attorneys and function as partisans rather than scholars. The role of the expert witness should be taught in medical and graduate school. Testimony should be treated as a scholarly endeavor and experts should be encouraged to seek peer review of their opinions and not to testify secretly and in isolation. It is suggested that greater visibility of experts and their testimony (light of day phenomenon) should raise the quality of expert witness testimony and encourage more qualified experts to participate as expert witnesses, thus removing the stigmata usually associated with unqualified expert witnesses.

When I entered the fields of pediatrics and teratology in the early 1950s, there were few professional fields that were more removed from the courtroom and negligence litigation. Following the thalidomide tragedy, there was an increased awareness of the potential for environmentally induced congenital malformations. In 1962, I received my first request to render an opinion as an expert medical witness concerning the etiology of a child's malformation. In a 1967 article, I indicated that the vast majority of human congenital malformations were not produced by drugs and radiation and that many nonmeritorious cases were initiated because of the ignorance of physicians and attorneys about the causes of human malformations (1). The two most important aspects of that article were the recognition that the number of negligence lawsuits involving malformed children was rising exponentially. Second, specific recommendations were made to decrease the number of nonmeritorious lawsuits and to arbitrate or settle meritorious lawsuits fairly.

Although my involvement with medical negligence litigation is a peripheral part of my professional life, it has had a tremendous impact on my view of medicine, the law, and our society. I view the judicial system as the cornerstone of a democractic society and the protector of human rights. My experience with medicolegal cases involving congenital malformations and radiation exposure has disillusioned me, as I find that justice is sometimes a distant by-product of the judicial system. Some of the lawsuits that I have dealt with are so technical that the jury has difficulty digesting all the information, and frequently the attorneys and judges have a difficult time evaluating the significance of the wealth of scientific material that may be presented. Frequently, the verdict is not based on the merits of the case, but is determined by unrelated emotional factors, such as sympathy for the injured plaintiff, anger about fabrication on the part of the plaintiff or defendant, or dislike for the attorneys on either side. Recently, at a national meeting of lawyers, Chief Justice Berger reprimanded attorneys because so many legal cases were being decided by technicalities, unrelated to the merits of the case (reference 2 and The Evening Bulletin, Feb 21, 1978, p 12). He wondered whether the judicial process has become an expensive game.

My experience with negligence lawsuits is in the field of congenital malformation causation and radiation injury. My views are

From an article published in Pediatrics 70:754–762 (1982). Reprinted with permission.

summarized in a series of articles (1, 3–5) and in the following quotation (3):

> The exponential rise in malpractice litigation is due to attitudes and happenings in the medical, legal and lay sectors of our society. Evaluation of congenital malformation lawsuits provides a unique opportunity to evaluate the process of litigation. Because the cases are rarely meritorious, the litigation process is detrimental to the plaintiff, society and frequently unfair to the defendant. There is no area of our legal system with such a high percentage of innocent defendants. When the family of a malformed infant becomes orchestrated by an attorney into a position of devoting their energy to winning a lawsuit, many high priority family responsibilities may be ignored and important ethical standards are distorted. To win at all costs may be appropriate for a football team but it can be detrimental to a family. The family enters the litigation arena unaware of the lengthiness of the litigation process and ignorant of the fact that only a small portion of the malpractice premium dollar ever reaches the patient. The plantiffs are not the only participants who lose their objectivity and lower their ethical standards. The quality and veracity of the testimony of expert witnesses has deteriorated to the point that drastic corrective measures have to be instituted. It is believed that recommendations for solving the malpractice crisis, which are based on the experience with congenital malformation lawsuits, should have applicability to the overall malpractice problem and must involve changes in the medical, legal and lay sectors of our society. It must be recognized that it is difficult to alter the laws and procedures that are not of benefit to the legal profession because so many legislatures are dominated by elected officials who happen to be attorneys. But it is emphasized that of all the recommendations put forth, the one having the greatest beneficial effect on the present malpractice crisis would be the elimination of the contingency fee system and replacing it with no-fault compensation or legal-fee insurance. The contingency fee system provokes and promotes negligence litigation. The process of litigation in congenital malformation lawsuits rarely solves the patient's problems and frequently develops into a disease of its own.

It is not very likely that the medical profession can change the views of a litigation-prone public, alter the judicial process, decrease the high representation of attorneys in the legislatures, introduce no-fault negligence insurance or national legal insurance, or eliminate the contingency fee system. One may believe that changes in these areas might improve our society, but realistically only lawyers and legislators can modernize the methods by which the injured are compensated and differences of opinion are settled.

Inasmuch as physicians and scientists do contribute in some measure to the phenomenon of increasing litigation (4), it would seem prudent to concentrate our efforts on the areas in which the medical-scientific community can exert some positive influence. There are four contributions to the increase in medical negligence litigation directly related to the performance of the physician-scientist: (1) deteriorating image of the physician in the public's mind, making him more likely to be sued; (2) improper communication with the patient by physicians, nurses, residents, and students; (3) failure to eliminate incompetent physicians from the practice of medicine; and (4) inappropriate testimony by expert witnesses. This article will deal only with matters pertaining to the expert witness.

THE EXPERT WITNESS

It is alleged that malpractice litigation was uncommon years ago because attorneys were unable to obtain expert medical witnesses to testify against other physicians (6). The allegation is correct but, today, the expert medical witness for the plaintiff is no longer a rarity. Robitscher (6) describes the plaintiff's expert medical witness as follows: "... a small fraction of medicine that relishes the attention and sometimes also welcomes the remuneration that results from court testimony ... who is ready to see causal connections—a blow by a taxi door and the resulting development of cancer.... Lawyers use these witnesses frequently, but they do not always respect them." They are a "few of the best doctors and most of the worst doctors."

Inasmuch as not all litigation involving malformed infants involves a physician defendant, it has been somewhat easier for the plaintiff's attorney to obtain an expert witness, especially if the defendant is a pharmaceutical firm, industrial firm, or branch of government. My experience in malpractice litigation is limited to areas of radiation hazards and the etiology of malformations, but in these cases, I have been amazed at the lack of veracity and objectivity of many expert witnesses (Table). As an example, a scientist who published a paper in which he listed a drug as nonteratogenic was willing to testify for the plantiff when the same drug was implicated as a cause of a child's malformations. A nonmeritorious suit that had been discontinued was reinitiated when the plaintiff's attorney was able to locate a general practitioner to testify as a medical expert witness in the field of teratology. Some medical experts demand and receive substantial fees, resulting in a sycophantic alliance between the expert witness and the attorney. This situation could worsen if expert witnesses were permitted to be paid on a contingency fee basis, as has been suggested by some attorneys.

Until I participated as an expert witness, I was not aware of the magnitude of the problem of the irresponsible or unscrupulous expert witness. My observation of many expert witnesses has been one of the most distressing and disillusioning experiences of my professional life.

Let me examine the role of the expert witness in two negligent law suits involving malformed infants. I selected these cases because they are not unusual and because there was no merit to the allegation that the child's malformations were related to the alleged malforming agent or incident.

TABLE 1. Source of expert testimony in medical negligence lawsuits (327 appearances)

Testimony	(%)
Practitioner testifying < 3 times	24
Practitioner testifying > 3 times	8
Academician testifying < 3 times	12
Academician testifying > 3 times	31
Full-time expert	4
Nonphysician expert	21

CASE REPORTS

Case 1

During the 11th week of pregnancy, an expectant mother was sitting in the rear seat of an automobile that was hit broadside by another car. Her car overturned and she sustained a comminuted fracture of the right femur. There was no obvious injury to the abdomen, no abdominal pain or tenderness, and no vaginal bleeding. Examination by her obstetrician over the next ten days revealed all aspects of the pregnancy to be normal. She was eating well in the hospital. Members of the family suggested that she obtain an attorney following her discharge from the hospital 11 weeks after the accident. A well known negligence attorney was retained who discharged the expectant mother's physicians and selected another physician. This physician, an obstetrician, examined the patient for the first time in the 29th week of pregnancy and admitted her to another hospital for the remainder of the pregnancy because "she appeared markedly undernourished" and the patient complained of a 10-lb weight loss. During the first and second hospitalization all of the records indicated that the fetal heart rate and movements were normal. During the 38th week of pregnancy she delivered the plaintiff. During the labor, meperidine hydrochloride (Demerol) was administered to the patient. Her blood pressure dropped precipitously and the fetal heart rate dropped simultaneously. With the infant in an arrested transverse position, vasopressors and oxytocin (Pitocin) were administered to the mother while a midforceps delivery was attempted. The transverse position was converted by fundal pressure and the infant was delivered 35 minutes after the maternal blood pressure dropped. The umbilical cord was within the birth canal during the second stage of labor and was compressed by the infant's neck and shoulder. At birth the infant was deeply cyanotic; she did not breathe for two minutes nor cry for 45 minutes. There was absence of muscle tone and failure to respond to painful stimuli; convulsions occurred on the second day of life. At the time of the trial this little girl was approximately 9 years old and had severe spastic quadriplegia.

First expert

The obstetrician who delivered the plantiff testified that in his opinion the cerebral palsy was due to the automobile accident in the 11th week of pregnancy, which resulted in damage to the placenta. He also testified that the placenta was 70% to 80% infarcted at birth and that these infarctions were due to the trauma of the automobile accident.

Second expert

An authority on the diagnosis and treatment of cerebral palsy testified that in his opinion the cerebral palsy was caused by the automobile accident in the 11th week of pregnancy.

Third expert

A pediatric rehabilitationist testified that in his opinion the automobile accident produced the placental infarctions and the resulting cerebral palsy during the 11th week of pregnancy.

Comments on merits of allegation that automobile accident caused cerebral palsy

The work of Windle (8) indicates that the lesions of cerebral palsy are predominantly produced in the perinatal period. In this case, there were at least four obstetric mishaps that are etiologically correlated with perinatal fetal brain injury. Furthermore, if the placenta was infarcted 70% to 80% by the accident in the 11th week, it would be impossible for the fetus to have reached 7 lb at the 38th week. One would expect severe growth retardation if the placenta was actually 70% to 80% infarcted and, in fact, the embryo probably would not survive. There is no clinical or experimental data to indicate that first trimester environmental insults of this type result in the brain lesions that are observed in cerebral palsy. If anyone contributed to the plantiff's cerebral palsy, it was the plaintiff's attorney and the obstetrician who delivered the baby.

What prompts physicians and scientists to provide the court with testimony that is unsound or untrue? It may be the ego gratification of being called an expert and the high level of remuneration received by some experts. I believe that the most important factor in many instances is that the expert is unaware of his or her proper role in the courtroom.

Case 2

A male infant weighing 7 lb 14 oz was born with assymetrical hemimelia and a nasofrontal capillary hemangioma. Several months after birth he was treated for hip dysplasia and several years later his condition was diagnosed as bilateral inguinal hernias. His intrauterine and extrauterine growth had been above the 50th percentile and his parents and doctors described him as having normal intelligence.

The mother was the employee of a large corporation and was the operator of an x-ray diffractometer that was used to orient silicon crystals. During her employment, the mother wore ring badges which revealed exposures below the maximum permissible exposure. In fact, most of the exposures were zero. Exposure was possible only for the first 50 days of pregnancy, as she no longer used the x-ray diffractometer after that time. The plaintiffs alleged that employee education about x-irradiation was inadequate and the quality of the health physics program was inferior. Although these are important matters, they are not related to the etiology of the child's malformations.

The facts of the case are as follows: The diffractometer sat on a table, the x-ray beam projected 180° from the operator and was only several millimeters wide and high at the ledge of the table opposite the operator. There is no way that she could operate the machine and be in the beam on the other side of the table. Even if someone else operated the machine and she stood in the direct line of the beam, her abdomen would be below the level of the table and, therefore, would receive no radiation. Furthermore, even if the abdomen could be placed in the beam, she would have to remain in one position to expose the embryo. This bizarre circumstance would result in an abdominal exposure of tens of thousands of rads before the embryo would receive an embryotoxic exposure. This is partly due to the fact that this x-ray diffractometer had a copper anode and, therefore, had a predominant x-ray energy of 9 keV. Any competent, objective radiologic physicist or radiation biologist, after examining the machine and performing the dosimetry, would have concluded that there was no way that the fetus was exposed to radiation, in this case.

Evaluation of the child's physical status confirmed that intrauterine radiation exposure was not responsible for the malformations. In spite of the fact that there were very serious malformations of the limbs, there was no intrauterine or postnatal growth retardation, no microcephaly, and no mental retardation. Human epidemiologic studies and case reports clearly indicate that one would not expect normal growth and a normal CNS if radiation had produced such severe malformations of the limbs. Animal studies support these findings. The CNS is the most sensitive developing organ system and maintains this sensitivity to x-irradiation over the greatest range of development. Not one of the plaintiff's experts adequately discussed the causes or incidence of limb reduction defects. There are many review articles dealing with the subject. Approximately 15% of the cases have a genetic etiology. A smaller percent are due to intrauterine constrictive phenomena, such as amnionitis, malformation of the mother's uterus, amniotic bands, or intrauterine infections. The remaining group are of unknown causes. Except for thalidomide, all other environmental etiologies are presumptive or hypothetical (9).

First expert

The first expert was a friend and colleague of the plaintiff's attorney who contacted many of the experts. He was a pediatrician with no training or experience in the field of radiation embryology. He did not examine or evaluate the child. He felt that a normal chromosome analysis means "There was no associated genetic abnormality on a hereditary basis." He stated that all of the plaintiff's malformations were caused by a radiation exposure between 100 and 200 rads, but that these malformations could be produced by 0.5 rad or exposures just above background radiation. Before any of the exposure estimates were available, this physician visited an English epidemiologist and he "described the anomalies, the exposure and [the epidemiologist] said . . . there was a causal [relationship] . . . to the radiation." This conclusion was arrived at without any report from the plaintiff's radiologic physicist.

Second expert

The second expert was a practicing radiologist who was contacted by the first expert. He was told the exposure to the embryo was 200 R by the plaintiff's attorney and that the plaintiff's mother was standing so that the abdomen was directly in the beam. He never examined the facility, spoke with the physicist who did the dosimetry, or reviewed the physicist's report. He testified that 2 to 5 R could produce major malformations, that background radiation was harmful, and that exposure to the fetal brain could cause hemimelia.

Defense Attorney: "Could you say with some certainty that it is exposure to the fetal brain that could possibly cause hemimelia?"

Expert Witness: "Absolutely. This is proven. The whole limb formation is directed by the brain. Spine and ribs also. This is a neurotropic growth concept. Incidentally, that's a science that is not practiced in this country. You have to go to Germany to learn that."

The expert testified that the cause of these defects was the radiation and that he had not considered other possibilities. He further stated that the plantiff had 30 times the spontaneous risk of developing leukemia and that hip dysplasia was the most readily produced malformation from intrauterine radiation exposure. This expert's statements are wrong (10,11).

Third expert

The third expert was an experienced radiologic physicist who rendered an opinion about the causation without performing dosimetry, without visiting the site of the alleged exposure, and without even seeing the report of the radiologic physicist who did the dosimetry. He obtained all the information about the dosimetry and exposure from the plaintiff's attorneys. He stated that he would not be surprised to see the malformations exhibited by the plaintiff at "doses as low as 5 R. It would not be surprising to find them at doses as low as 1 R or maybe even 0.5 R." He admitted that there were no absent limbs in the children exposed in utero in Hiroshima and Nagasaki, but that these children, besides exhibiting an increased incidence of microcephaly, "they had quite a burst of leukemia . . a few years later. . . ." He stated that background radiation or slightly above background exposure could not be responsible for the plaintiff's malformations.

(Prenatal exposure did not result in a "burst of leukemia" in Hiroshima and Nagasaki. The statement is wrong) (10,11).

Fourth expert

The fourth expert was an English epidemiologist with no experience in the fields of congenital malformations, genetics, radiation embryology, teratology, radiation biology, or dosimetry, but with expertise and experience in the field of radiation oncogenesis. The expert stated that an exposure of 100 R caused the plaintiff's malformations.

Defense Attorney: "Do you have an opinion as to how much the dose would have to be in order to cause this type of malformation?"

Expert: "Yes, I have an opinion . . this implies a single hit theory that all you need to do is cause one known lethal mutation [which] could be enough to cause a defect."

Defense Attorney: "Could one photon in your judgment cause the . . . malformations you know he (plaintiff) sustained?"

Expert: "It would be sufficient."

This expert stated that the incidence of limb reduction defects is 1 per 1,000,000 (not true, 1:2,000) (12). This expert did not review the dosimetry report or the x-ray diffractometer facilities, nor did she determine whether the plaintiff was ever exposed.

When asked "What is the background radiation in England?", the expert replied, "It's never been revealed to me."

Defense Attorney: "Do you believe in the linear or threshold theory with regard to malformations?"

Expert: "There is no question that the threshold theory doesn't pertain to congenital defects. Threshold [phenomena] are two stage processes . . . you need an initiator and you need a promoter and these can be separate events, but in the case of teratogenic effects . . . single damage to the cell is enough, because this was the finding of Dr. Mueller in relation to the fruit fly."

Defense Attorney: "Do you accept the threshold concept for radiation induced malformations?"

Expert: "No. I don't think many people do." This expert is unfamiliar with the literature which supports the threshold hypothesis for teratogenesis (11,13,14). Confusion between genetic effects and teratogenic effects frequently occurs when scientists not familiar with genetics and teratology testify in malformation cases. Dr. Mueller's work has nothing to do with teratogenesis. His work deals with mutagenesis of germ cells before conception.)

Fifth expert

The fifth expert was a radiologic physicist with good training and good credentials. He performed dosimetric measurements on the actual diffractometer and on an x-ray machine at another site. The kiloelectron volts of the second machine were adjusted to be similar to those of the diffractometer. (He was unaware and never determined that the two machines were not comparable because the diffractometer had a copper target whereas the x-ray machine had a tungsten target.)

Although he calculated the exposure that an individual would receive if he placed himself in the primary beam of the diffractometer, and he submitted this dose as the exposure to the embryo, he never determined whether this was possible.

Defense Attorney: ". . . have you ever heard her [plaintiff's mother] make any statements about how she operated the machine? [x-ray diffractometer], what position she stood in and so forth?"

Expert: ". . . I was not going to concern myself with who was standing where and when. I was interested in getting what we call the pattern of radiation around the machine."

Defense Attorney: "Did you try to determine whether [plaintiff's mother] was ever exposed to the primary beam?"

Expert: "No."

Defense Attorney: "Do you know whether any part of her person was ever exposed to the primary beam?"

Expert: "I have no idea."

Defense Attorney: "Are you prepared to express an opinion as to the causation of the [plaintiff's] malformations?"

Fifth Expert: "No, definitely not." (Furthermore, he refused to commit himself with regard to causation because he knew the patient was never exposed to the primary beam, yet the calculation he prepared from the plaintiff's attorneys was the absorbed dose of a dosimeter in the primary beam.)

Defense Attorney: "What was the highest reading that you obtained of the scattered radiation outside the primary beam?"

Fifth Expert: ". . . 8.2 mrem/hr."

Defense Attorney: "Could you measure any radiation below the table top level?"

Fifth Expert: "No."

Defense Attorney: "Did you try?"

Fifth Expert: "Yes."

Defense Attorney: "Do you have any opinion as to whether these [the plaintiff's] malformations were caused by scattered radiation?"

Fifth Expert: "I have no opinion."

Defense Attorney: "Does any conclusion that you reach about radiation safety with respect to the measurements you did take, rest on the conclusion that someone might be in the primary beam of the x-ray machine?"

Fifth Expert: "Let me make it clear. I cannot escape knowing if we are talking about the possibility of being irradiated and the question of some damage having been done, but as far as I'm concerned, I made physical measurements. In particular, I made some measurements trying to evaluate what the dose rate or exposure rate might have been at a particular depth or range of depth in human soft tissue placed at a particular location, but I don't wish to be placed in the position of evaluating whether those measured exposure rates may not have produced any particular effect."

During the course of the deposition the radiologic physicist made the following statement in response to the attorneys for both sides discussing how long the deposition was going to continue.

Fifth Expert: "I would like to think of myself as an impartial witness trying to help everybody see the truth."

Sixth expert

The sixth expert was a radiologist with good training who is presently director of radiation therapy at a large hospital. This expert was contacted by the radiation physicist (fifth expert). He testified that the plaintiff's attorneys told him that the plaintiff's mother stood in the primary beam of the x-ray diffractometer when operating the machine. At one point in his deposition he testified that he did not speak with the radiologic physicist (fifth expert) about the position of the plaintiff's mother, but at another time he stated that the radiologic physicist had informed him "the patient's work position was such that she stood in the primary beam so that it struck her in the lower abdomen. . . . The uterus received a dose of approximately 1 rad/hr during this working experience."

(This is of interest because the radiologic physicist never determined whether the plaintiff's mother was exposed, but only prepared a theoretical maximum exposure if someone had remained continuously in the primary beam. This expert was told by the plaintiff's attorneys that the woman was in the primary beam and the uterus did receive the exposure. If one might wonder about communication difficulties, it should be pointed out that the radiologic physicist worked in the same institution with the radiologist.)

Question: "Based on the information given to you, do you come to an opinion, Doctor, as to the cause of [plaintiff's] malformations?"

Answer: "Yes, I did."

Question: "What was the opinion?"

Answer: "I think that the irradiation (plaintiff's mother) received during the operation of this machine was the probable medical cause of these malformations."

Question: "What malformations do you include."

Answer: "I include the malformations of the arms as the most central issue here. He had several other congenital malformations which I think have a more tenuous relationship with radiation. . . hemangioma, hernia and hip dysplasia."

Question: "Is your opinion based on reasonable medical certainty, what radiation exposure to the fetus would be necessary to cause limb malformations found in [the plaintiff]?"

Answer: "I think it would be generally accepted that 25 to 50 rads could cause this malformation."

Question: "Would that be necessary in order to cause such malformations in your opinion?"

Answer: "Less might do it."

Question: "How much less?"

Answer: "I don't know. As I mentioned previously a figure of 10 rads has been given as a safe lower level. Again, one has the problem of probability. There just are not enough mice and buildings available to test the probability of any specific given dose to do this. How many bullets do you have to fire to shoot one person. It is the same phenomena. For the specific target to be hit, I believe it is an all or none phenomena. It doesn't matter whether it is hit once. One portion might be enough to do it, but it doesn't matter how many other protons are in the environment. It doesn't matter how many missed it. You have a critical mass here, a critical cell."

Question: "Is a human fetus less susceptible to radiation than a mouse or rat fetus?"

Answer: "I don't believe so. I think that it might be more sensitive."

Question: "What do you base that on?"

Answer: "The atomic bomb casualty reports. The Atomic Bomb Casualty Commission reports that there are reports in the literature of anomalies occurring at very low doses of radiation or a few roentgens."

Question: "It is your understanding of the atomic bomb studies that the human fetus is more or less susceptible than the mouse or the rat."

Answer: "It is my understanding that the

human fetus is more susceptible" [No basis for this statement.]

Question: "Do you know how much above background radiation exposure might be necessary to cause malformation to the human?"

Answer: "I think that there is evidence to indicate that background radiation could conceivably cause malformations and may in part be responsible for what we call spontaneously occurring malformations, but subjecting this to statistical proof is altogether a different matter. Again, we are talking about that single bullet theory. A single bullet, no matter where it comes from might be sufficient to do the job. Proving that the bullet did it to the exclusion of everything else is quite a different matter."

Question: "Do you subscribe to the single bullet theory?"

Answer: "This is my personal belief."

Question: "Your entire opinion as I remember it is based on the assumption that her abdomen (. . . the position of the embryo) was above the level of the table."

Answer: "This is correct."

(This radiologist ignored the deliberations of the National Council on Radiation Protection and the American College of Radiologists which indicated that the risks of malformations from intrauterine radiation were either zero or so small as not to be of clinical significance when evaluating the risk-benefit of diagnostic radiography) (15).

Comments

As with the first medicolegal case, these experts displayed ignorance and irresponsibility. They did not function as scholars, but as partisans who felt that it was their job to win the case, rather than provide the court with an objective evaluation. It is an untenable position for an expert witness when he: automatically sorts the facts newly brought to light. He retains those, even the modest ones that seem to prove him right and neglects the others, even the clearest and most precise and convincing ones if they appear to indict him. Blinded by his passion, that is, by his immoderate love for his theory, he has recourse to all means, honorable or not, in order to define it, for to him all means have become legitimate. He has ceased to be a scientist and has become a partisan (16).

Besides being partisans, what are some of the errors that expert witnesses made in these cases?

They obtained sophisticated data from the attorneys rather than obtain the data directly. One of the radiologic physicists in the second case obtained the patient's radiation exposure from the attorneys for the plaintiff. He never reviewed the dosimetry report, examined the facility, or communicated with the individual who performed the dosimetry. He rendered an opinion on causality of congenital malformations, a field in which he was not an expert and ignored evaluating the exposure and dosimetry, a field in which he was an expert.

The fifth expert, a radiologic physicist, functioned as a partisan. He refused to answer questions that he knew were damaging to the plaintiff's case and ignored dosimetric evaluations that would indicate that the plaintiff's mother did not receive any radiation. He told the truth whenever he thought it assisted the plaintiff's case. Whenever a line of questioning was damaging, he said that he was not an expert in that field or he did not investigate that area. Can you imagine performing a dosimetric evaluation for possible radiation exposure and not bothering to find out where the individual was positioned? The other experts displayed an ignorance of the fields of radiation embryology, genetics, and teratology.

In the first case, the extensive literature on the etiology of cerebral palsy was ignored. In the second case, the experts were testifying in the fields of radiation embryology, genetics, and teratology, and they demonstrated lack of scholarship and unfamiliarity of the literature in these fields.

FAILURE OF EXPERT WITNESSES TO MEET THEIR RESPONSIBILITIES

Some of the responsibility for the inadequacy of expert witness testimony is that the court's definition of an expert is far different from medical science's definition of an expert. Any medical scientist who has an advanced degree and has reviewed the subject may be acceptable to the court as an expert.

If an attorney cannot find a scholar in the field to be his expert witness, than he can "groom" any medical scientist to perform as his expert. Scientists might perform in this capacity for ego titillation or for remuneration. Many experts, once having partaken of the lucrative fees, offer their "expertise" in a variety of fields.

The educational community also bears some responsibility for the phenomenon of the irresponsible expert witness. Few medical schools, residencies, or graduate schools prepare their graduates for participation in the judicial process. The qualities of the ideal medical expert witness are as follows.

1. The testimony provided should be similar regardless of whether one is testifying for the plaintiff or defense, otherwise, one is presenting partisan testimony.

2. The expert witness should be a scholar in that field or related fields, being familiar with and having contributed to the literature in that field.

3. He should be an active or recently active investigator in a particular field if testifying on research matters. He should be an active or recently active clinician in a particular field if testifying on clinical matters.

4. His activity as an expert witness should be a minimal part of his professional activity. One cannot be a professional expert witness, inasmuch as the main activities of an expert witness should be a scholar, clinician, teacher, or investigator in the field of his expertise. (A letter to the author had as part of the letterhead "practice limited to forensic neurosurgery." This is a contradiction of terms.)

5. He should be aware of the legal and ethical impact and importance of his testimony.

6. He should be aware of the basic elements of the law and the legal procedures with which he will be involved.

7. He must understand that it is not his job to win the case, and, therefore, he must avoid becoming consumed by the protagonistic atmosphere of the litigation process.

8. He is obliged to obtain all the facts from the attorneys and clients so as not to be surprised by information late in the litigation process. Frequently, attorneys are reluctant to provide expert witnesses with damaging information. It is more important that the expert witness makes it clear to the attorney that he must have all the information.

9. He must avoid being manipulated by the attorney into becoming a partisan. It is the attorney's role to win a case by any legal means. The expert witness must refrain from becoming involved in this process.

10. He must remember that his improper testimony may prevent injured parties from receiving compensation, may ruin the lives of innocent defendants and their families, may destroy the reputations of individuals or companies, or may financially destroy an individual or company. The expert witness should never forget this burdensome responsibility.

11. Above all, he must remember that he is an expert—a scholar; not a lawyer, not a judge, and not a jailer.

IMPROVING THE QUALITY OF MEDICAL-SCIENTIFIC EXPERT TESTIMONY

As I indicated earlier in this presentation, there are only a few areas of the judicial process that the medical-scientific community can affect. The quality of expert testimony is one of these areas. The following methods are suggested for improving the quality of expert testimony.

1. An educational program should be instituted in medical and graduate schools in order to inform the students about the proper protocol for providing expert witness testimony to the courts. It is amazing how many physician-scientists are unaware of the role of the expert in the courtroom. They are especially unaware of the tenet that a true expert should not be a partisan and should provide similar testimony regardless of whether he is assisting the plaintiff or the defendant. Most moral, competent, ethical scientists will benefit from being made aware of the pitfalls, errors, and proper guidelines when providing the courts with expert testimony.

2. Depositions and court testimony should be treated as scholarly endeavors. Academic medical-scientists should be encouraged to report all medicolegal activities to the chairman of their department and review their expert opinion and analysis with their supervisor, colleagues, or peers. If employed in an industry, the expert should be encouraged to submit his testimony for review by his or her supervisor and peers. Practicing physicians should be encouraged to submit their case analysis to their colleagues for peer review. I call this the "light of day phenomenon" inasmuch as I believe that, if experts learn to consult with their peers, their testimony will become more accurate and scholarly.

It is of interest that most medical experts who function as partisans deny their frequent participation as an expert witness. They would rather not be known as a plaintiff's expert witness by their colleagues. I reviewed the depositions of cases with which I have been involved, and there are a surprising number of academicians performing surreptitiously as expert witnesses. A breakdown on the source of expert witnesses is listed in the Table. We must discourage experts from functioning in an isolated and secret manner. By raising quality and accuracy of expert opinions, we can expect a greater willingness on the part of highly qualified experts to participate as experts for the plaintiff or defense.

3. Universities and employers should recognize that medicolegal consultations can be very remunerative and, therefore, formal policies should be developed for monitoring and handling these monies. These policies should be formulated on the same basis as the institution's regulations pertaining to honoraria, practice plans, or research and development funds.

In this country many businesses have been formed to obtain expert witnesses primarily for the plaintiff. They provide the experts with fees up to $2,000 a day. In a recent trial, one expert witness for the plaintiff charged $5,000 per day. Information on these organizations may be obtained by writing to one such organization: Medical Expert Witness, PO Box 843, Vienna, VA 22180; toll-free number 800-336-0332. The preamble to their brochure reads: "Experts to render the plaintiff honest medical opinions in medical malpractice suits. . . . Our goal is to improve the quality of medical care by making each doctor police himself."

At the present time, medicolegal fees are much greater than lecturer honoraria and National Academy of Science or National Institutes of Health (NIH) consultations. Medicolegal consultations should not be considered as separate and secret activities of physician-scientists. It is the "moonlighting" or secretive nature of these activities that permits some physician-scientists to make statements that they would never publish in a scientific journal or repeat at a seminar.

4. The courts should modify their definition of an expert witness in order to eliminate the unqualified and the so-called professional expert witness. This will be extremely difficult to accomplish without the cooperation of the legal profession. There is no question that unqualified and disreputable experts can contribute to nonmeritorious decisions for the plaintiff or defendant.

5. Encourage the preparation of scholarly review articles in the fields that are presently involved in frequent malpractice or negligent litigation (L.S. James, personal communication, 1982). These review articles or consensus documents should be prepared under the auspices of professional biomedical organizations by a group of experts. The document prepared by the American Academy of Pediatrics on retrolental fibroplasia is a model (17). This type of document can be used by experts and attorneys for obtaining objective, accurate information on the "state of the art," history and progress in a field. Such a document can raise the quality of expert testimony, discourage nonmeritorious suits, and precipitate pretrial settlements in meritorious suits. Although most courts do not encourage testimony or reports by neutral "friends of the court." (1) such scholarly review articles could truly be "friends of the court."

ACKNOWLEDGMENTS

The Stein Research Center Developmental Biology Laboratories are supported by NIH HD 7075, HD 18396, HD 19165, HD 18167, HL 7497; the Foederer Foundation, and the Harry Bock Charities.

LITERATURE CITED

1. Brent, R.L. (1967) Medicolegal aspects of teratology. J. Pediatr., *71:*288–298.
2. Wessel, M.R. (1978) Medical ethics in litigation. Bull. NY. Acad. Med., *54:*808.
3. Brent, R.L. (1977) Litigation-produced pain, disease and suffering: An experience with congenital malformation lawsuits. Teratology, *16:*1–14.
4. Brent, R.L. (1979) Physician, protect thyself. Jefferson Med. Coll. Alumni Bull., *28:*22–26.
5. Brent, R.L. (1980) An analysis of congenital malformation lawsuits: The role of the medical practitioner and academician in providing inappropriate testimony. Teratology, *21:*29A.
6. Robitscher, J. (1967) The doctor as an occasional witness. Mod. Med. June 30, p. 78–81.
7. Rubsamen, D.S. (1975) The evolution of medical malpractice litigation in the United States. Can. Med. Assoc. J., *113:*334–341.
8. Windle, W.F. (1966) Role of respiratory distress in asphyxial brain damage of the newborn. Cerebral Palsy J., *27:*3.
9. Temtamy, S., and V. McKusick, (1978) The genetics of hand malformations. Birth Defects, *14:*619.
10. Okada, S., H.B. Hamilton, N. Egami, et al, (1975) A review of thirty years' study of Hiroshima and Nagasaki Atomic bomb survivors. J. Radiat. Res., *16* (suppl):1–164.
11. Committee on the Biological Effects of Ionizing Radiations: The Effects on Populations of Exposure to Low Levels of Ionizing Radiation, 1980. Washington, DC, National Academy Press, 1980, pp. 1–524.

12. Congenital Malformation Surveillance Bulletin. Atlanta, Center for Disease Control, US Department of Health, Education and Welfare, April 1978 to March 1979, pp 1–14.
13. Brent, R.L. (1980) Radiation teratogenesis. Teratology, *21*:281–298.
14. Wilson, J.G. (1978) Current status of teratology: General principles and mechanisms derived from animal studies, in J.G. Wilson, and F.C. Fraser (eds): Handbook of Teratology. New York, Plenum Press, chap 2, pp. 47–74.
15. Medical Radiation Exposure of Pregnant and Potentially Pregnant Women, National Council on Radiation Protection (NCRP) and Measurements, Report No. 54, Washington, DC, July 15, 1974, pp. 1–32.
16. Arthus, M. (1943) Philosophy of Scientific Investigation. Sigerist H (trans). Baltimore, The Johns Hopkins Press.
17. James, L.S., J.T. Lawman (eds) (1976) History of oxygen therapy and retrolental fibroplasia. Pediatrics, *57*(suppl):591–654.

Index